THE CAPITATION SOURCEBOOK

A practical guide to managing at-risk arrangements

Peter Boland, Editor

BOLAND HEALTHCARE • BERKELEY

This publication is designed to provide accurate and authoritative information in regard to the subject matter covered. It is sold with the understanding that neither the authors nor the publisher is engaged in rendering legal, accounting, or other professional service. If legal advice or other expert assistance is required, the services of a competent professional person should be sought. (From a *Declaration of Principles* jointly adopted by a Committee of the American Bar Association and a Committee of Publishers and Associations.)

Text and cover design by Seventeenth Street Studios

The Capitation Sourcebook: a practical guide to managing at-risk arrangements
edited by Peter Boland
Library of Congress Catalog Card Number: 96-85011
ISBN: 0-9652717-0-6

To Autumn

Contents

Preface

*T*HE CAPITATION SOURCEBOOK describes how physicians, medical group managers, hospital administrators, and managed care executives can promote cost-effective care by balancing financial and nonfinancial incentives. Capitation affects how medical services are organized and delivered as well as how providers are paid. It is a unique payment system and a philosophy of care management that requires managing people and services differently than under traditional fee-for-service or cost-plus reimbursement.

Due to market pressure for cost reduction, practitioners are being forced to share more and more financial risk for delivering care. This is motivating stakeholders throughout the industry to reassess how to structure both risk sharing and financial incentives in compensation. In short, compensation design must be easy to understand and perceived as fair to foster more cooperation and better performance. When the pros and cons of prepaid medicine are clearly understood and accepted by each stakeholder, the business relationship is more likely to succeed. Such a common sense approach is the basis for this book.

Trust is at the heart of a successful business relationship. This book draws upon the expertise of numerous practitioners around the country regarding how to build business trust among providers, payers, and purchasers through accountability and mutual respect. It is a sourcebook of practical tools and techniques to manage at-risk arrangements, measure results, and improve care. This volume provides answers to many of the most difficult issues facing providers and health plan managers regarding aligning financial incentives and promoting cost-effective care. The book was written for practitioners by practitioners and can be used as a practical resource for operations management as well as strategic planning and product development. Each section presents material that focuses on the critical building blocks of successful capitation and is designed to help healthcare professionals to

- Assemble organizational and service components for integrated care delivery

- Design income distribution models to improve medical group financial and clinical performance

- Align risk-sharing incentives with performance objectives

- Identify data requirements and report formats for monitoring provider and health plan performance

- Build different compensation models for phasing in capitated revenue

- Develop network financial management controls

- Measure hospital resource consumption

- Create organization infrastructure to manage hospital capitation

- Combine quality improvement and utilization management functions

- Create risk-sharing formulas and bonus incentives to manage ambulatory care

- Analyze contracts based on actuarial cost models

- Assess and decrease the financial impact of high-risk individuals on capitated provider payments

- Identify disease life cycle implications for aging populations

- Compare the advantages and disadvantages of subcontracting with specialty providers

- Establish organizational requirements for integrating behavioral health capitation with general medicine

- Purchase ancillary medical services

- Address ethical dilemmas in the organization and delivery of care

Section one presents an overview of industry dynamics and the influence of managed care on payment systems. It describes how capitation can improve care through the use of performance strategies, provider accountability, system integration, and population-based care. Section two describes physician compensation design in terms of payment methodologies, a framework for balancing financial and nonfinancial incentives, and performance-based compensation criteria.

Section three demonstrates techniques for managing the transition from fee-for-service to risk-based payment. This section illustrates reimbursement models for phasing in capitation, pros and cons of budgeted payment, and a global capitation approach for integrated delivery networks. Information system requirements for Medicaid capitation are detailed as well as a case study on how to allocate risk for a community of physicians rather than individual providers. Section four illustrates network financial management controls and reporting formats for monitoring inpatient and ambulatory care services.

Section five covers resource management issues in relation to hospital services, ambulatory care utilization, and care management programs. Section six discusses contract negotiation principles and includes actuarial cost models for evaluating capitation contracts, risk adjustment caveats for high-risk individuals, and measures that can minimize employer liability in managed care arrangements. Section seven describes specialty and ancillary services contracting options. The book concludes with a discussion of ethical issues involving risk-sharing arrangements and the capacity of economic incentives to do good or harm. A glossary of capitation and managed care terminology is also included.

This is a comprehensive book and is meant to serve the diverse day-to-day needs of varied healthcare professionals. The goal of this publication is to stimulate critical thinking about capitation and to initiate a dialogue among industry stakeholders about how financial incentives can be structured to best serve the needs of the community. Reader feedback is an essential ingredient in this process and is highly valued by Boland Healthcare. Readers should point out what further learning material would enhance their knowledge base, job skills, and career development and are encouraged to send suggestions to:

Peter Boland, PhD
President and Publisher
BOLAND HEALTHCARE, INC.
1551 Solano Avenue, 2nd Floor
Berkeley, California 94707
Telephone: 510-524-4521
Fax: 510-524-4607
E-mail: bolandinfo@aol.com

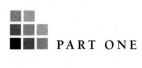
PART ONE

INTRODUCTION

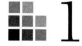 1

The power and potential of capitation

Peter Boland, PhD
President and Publisher
Boland Healthcare, Inc.
Berkeley, California

CAPITATION CHANGES EVERYTHING in healthcare. It affects corporate strategy, financial incentives, operations, access, quality, and profitability. Most of all, it challenges traditional notions of patient care, physician autonomy, and accountability. Many physicians and hospitals view capitation as the single biggest threat to American medicine. Others perceive it as a powerful vehicle to improve clinical and service quality as well as efficiency.

There are numerous factors that help explain the role of capitation in healthcare delivery today. This chapter describes seven of the most important factors to establish a context for capitation: market forces and the managed care industry's development cycle; business strategy; aligning financial incentives and the continuum of reimbursement mechanisms; changing attitudes and behavior; reengineering imperative; population-based risk management; and chronic care management.

Capitation is both a financial management system and a philosophy of care; one without the other will not produce long-term savings and better patient care. As a stand-alone reimbursement strategy, capitation is neither good nor bad. It should be evaluated in terms of meeting the demand for high-quality care at predictable and acceptable costs. How it is understood and managed, however, often means the difference between success and failure for both providers and patients. As a payment mechanism that drives the HMO delivery model, capitation plays an increasingly important role in the development of managed care for

both providers and payers. Managed care companies and the government, pressured largely by costs, are employing capitation to stabilize
medical costs and to remove excess capacity from the healthcare system.
Delivery systems are using capitation to align financial incentives among
network providers. Medical groups and hospitals are using it as a support mechanism to redesign care to maintain quality with reduced revenue. And other stakeholders, such as employers and healthcare reform
advocates, are proposing capitation as a vehicle to control cost while
using other strategies to improve the health status of individuals and
population groups.

Market forces

Managed care is the most powerful force responsible for reshaping
healthcare today. The growth of capitation as a payment mechanism mir-
rors the evolution of the managed care industry on a market-by-market
basis. Its stages of development vary across different markets, and the
type and pace of change is defined locally. As shown in Table 1, cost control, network management, accountability, and customer focus are powerful forces that influence change depending on the stage of the
particular market.

DEVELOPMENT STAGES

The development cycle is an evolutionary process, yet each market does
not necessarily go through each stage in a logical stepwise manner. During the past two decades, there has been a concerted effort by health
plans to decrease costs by using treatment preauthorization, case management, and negotiated discounts from fee schedules. Generally, these
techniques were followed by the development of primary care networks
of providers and additional attempts to exert more systematic cost and
quality controls on them and on physician specialists, hospitals, allied
health professionals, and ancillary services vendors. Many payers have
placed increasing financial risk on individual providers by capitated or
budget-based reimbursement.

   As cost pressures intensified and reimbursement levels decreased,
providers and health plans began to consolidate for economic survival.
Hospitals and health plans increasingly purchased physician practices.

TABLE 1
Managed care industry development cycle

Driving forces	Stage 1	Stage 2	Stage 3
Cost control	Contain costs case by case Achieve economies of scale: ■ membership size ■ geographic concentration ■ service volume Transition fee for service to budget-based reimbursement	Consolidate vendors and distribution channels: ■ hospitals ■ medical groups ■ ancillary services ■ health plans Contain continuum of cost throughout care delivery	Manage at-risk groups Integrate patient care delivery and health plan administration functions
Network management	Build primary care networks	Integrate continuum of services and providers through multidisciplinary care teams: ■ primary care ■ specialty care ■ behavioral healthcare ■ allied healthcare	Establish interdependent alliances across and within industry sectors
Accountability	Develop aggregate cost reports	Document service and clinical quality	Consolidate information services and reporting functions: ■ administrative ■ clinical ■ financial Document treatment outcomes
Customer focus	Offer comprehensive employee benefits packages and covered services	Increase customer value: ■ medical management ■ treatment outcomes ■ member focus	Improve health status: ■ members ■ population groups

Many hospitals merged or were purchased by larger hospital management companies that, in turn, pressured suppliers for lower prices as a trade-off for greater volume. This activity led to streamlined distribution channels. Another benefit of this consolidation was the opportunity to use multidisciplinary patient care teams to integrate a continuum of services across providers and, thereby, improve quality and cost control. But again, this progression did not occur in lockstep fashion in every locale, and some markets have not yet experienced all of these developments.

Quality recently became an issue because payers and purchasers, particularly large employers, demanded it and clinicians embraced continuous quality-improvement methodologies to improve and document care provided. Clinical and service quality are now the object of data collection and reporting efforts for providers and health plans, in addition to cost profiles. Purchasers are increasingly demanding more value from their healthcare providers and delivery systems. Perceived value, not just cost control, has become an important criterion for judging health plan adequacy. Value means effective medical management, better treatment outcomes, and improved customer satisfaction—all of which must be documented as a justification for purchasers' premiums and ongoing business trust.

As more risk continues to be transferred from public payers and employers to health plans, the plans and providers will be called upon to manage the care of high-risk, high-cost groups such as the frail elderly, AIDS patients, and chronically ill children on a capitated basis. Here, an emphasis on risk management encourages delivery systems to focus on containing costs and monitoring the impact of care to measure improved functioning of patients and health status of plan members. Risk management also calls for increased care coordination—seamless patient care along a service continuum—to reduce overlapping functions and duplicated services among provider organizations and delivery systems. This requires increased functional integration and tighter working relationships among employers, insurers, delivery systems, and providers. These interdependencies are created among stakeholders for a reason: such seamless care is more cost effective and increases value for customers.

A growing emphasis on accountability dictates that delivery systems consolidate most of their data repositories, information services, and reporting functions. This consolidation will enable them to better integrate administrative, clinical, and financial data into easy-to-understand yet comprehensive reports. Still, employers need more "actionable data" to make better decisions about designing employee benefits. What health plans need is more flexible and focused information systems to manage provider networks and document the effect of services on the status of enrollees.

As part of the transition from fee for service to capitation, managed care organizations continue to evolve and change in response to underlying market trends, financial constraints, and innovative medical treatments. The most pressing agenda for healthcare delivery systems is to meet customer needs, improve health status, and lower costs. Payers have begun to force providers to more aggressively manage risk in order to increase their profit margins and provide better care. Some delivery systems are also moving from a focus on individual episodes of acute care to include broader population-based attempts to improve the health status of enrolled groups. That is an important step, because payers and patients are best served when their delivery systems adopt a systematic approach to manage overall health risk for a defined population.

Business strategy

Capitation is a double-edged sword hanging over the future of healthcare delivery. If it is used effectively, capitation can be a stimulus to streamline and better integrate healthcare services, improve patient care by reducing inappropriate utilization, and reward providers for good clinical performance. However, because providers under capitation are placed on a fixed budget, some delivery systems have responded by arbitrarily ratcheting down service levels, thus undermining quality while generating large profits for health plans at the expense of physicians, hospitals, and other providers.

Capitation is not a panacea. It cannot turn around poorly managed medical groups, floundering hospitals, or stagnating health plans. It is, however, a vehicle for each of these stakeholders to redefine their business relationships with each other and realign their financial incentives to accomplish specific strategic goals. The goals of capitation can be as diverse as gaining market share, reducing operating costs, or improving patient care. Accomplishing such objectives requires stakeholders to define explicitly their individual roles and responsibilities in relation to each other.

Capitation fosters new business relationships and interdependencies because it forces aggressive patient management at each point along a continuum of care. Thus, the assumption is that collaboration can work better than adversarial competition if the process is thoughtfully managed. Capitation can present a unifying theme (e.g., cost-effective care) and a common frame of reference (e.g., fixed payment) for aligning different organizational strategies and financial incentives among business partners. Successful capitation requires a true partnership among health plan members, health professionals, and payers or delivery systems.

Because capitation joins healthcare delivery and financing, it also poses a potential ethical challenge, but not an insurmountable one. How can the clinical practice of medicine, which formerly operated at arm's length from cost management, balance the patient's interests against the health plan's interests to economize and maintain profit margins? The integration of provider and payer functions presents a unique challenge to develop compensation and reward systems to serve both ends. Capitation can do this if the delivery system's business values are founded on a philosophical commitment to four practices: preventive care, early detection and appropriate treatment of disease, health promotion and education services, and objective performance measures.

By keeping members healthy as long as possible and targeting appropriate treatment goals for specific illnesses, delivery systems can serve the needs of patients and be financially accountable at the same time. It is a practical strategy that creates a win-win result if stakeholders share the same overriding business goals and values. Thus, identifying shared values and developing common business strategies is essential for success in managing risk arrangements under capitation.

Aligning incentives

Capitation payment techniques evolve in response to the needs of particular provider groups and delivery systems. The more competitive a local market is in terms of managed care penetration, the more sophisticated and aggressive the form of capitation is likely to be. Capitation payment mechanisms range from individual productivity-oriented approaches based on volume to salary-oriented models based on group performance. Each can build in bonus payments or other performance factors such as referral management, clinical quality indicators, and patient satisfaction measures.

TABLE 2
Reimbursement continuum

Low risk	Medium risk	High risk
Fee for service	Performance-based fee for service: ▪ primary care ▪ specialty care	Combined physician and hospital services capitation
Discounted fee for service or discounted charges	Capitation: ▪ primary care ▪ specialty care	Global capitation: ▪ physicians ▪ other practitioners ▪ hospital services ▪ ancillary services
Bundled fee for service	Institution case rates	
Single and multiple per diem rates		

At-risk arrangements, which put providers at some financial risk for the cost of patient care, cover a variety of payment mechanisms from modified fee for service to global capitation as shown in Table 2.

One of the goals of capitation is to align the incentives of primary care physicians, specialists, hospitals, and other practitioners to provide better care to more people at less cost. This can be achieved by designing a compensation strategy with financial risks and rewards that are mutually shared. An effective compensation strategy aligns individual physicians, medical groups, and hospitals with the long-term strategic objectives of the health plan, delivery system, or purchasing group. A properly structured compensation system can achieve specific goals and objectives by motivating healthcare practitioners and institutions to change day-to-day clinical behavior and administrative procedures by rewarding greater efficiency and effectiveness.

This means that stakeholders, including employers, must identify their business goals before proposing, designing, or accepting a capitation payment strategy. It also suggests that buy-in will occur, particularly among physicians, only if the capitation distribution formula is simple, easy to understand, and fair. Likewise, it must support the key values (such as quality care) of each stakeholder group in order to become part of its corporate culture.

Capitation works best when stakeholders, including patients, clearly grasp their respective roles and responsibilities in advance. Practitioners must understand and accept any performance standards (e.g., productivity requirements, patient satisfaction measures, and quality indicators) that define accountability as a basis for compensation. Setting explicit performance goals with measurable objectives that are shared and discussed with providers and health plans in advance is a key to improving performance. Accurate information and timely feedback on individual and group performance are essential components for making a positive impact on provider behavior and practice patterns.

As a compensation system, one of the purposes of capitation is to motivate practitioners to provide medically necessary care in the most appropriate setting and at the right time. This rewards good clinical care and discourages unnecessary or inappropriate care that does not result in desired treatment outcomes. With an effective reimbursement mechanism, the focus of clinical decision making and care coordination becomes what is best for the individual patient—the plan member. This is fundamentally different than responding to the organizational needs of hospitals, physicians, or delivery systems.

Changing attitudes

Capitation transfers risk from the purchaser, insurer, or health plan to any participating provider, starting with physicians. This brings a provider's financial incentives in line with the delivery system's. Economic reward comes from lowering total healthcare costs rather than unit costs or the amount of resources used by any one practitioner for a particular patient. For example, if a provider contract is structured so that physicians in an HMO network have a direct stake in the financial performance of the plan, then they are at risk for how their colleagues manage patients. This changes how physicians relate to one another, the hospital, and the health plan. In fact, it can encourage IPA physicians to behave more like group practice physicians—a desirable effect. As a result, such a contract establishes a fundamentally different relationship among major stakeholders.

Capitated payment requires greater administrative and clinical integration than fee for service, enhancing the potential to bring together different care facilities and professional disciplines. Integrating payment leads to integrated practice among practitioners in a delivery system's network of providers, changing the orientation and behavior of providers. Practitioners are also encouraged under capitation to recognize what the patient needs rather than the services the hospital, medical group, or health plan is accustomed to providing. The latter focus is internally generated, not externally oriented or market driven. Furthermore, maintaining an organizational rather than a member focus is a serious mistake in providing care to defined populations under capitation. Successfully managing risk requires meeting patient needs and preferences as well as providing cost-effective care.

Each of these factors represents a tremendous cultural change for providers entering capitated healthcare and for health plans struggling with the requirements of managing risk-based groups. It means doing business differently.

To successfully incorporate capitation, hospitals and medical groups must demonstrate their capitation readiness by developing the necessary expertise to actually manage risk and prepaid revenue. For example, making the transition from gross charges from fee for service to net revenue from capitation involves changing provider perceptions about accountability, customer service, use of resources, and day-to-day patient management. It often takes hospitals and physicians two to three years to learn how to incorporate the operational requirements of capitation, such as actuarial analysis and forecasting, fixed budgets, utilization management procedures, data processing and medical informatics, and claims payment.

Moreover, the shift to measuring improvement in health status as a primary measure of performance requires an even bigger change. Implementing a change of this magnitude requires a fully developed cultural strategy to influence an organization's corporate culture. Corporate culture is generally not seen by health plans as a critical factor that determines success in capitation but is often regarded as a soft, free-floating notion that cannot be readily defined and translated into concrete management actions. As such, corporate culture often goes unrecognized and unchallenged despite its pervasive influence throughout an organization.

It is the cultural strategy that connects the overall business strategy with the day-to-day operating strategy and reimbursement strategy. How this work is accomplished depends on motivating employees, rewarding desired behavior, and reinforcing the need for organizational change. Changing how people think and act and overcoming their resistance to change is a prerequisite for implementing a new reimbursement system or different business and operational strategies. Such a change in direction means that providers (including delivery systems) must critically assess how healthcare work is structured, organized, and delivered. Whose needs are being served and what results are being achieved must be considered. Such questioning inevitably leads to the conclusion that fundamental change—structural, cultural, and personal—is necessary to provide better care and services to individuals, to payers, and to the community.

The healthcare delivery system must be fundamentally redesigned in order to improve patient care within fixed budgets. This is the biggest challenge of healthcare reform at the local, state, and federal level. It means that delivery systems must reengineer their organizational and service components to be successful under capitation.[1]

Reengineering imperative

Price competition, capacity consolidation, and capitated risk arrangements are powerful market forces responsible for restructuring the healthcare industry from top to bottom. The market's need for substantially lower healthcare premiums compels providers—including hospitals, physicians, and other practitioners—to face the stark reality that industrywide consolidation will result in few clear winners and many losers. At a minimum, there will be much more service integration between health plan administration and patient care delivery functions, among facilities and practitioners, and within institutions through comprehensive case management and individualized care protocols. Widespread merger and acquisition activity in the industry will leave few organizations untouched and will provide further rationale to integrate fragmented services and operations with reengineering tools and to change management techniques. Therefore, just doing more of the same but better will not meet customer demands for significant cost reduction and improved service quality, which means doing more for less.

Market forces and industry dynamics are generating an unprecedented level of change, resulting in reduced need for acute care facilities, providers, and healthcare vendors. Managed care has cut the utilization rate for inpatient services to such an extent that most markets now have a significant excess of hospital beds and physician specialists. Thus, both successful and challenged organizations are being forced to reassess their future in light of decreasing revenue, increasing competition, and the demand for more accountability and documented results. These factors make fundamental change a requirement for survival; incremental change on a piecemeal basis will not enable healthcare organizations to succeed. Much more serious intervention is required. Organizations must rapidly rethink what they do and how they do it to remain competitive.

As market forces define stringent cost and performance targets for healthcare organizations, reengineering methodologies become essential survival tools to manage change and improve service. Cost reduction demands by purchasers and payers have been driving down provider reimbursement rates each year, but this is not a viable long-term strategy. Rates can be ratcheted down only so far before payment no longer covers real costs and provider resentment negatively affects the physician-patient relationship. At that point, quality is jeopardized. Fundamental delivery system redesign is necessary, because capitated healthcare organizations cannot sufficiently reduce their ongoing operating costs without sustained efforts.

Capitation can be a means to achieving increased volume and improved quality, as well as better cost management. Thus, capitation requires gaining mastery over new skills and molding new values. Providers must clearly understand how capitated reimbursement can help realize common strategic and operational goals to make the difficult learning process palatable. This is neither quick nor easy, just necessary.

Population-based risk management

Advanced capitation strategies change the focus of health plan activities from a single incidence of patient care to managing the care of all enrollees covered under a contract. Called "population-based" care, it incorporates all the necessary services, practitioners, and treatment settings needed by health plan members.

Managing populations requires a broader perspective than caring for individuals. It means changing the emphasis from being event driven to risk driven (e.g., reducing the likelihood of illness with preventive services or intervening sooner in the illness cycle through early detection and screening services) and matching specific medical and social services to target groups. The objective is to better manage the health risk of target groups, which extends well beyond acute care patients and chronically ill members.

To identify and manage population-based risk, new information systems, tracking mechanisms, and medical management procedures must be developed and established. To better manage aggregate costs as well as unit costs, multidisciplinary care teams must concentrate on the causes of acute care episodes—the underlying psychological, economic, and sociological factors that affect the incidence and prevalence of disease and injuries. Care teams can then use treatment protocols that identify the least costly and most clinically appropriate settings to direct patient care. This shift in treatment strategy calls for delivery systems to take more responsibility for providing care in three ways: providing care that best fits the medical, social, and cultural profile of the enrolled population; maintaining and improving the health status of at-risk groups; and lowering the cost of care for individuals and the community.

The role of delivery systems and partnering organizations such as medical groups, hospitals, ancillary services vendors, and allied health professionals must change in order to intervene in illness sooner and more effectively. It is too costly for customers and health plans, particularly capitated arrangements, to wait until a member is acutely ill or in need of chronic care services. At the same time, it is not known how long it takes for most illness prevention services to make an impact in terms of reduced need for acute care services. As a payment system, capitation creates powerful economic incentives to move the focus of care away from high-cost settings (e.g., hospitals) and types of treatment (e.g., acute) to community-based services that can better affect the incidence and prevalence of disease in the first place. Reducing the need for medical care—inpatient, outpatient, and ambulatory—is the key. However, because hospitals and most physicians only treat patients once they are sick, providers have little ability to influence the course of events that leads up to the episode of care itself.

An effective capitation strategy avoids, or at least minimizes, the need for high-cost medical services such as hospital admissions. By influencing the underlying causes of acute care episodes that can be controlled, such as preventable accidents and injuries and behaviorally linked illnesses, health plans realize financial savings and members develop and maintain better quality of life. This requires intervening at the right time before acute or chronic care management is necessary. However, it is still unclear how long it takes for most illness prevention services to reduce the need for acute care services.

As shown in Figure 1, the progression from "healthy" to "chronic" is both a function of controllable factors and factors beyond an individual's direct control. However, with appropriate and early intervention, an individual's health status can be influenced toward the healthy end of the continuum even if his or her current status is at-risk or acute.

Capitation presents a compelling economic case to intervene in the social and economic fabric of the community to prevent illnesses and avoid hospital admissions. In order for health plans to realize significant long-term savings, a genuine public-private sector partnership is required. This approach blurs the distinction between for-profit and not-for-profit providers, traditional and complementary medicine, and institutional and alternative settings for care.

By making an investment in community- and neighborhood-based services, health plans and delivery system partners demonstrate an

FIGURE 1
Life cycle stages and health status factors[2]

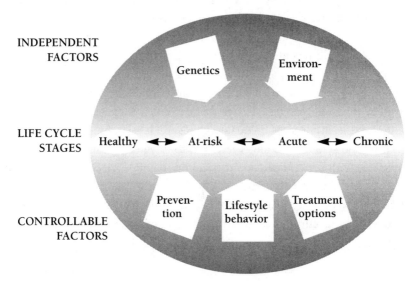

ongoing commitment to local stakeholders and to improving the health status of the community. This requires health plans to commit capital over a multiyear period. Such a partnership approach enables community-based agencies—public health centers and clinics, social service agencies, school systems, and self-help organizations—to develop broad-based prevention and early intervention techniques that decrease the incidence and prevalence of disease, which, in turn, reduces avoidable costs to the health plan and members.

Capitation provides the economic rationale and the financial incentive for delivery systems to target services in order to accomplish an overriding objective: to help members stay healthy and regain optimal functioning as quickly as possible. That is the power and potential of capitation.

Chronic care management

One of the most far-reaching economic and clinical challenges facing managed care is the growing demand for chronic care services. As the current demographic bulge passes from middle age into the 65-plus age group, delivery systems will be overwhelmed by the prevalence of chronic illness and the accompanying cost burden. Reengineering the current approach to care is an economic necessity for healthcare delivery systems and society.

Managed care delivery systems are deeply rooted in the acute care model of curative medicine. This model is not geared to an aging population whose chronic illnesses cannot be cured, but who need relief of symptoms and prevention of further dysfunction. It calls for a biopsychosocial model (i.e., medical, social, and community orientation) that encompasses far more than physiological factors commonly associated with acute care treatment. The goal of chronic care management is not curative; the emphasis is on quality of life and level of function.

A multidisciplinary team is required to integrate primary and specialty care with home-based and community-based services. Both patient and family perspectives must be integrated into the care process for treatment to be effective and valued. This approach means reengineering and reorienting current medical management practices—including capitation—that are often based more on the needs of healthcare organizations and providers than on patients or health plan members.

Capitated delivery systems have the potential to improve care for members with chronic conditions because they can intervene at a system level as well as at the individual patient or provider level.

Conclusion

Capitation creates a financial incentive to deliver care in the most appropriate setting, often within the community or at home. It offers programmatic flexibility and rational economic incentives for stakeholders to take effective action. All major stakeholders in the healthcare industry—members, employers, practitioners, delivery systems, community organizations, and the government—share a common interest in managing care more effectively by managing risk sooner and better. Capitation can be a catalyst that encourages and reinforces this commonality of purpose.

NOTES

1. P. Boland, "The Role of Reengineering in Healthcare Delivery," in *Redesigning Healthcare Delivery* (Berkeley: Boland Healthcare, 1996).
2. This model is adapted from New Century Healthcare Institute, San Francisco, California.

2

Components of a vertically integrated system

Javon R. Bea
President and Chief Executive Officer
Mercy Health System
Janesville, Wisconsin

WHILE THERE ARE STILL numerous healthcare organizations operating under traditional fee-for-service
financial models, the healthcare industry is increasingly moving toward
capitation. Whether it be full capitation or balancing a mixed fee-
for-service and capitated payment system, the movement toward this
new financial model presents a myriad of challenges.

In a capitated system there are two concerns crucial to its success:
controlling provider cost and promoting quality care. Both require creating a new organizational vision. The challenge is to create an infrastructure and support system to successfully convert fee-for-service
organizational structures to a workable capitated environment that max-
imizes cost savings and increases quality.

This chapter examines an organizational model that has succeeded
thus far: capitation implemented through a vertically integrated full-
service provider network, with particular emphasis on the role physician integration plays.

In an integrated system, the goal is to provide seamless delivery of
patient care in the most cost-effective way, bringing together all major
components of a healthcare system including an insurance product.
This type of system enables providers to better manage the delivery of
care while simultaneously controlling the costs typically unaccounted

for when services are contracted from unaffiliated providers. When all providers are part of the same vertically integrated system, the financial pressures on each individual component within the system are reduced.

The turf battles often seen in loose affiliations are eliminated. Ideally, when individual organizations are merged, a central mission is created that permeates the entire organization. With loose affiliations, each component has its own mission that can conflict with the mission of the whole, creating a power struggle. For example, a loosely affiliated organization may not be able to decide which managed care companies to affiliate with due to conflicting wants; the physicians may like the financial rewards associated with one managed care organization, while the hospital finds another more beneficial for other reasons. In a commitment to one single mission, all parts of an organization are moving toward one goal.

A commitment to integration, however, generally revolves around one key component: the physicians. The first step to develop an integrated delivery system (IDS) is to bring the physicians into the system, most importantly, the primary care physicians (PCP). In an IDS, the PCPs are the entry point to the system. Thus, the degree to which an integrated healthcare provider can hire a sufficient number of PCPs and distribute them appropriately will be crucial to its ability to capture market share in a managed care environment.

Putting the pieces together

To make capitation work, a number of components are necessary. First, providers need to develop a new way to identify and solve problems. Perhaps the most important thing a provider must do initially is to change its emphasis to system effectiveness rather than component effectiveness. In capitation, the whole must be greater than the sum of its parts.

As healthcare providers attempt to put an IDS together, there are established guidelines to follow. A vertical integration model that defines these steps can be helpful in pinpointing initial goals. In order to create a fully integrated system that covers the spectrum of care, an organization must secure

- Acute inpatient hospital care services

- Tertiary subspecialty care services

- Secondary specialty care services

- Outpatient care services

- Long-term care services

- Rehabilitation services

- PCP services

- Health promotion and disease prevention programs

A vertical integration model suggests that providers expand their services to offer a full continuum of care, in addition to developing a complete array of hospital services that are based on need. This need is defined through a service-demand analysis that assesses the health status and trends of the community on an ongoing basis. Data compiled from the demand analysis can also be used as a cornerstone in physician recruitment. If a proper demographic analysis is done, a correct primary-speciality care physician mix can more effectively be recruited (providers can document the need for particular services) and retained (by ensuring a sufficient patient base exists to support current physicians). In this demand analysis, the IDS must not forget to examine mental health and substance abuse programs, inpatient and outpatient services, home care services, and disease prevention and wellness initiatives as potential service areas. In addition, to keep up with and regularly update changing health trends, a demand analysis should be done at least every 18 to 24 months.

The move toward vertical integration is also in harmony with a capitated environment's new emphasis on the system. Under capitation, it is not enough to work on hospital, physician, or insurance product efficiency alone. For true effectiveness, all three pieces must function in concert, as part of a single integrated organization with a unified mission. An infrastructure that provides and controls a continuum of care will allow a capitated financial structure to work.

Under capitation, the provider must rely heavily on the community for organizational direction as the community needs will largely dictate the services an organization provides.

Analyze, analyze, analyze

In the transition from a fee-for-service to a capitation arrangement, a detailed plan of action is essential. When determining which direction will best suit an organization's member population needs, it is crucial that providers analyze three things: community demographics, prevalence of various diseases, and convenience of patient access. By incorporating these three pieces of information into the design of a vertically integrated system, providers can accurately reflect member needs.

Planning for personnel requirements, particularly physicians, based on analysis of the community's needs is critical and cannot be overstated. As with any market sensitive system, health systems need a salable product to survive. In essence, vertical integration allows healthcare to engage the consumer-driven market. Community needs determine what role a provider plays, the number and type of services delivered, and the proper primary-specialty care physician mix. Proper analysis of these needs requires a diverse array of research skills, which are typically found in such organizations as insurance companies and market research firms that use computerized systems to establish premium rates, physician supply and demand analysis, prevalence of disease statistical analysis, patient access analysis, and other sophisticated analysis. Typically hospitals do not have these resources available, so a consultant may be hired to help develop the necessary research skills.

The results of this research analysis then forms the system's physician hiring plan, a comprehensive evaluation that consists of in-depth analysis of present and future population demographics, age distributions, and other significant numbers. From that information a supply-and-demand report of physician needs broken down by physician specialty and geographic location is created. This plan is then used to establish hiring needs.

An action plan alone does not result in a good system. Providers need to follow the plan and recruit and retain the necessary physicians and support staff to meet the market demand they have discovered. They also need to continue to monitor the healthcare pulse of their community and allow for changing needs while maintaining flexibility. If service demand wanes or increases, appropriate measures need to be taken to reflect that change.

Gathering the tools

Successfully analyzing the market and implementing an infrastructure that facilitates capitation takes a variety of tools. These include a new management culture, population-based needs assessment, patient care management systems, technical assessment systems, a continuous quality improvement (CQI) process, information linkages, and incentive systems.

- *New management culture.* The new culture must be market driven. The delivery system must respond to the market's needs rather than reflect a service-specific orientation. It also must be entrepreneurial, market assertive with a high tolerance for change (e.g., there must be a recognition that care is moving from the inpatient to the outpatient setting. This may be a difficult transition for hospital managers steeped in the inpatient tradition)

- *Population-based needs assessment.* A community analysis, to determine necessary services, must be based on the population served and the healthcare trends likely to occur in such a population. An actuarial analysis is often required. Population-based assessments should be done on a regular basis and at least every two years to maintain accuracy (e.g., an aging population may require more internists, while a younger population may require more family practice physicians)

- *Patient care management system.* A patient care management system should recognize that entities making up the health system do not stand alone and that preserving a continuum of care is vital to maintaining its health. The patient care management component should be designed to support and enhance this continuity of care. When developing guidelines, a multifunctional approach must be taken to ensure physician and organizational goals are kept in sync (e.g., the hospital cannot develop guidelines in a vacuum without input from and participation by the physicians covering the primary care clinics)

- *Technological assessment systems.* Outcomes management and physician practice guidelines should be developed. These should cover the entire spectrum of care a patient receives throughout the integrated system (e.g., a physical a patient receives in one clinic location should be identical to a physical performed in another clinic location 15 miles away)

- *Continuous quality improvement processes.* On one level, continuous quality improvement ensures that the quality of care is equally balanced with utilization and cost conservation measures in managed care. On another level, quality improvement is a key component in controlling utilization internally. From implementing programs that meet the National Committee for Quality Assurance (NCQA) standards (necessary for HMO accreditation) to self-imposed CQI initiatives—such as membership satisfaction surveys, membership health status surveys, and physician resource use reports—all quality improvement initiatives aim to raise the standard of care and decrease unnecessary utilization. The result: members stay healthier and require less extensive and costly care

- *Information linkages.* A central computer system to link all components of the health system is essential. Everyone in the organization should be well informed of organizational goals. On an organized basis, it is useful to have frequent meetings with physicians and employees on both the direction of the organization and the technological approaches to capitation management. Such meetings make the medical management activities required for success easier to implement

- *Incentive systems.* For physicians, incentive systems should be based on productivity, patient satisfaction, and quality measurements. All three components encourage a different range of behaviors that are crucial to overall success. For example, a basic salary based on productivity can be coupled with a set of quality and utilization targets that encourage cost-effective behaviors. The attainment of these targets can be used as the basis of further compensation bonuses

Integrating physicians

Physicians form the foundation of a successful capitated organizational model. They are the gate through which the patient enters the system and the road the patient uses to travel the system. Encouraging physicians to move to a capitated way of thinking and actively encouraging them to create an effective system may take daily effort by managers as well as physicians. To ensure that vertical integration and capitation work, physicians need to be involved at every stage, from recruitment to day-to-day management.

It is important that physicians understand and accept the organization's mission, beginning with physician recruitment. Because IDSs need to keep up with current market needs, it is crucial to perform a demand analysis to gauge what type of physicians are necessary and to estimate to what extent their services will be used.

The next challenge is to recruit physicians to the organization as partners, rather than independent contractors who may not share the organizational vision. There are a number of steps a healthcare provider can take to effectively recruit physicians who will positively contribute to this new integrated healthcare system.

Recruit with high expectations

- Make the physician want to become a part of the organization and a partner

- Give each physician positive news about the organization, its location, and the area's economic climate (e.g., its profitability, success with new programs and new locations)

- Let the physician know the organization is an aggressive player in the marketplace and intends to be around in the next century. In a market-driven system, market assertiveness is one of the keys to create and sustain a successful organization

- Show the physician the organization is concerned with quality of care provided to members as well as the quality of a physician's relationship with the organization. It is also important to cover the personal concerns of the physicians and their families (e.g., school quality, community safety, recreational and cultural activities in the area) and the physician's professional concerns (e.g., who handles administrative tasks—the physician or support staff, who takes responsibility for management issues). To best address these potential concerns, as much information as possible should be gathered on the physician before and during recruitment

- Introduce the physician to other key physician partners

- Provide a carefully planned tour of the facilities and communities, illustrating state-of-the-art facilities, equipment, and services. This will demonstrate the organization is committed to quality. Facilities and equipment expenditures are a relatively small price to pay for the degree to which they can enhance an organization's volume and geographical spread

- Provide a competitive package of compensation and benefit incentives (e.g., a standard benefits package should include provisions for pension, relocation, vacation, time off for continuing medical education, reimbursement for certification, and membership in professional groups; plus life, disability, and family health and dental insurance). Compensation figures should reflect up-to-date physician salary standards

- Answer questions honestly and share the organization's vision for the future

The organization should
- Check physicians' references thoroughly

- Ask the physicians what type of practice they want (e.g., ideal hours and days, on-call schedule, compensation goals). The more specific the information, the easier it will be to match the physician

- Seek physician expectations

- Ask about personal considerations, such as schooling considerations for family and housing preferences. This information can aid recruiters to direct physicians to available resources during the recruitment phase

Be fearless in seeking to meet goals
- Provide contracts with an initial limited term (e.g., one- to two-year contracts with defined renewal mechanisms) and retain the right to

terminate for cause (e.g., loss of license, Medicare/ Medicaid certification, or medical staff privileges)

- Do not be afraid to be bold and take calculated risks. Developing an integrated delivery system and instituting a capitated payment structure is risky and cannot be developed halfheartedly. Those who take the challenge must believe in themselves and meet the opportunities that arise head on

In order to make capitation work, a cadre of dedicated physicians must be in place. To assure the ongoing dedication of this group, it is important that the following contract and compensation components exist.

Important contract components
- Determine the contract's initial term provisions and provisions for contract termination, renewal, or renegotiation

- Develop future employment agreement follow-up before the contract expires

- Define the physician reporting mechanism, which should define whom the physician should report to regarding operational matters (i.e., the CEO or a mutually agreed upon designee)

- Determine an accurate job description including all physician responsibilities and expectations

- Define maintenance of all licenses and medical staff privileges, obtaining board certification and compliance with pertinent regulations

Compensation
- Determine structure of salary and the extension of any initial practice development supports (e.g., advertising, marketing, and staffing assistance)

- Develop production objectives and incentives and how these are calculated

- Develop a clear description of bonuses or other incentives

- Determine salary or production incentives to be paid following the initial contract term (e.g., x percent of revenue generated over a specified amount, as long as utilization targets are met)

- Establish formulas and examples to illustrate the terms as precisely as possible

Termination
- Outline types of termination scenarios (i.e., illness or disability, cause, voluntary, and mutual agreement)

- Detail any competitive restrictions

Benefits
- List in detail all vacation, sick days, and continuing medical education time

- Define medical, dental, life, and disability insurance provisions

- Define credentialing, licensing, board certification, medical societies, retirement, and pension plan payment availability

Hiring committed physicians, however, is only the first step toward physician integration. This new system replaces long-standing patterns, such as informal referral procedures, with formal, in-house processes—something that may initially appear too confining when taken out of context of the system.

Perhaps most importantly, capitation means physicians' salaries are no longer affected exclusively by the number of patients they see or the type of procedure they perform. In contrast to fee-for-service medicine, physician payment is the same regardless of the number of patients seen or the various procedures performed. Some specialties have characteristics that make them easier to capitate than others. Since PCPs, for example, generally see the patient first and on a more predictable basis, they may be more accepting of capitation than specialists who traditionally care for high-risk patients with large variations in care needs.

Capitation will also require physicians to change their behavior. It changes the way physicians practice and are paid. If the physician does not understand that preventive healthcare, resulting in fewer visits, tests, and procedures, actually generates higher profits, overutilization may be the result. This means that the attendant cost risk is shifted entirely to the healthcare organization using the capitated payment system.

Because striking a balance between utilization and quality is an operational goal under capitation, peer review among physicians is often used to encourage physicians who are not meeting established guidelines. A true understanding and participation in this process, coupled with education designed to improve outcomes, will make capitation more acceptable to physicians.

Organizations that use capitation have developed a number of other ways to encourage physicians to be more effective, including merit or bonus systems and performance measurements. Organizations should examine problems situationally to create a unique model that works for them, maintaining flexibility. Staff members should be empowered to solve problems creatively and offer constructive suggestions.

Physicians need to understand that they can actually earn more by better management of patient care in a capitated system than under fee for service. A merit or bonus system can capitalize on this idea because it is tied to the overall success of the organization responsible for managing the risk arrangement. The more actual costs fall below the capitated target costs, the larger the bonus.

Another physician compensation issue that arises is the production measurement or standard now imposed on physicians. Providers have instituted a variety of compensation packages based on particular measurements. The more specific the measure, however, the harder it is to implement and perpetuate. The goal should be a workable, easily measured behavior or goal (e.g., financial success of the organization overall, meeting utilization targets). Devising such a measure, as well as a system of measurement, will be one of the greatest challenges administrators face as healthcare organizations move from fee for service to capitation.

To preserve revenue, however, providers must prevent both over- and underutilization. They must encourage preventive care and wellness, both to keep members from serious, long-term care and to prevent a common illness from reaching a critical and costly stage of treatment. Thus, physicians must be taught how to be efficient and motivated to function efficiently.

Both of these goals can be accomplished by using inpatient, outpatient, and follow-up guidelines providing feedback and communication and working with the physicians on a day-to-day basis to gain an understanding of how an integrated system functions. This foundation communication will do more than any financial incentives or disincentives an organization could create to foster physician acceptance.

Importance of outcomes

Outcomes are critical to preserve the quality of care. Because IDSs are dependent on the number of people in their risk pool, member quality and value are critical.

Issues such as quality of care, quality of service, and provider choice will emerge as the top member motivators. A foremost concern will be how to keep member satisfaction high. It is important for providers to remember that general member satisfaction is a top priority for membership, thus, motivating staff members—from reception to checkout—toward the central mission of an IDS is critical. How each staff person treats a member will formulate how that member perceives the quality of care received.

Inpatient versus outpatient

In an effort to control costs, healthcare organizations have already begun to encourage more outpatient procedures and fewer hospital admissions. Technology has helped to facilitate this trend by allowing a large number of procedures previously available only on an inpatient basis to be safely performed as outpatient procedures.

In a capitated environment, the trend toward outpatient procedures will only increase. Some experts predict this will increase by as much as 50 percent of current utilization rates, if not more. By the year 2005, a 35- to 40-member physician multispecialty group may be performing 85 to 90 percent of the procedures now performed in a 300-bed hospital.

Therefore, to manage capitation in the future, a successful integrated healthcare delivery system will also need updated ambulatory and outpatient surgery facilities to reduce costs and stay market competitive. For example, consider a procedure that can be done both outpatient and inpatient. While performing a procedure on an outpatient basis may require technologically advanced and more costly facilities, in many cases this is far less expensive and more efficient in the long term. The cost of a hospital stay hurts an IDS' bottom line and may be less attractive to the patient. By investing upfront in necessary technology, healthcare providers will be better equipped for the future and increase member satisfaction at the same time.

Managing care and costs to minimize risk

Capitation revolves around controlling the inherent risks of adverse selection. An insurance product owned by the providing network is a unique and effective way to complete the circle of integrated care and cost management.

In a fully integrated provider network spearheaded by an insurance product, the network owns and provides all the services and, therefore, does not have to contract for services from unaffiliated parties. The major benefit lies in the ability of this system to effectively control costs. Contracting with independent sources makes managing care and utilization far more difficult, if not impossible. Of course, there is always financial balancing involved when an organization decides to provide care directly rather than contract for services from another organization.

Analysts faced with a choice typically select the least costly option. However, the best advice is to avoid being shortsighted. What saves an organization some money today may be the undoing of the system when that contracted service engages in overutilization or raises its rates and becomes inaccessible (e.g., employing versus contracting emergency room physicians or providing addiction treatment services in-house rather than outsourcing these to a provider outside the health system).

Caring for the machine

In a vertically integrated system, healthcare providers can be compared to a well-oiled machine providing for 100 percent of the healthcare of their patients. Yet, as with any machine, there must be support mechanisms to prepare for and prevent malfunctions. To ensure an IDS has an infrastructure capable of handling whatever the future of healthcare may hold, two features are necessary.

First, a new measure of cost is required to accurately reflect the cost of providing care per member per month (PMPM) on an extended basis. Because historical data is scant or nonexistent, an actuarial analysis can help. Actuaries are able to make projections that take both past and potential future trends into account when creating budgets. Until more hard data is gathered, this is often the best method to determine a workable cost PMPM.

Second, the entire organization must be postured toward emphasizing good health, and IDS members must be active participants in this pursuit. The emphasis on health and wellness ensures plan members will require less costly care and will have fewer critical illnesses.

Assuming risk

Under capitation, cost-effective utilization is dependent on spreading and managing the risks a provider assumes. Today, there is no longer any pressure to keep hospital beds filled, and every visit or admission will cost the organization money. A continuum of care that can effectively spread the financial risks and improve the standard of the population's health minimizes the risks of a capitated system. Current industry HMO standards reveal that between 25,000 and 35,000 members are needed to achieve this ideal low risk. Thus, in theory, an integrated delivery system that offers an HMO product with 30,000 members could safely operate on a fully capitated payment model and survive. However, below that number, the risk could outweigh any potential gain. Any significant increase in the cost of care could financially break the organization. That is not to say that integrated delivery systems with small HMO memberships do not prosper. They can and do, but rarely on a fully capitated basis.

Integrated healthcare delivery systems building an HMO product should initially seek long-term contracts with businesses that are willing to work closely to reduce costs while continually developing and evaluating their guidelines and outcome measurements.

Final comment

Healthcare organizations are attempting to create more cost-effective delivery systems—through integration and capitation—that improve quality of care. It is a balancing act that involves managing financial incentives and quality determinants in order to create a win-win situation for everyone

Mercy Health System of Janesville, Wisconsin, was transformed from a single, stand-alone community hospital to a vertically integrated healthcare system. The new Mercy Health System has 27 locations in 13 different communities across five southern Wisconsin and northern Illinois counties. In 1989, Mercy had no employed physicians. Today, over two-thirds of its 195-physician medical staff are employed. These physicians participated in every aspect of the system's development, including their new insurance company, MercyCare HMO Health Plan, which has a network of 12 hospitals and more than 450 physicians. The vertically integrated health system includes all major aspects of the healthcare continuum.

3

Performance metrics and capitation strategies

Edward Thomas
Manager of Clinical Information
Blue Shield of California
San Francisco, California

BUSINESS AND CLINICAL MANAGEMENT strategies often take significant shifts of architecture or structure under capitation. Although some aspects of capitation may not be palatable to medical groups, it is a reimbursement system where a well-managed medical group can thrive.

This chapter discusses specific design requirements for building a capitation program based on efficiency, quality, and continuous improvement. It focuses on staffing requirements, utilization and quality targets, delegation, and a glimpse of future considerations. All ratios and rates are stated as per 1,000 and per member per month (PMPM). Targeted rates are based on assumptions of standard risk, health status, and age/gender distribution. It is this spirit of continuous quality improvement (CQI) that gain and enhancement strategies are based on.

Staffing requirements

Strategies focusing on appropriate staffing ratios have moved rapidly into most practice settings. It is evident for large multispecialty groups that a target primary care to specialty ratio is 60/40 to 70/30. To staff within this model the following specific ratios are recommended. Medical groups quickly notice that, based on these ratios, a community may be significantly overserved by specialists (see Table 1).

TABLE 1
Physician ratios to population

Medical specialties	FTE to members
Allergy	50,000
Cardiology	35,000
Dermatology	35,000
Endocrinology	100,000
Gastroenterology	50,000
Internal medicine and family practice	2,700
Neurology	55,000
Pediatrics	6,000
Rheumatology	100,000
Oncology	50,000
Surgical specialties	
Ear, nose, and throat	35,000
Obstetrics and gynecology	7,000
Ophthalmology	25,000
Orthopedics	20,000
General surgery	15,000
Urology	40,000
Other	
Anesthesiology	17,000
Psychiatry	20,000
Radiology	20,000

If staffing strategies are slow to reach ratio targets it is recommended that at least one full-time equivalent (FTE) per specialty be brought into the group, where that specialist would have the responsibility to manage that area of care.

For instance, a single urologist would manage his or her practice and the entire urology practice of the group to include all referrals. It may be useful to simply subcapitate this person for all urologic care, inside and outside of the plan. This provides for a direct incentive for the specialist to manage care in a manner that builds collaboration among other physicians in the group and the community specialists.

This collaborative approach assists with building internal guidelines of care and referral guidelines for primary care. The educational component of this may take the form of the urologist educating primary care physicians about appropriate referrals based on the American Urologic Associations scoring guide. Also, education for the medical community may help build guidelines of care for conditions such as incontinence and impotence.

Also, the group must make an important and difficult decision regarding inpatient staffing. The move to managing inpatient care with a handful of intensivists or internal medicine specialists is a sound and practical management decision. This allows for a tightly managed inpatient program but still considers the needs of the family practice physician by encouraging a partnering in the care or social visits to reinforce to the patient that strong communication between physicians is in place. Inpatient management practice variation is reduced, and critical pathways of care and guidelines of practice are easier to develop and implement because the group of physicians is built on a team concept and the number of inpatient physicians is small.

Groups adopting this approach have elicited favorable responses from their physicians and patients, citing more time for outpatient care, fewer after-hours telephone calls, and increased confidence in and accessibility to physicians respectively. The burden of inpatient management is lessened for the group overall, but a flexibility exists that does not eliminate the role of the primary care physician.

A favorable product of dedicated inpatient physicians is a dramatic decrease in cesarean sections, bed days per 1,000, and untoward events such as unexpected death or infection. This is especially important when quality improvement activities are undertaken that allow measuring performance for a small group of providers. Shifting to a dedicated inpatient team requires that an interested group of physicians be identified, policies, schedules, and guidelines of care be established, and, finally, a target date for finalizing the dedicated team be set. It may take six months to a year for physicians to go through the weaning stage from believing that inpatient management is the center of their practice to understanding that outpatient management is where their focus should be.

Utilization and quality targets

The healthcare industry is beginning to identify performance standards in the areas of utilization and quality monitoring. Bed days per 1,000 for the less-than-65-year-old population is acceptable at less than 170. cesarean section rates of 15 percent of deliveries is another example. The difficulty with this approach is that the rapid gains of operational improvement and new clinical knowledge not only narrow variation but also continuously shift the mean to improved standards. This constant

TABLE 2
Inpatient bed days per 1,000

	Non-Medicare days per 1,000	Medicare days per 1,000
Medicine	55	582
Surgery	40	404
Pediatrics	11	NA
Neonatal	10	NA
Mental health	6	19
Rehabilitation	7	NA

shifting of a standard makes implementing improvement programs tenuous as further improvements may mean significant and costly short-term changes. The rates in Table 2 are based on what has been accomplished by groups throughout the country rather than a theoretical target.

Because of the continuous gains in managing inpatient stays, it is projected that current inpatient targets will be halved within the next five to eight years. This trend is supported by more recent moves from inpatient to outpatient or alternative settings of care. Already, nearly 60 percent of surgeries are performed in the outpatient setting. With further technological advances on the horizon, such as improved laparoscopic and cryosurgery techniques, a further erosion of inpatient surgery will take place. Similarly, the home care industry has greatly improved its medical management techniques so that more medically ill patients can be treated at home with chemotherapy and other intravenous therapies such as anticoagulation and antibiotic. Table 3 illustrates rates for selected diagnosis related groups (DRGs) and surgical procedures.

Healthcare delivery has evolved into a complex strategy of balancing inpatient and outpatient management of patients. Admitting moderately ill patients is long gone and has been replaced by aggressive outpatient management.

For example, asthma admissions today act as a gauge for potential mismanagement because the standard of care is that most asthmatic patients should be managed in the outpatient setting. Such an admission is considered a failure of the outpatient system. Also, literature has commonly referred to the hospital as a germ-ridden environment that most people would be much better off avoiding.

As the shift to the outpatient setting increases so do the demands on that system. Demands for care, especially preventive care such as mammography and cervical cancer screening, are increasing. To meet this

TABLE 3
Target DRG and procedure rates

	Sample DRGs		
	Discharges per 1000	*Average length of stay*	*Cost per day*
14—Specific cerebrovascular disorders, except TIA	.22	3.9	$3,400
15—Transient ischemic attack and precerebral occlusion	.06	2.2	2,800
81—Respiratory infections and inflammations, age 0–17	.1	1.8	2,800
91—Simple pneumonia and pleurisy	.8	2.7	1,800
98—Bronchitis and asthma, age 0–17	1.5	2.0	2,200
140—Angina	.5	2.0	2,500
143—Chest pain	1.1	1.5	2,000

	Selected procedure rates	
	Age adjusted rate per 100,000	*Average length of stay*
Lumbar laminectomy	33.6	2.6
Cholecystectomy	71	1.8
Hysterectomy	156	3.4
Appendectomy	70	2.2
Percutaneous transluminal angioplasty	17	2.5
Coronary artery bypass graft	35	8
Hip replacement	31	5.5
Knee replacement	35.4	5.5

increased demand for resources, without increasing expenses, creates a need for bold strategies to build efficient delivery systems. The first step is to set efficient performance targets in order to reinvest financial and practice improvement gains. Performance targets are the base for discussions about capitation. To work successfully under capitation, a medical group must understand its business and, more importantly, its ability to improve the way it delivers care. The ability to measure targets and develop strategies to improve deficiencies becomes the medical group's underpinnings to success.

Open access, meeting the visit demands of the membership, is a common expectation of performance targets. Same-day scheduling is one example of supply modification strategies to meet demand.

TABLE 4
Patient visit rates

	Physician office visits per MD FTE per month
Medicine	348
Pediatrics	408
Obstetrics and gynecology	281
Surgery	250
Dermatology	629
Allergy	347
Neurology	208
Urology	237
Ophthalmology	383
Ear, nose, and throat	363
Orthopedics	354
Psychiatry (MD only)	156

For some groups the patient visit time has been shortened from 15 to 10 minutes to accompany analyzed demand. Over time, a year for instance, the demand for care can be mapped out into seasonal fluctuations and weekly demand expectations because the appointment demand changes by the day of the week.

Considering this predictable demand variation, it is also prudent to measure and map the type of appointments needed and booked. For instance, appointments may be categorized, for simplicity, into new, short-term follow-up, long-term follow-up, and routine (complex and simple). The idea of meeting daily demands for same-day service is to plan sessions for the month and to look at the percent of return appointments that flood the system. Many return appointments may be planned as same-day appointments instead of filling future bookings that often get canceled. Return appointments are usually defined as follow-up for such things as ear infections or laboratory results. A test is to measure the number of canceled and no-show appointments for a quarter. The result is often surprising and usually can meet the same-day demands of patients. Table 4 cites some office visit benchmarks.

When setting performance targets for settings such as office visits, cost targets for selected specialties must be determined. The PMPM for office visits includes midlevel practitioners such as in Table 5.

Preventive screening services are another prerequisite for effective capitation programs. Preventive screening targets can be illustrated in numerous contexts. Using Health Plan Employer Data and Information

TABLE 5
Office visit costs

Specialty	PMPM costs
Allergy	$0.44
Pediatrics	$5.00
Obstetrics and gynecology	$5.15
Primary care and specialty total	$30.00
Ear, nose, and throat	$.95
Orthopedics	$2.00
Urology	$.85
Surgical specialties total	$8.70
Anesthesiology	$1.25
All costs	*$54.34*

TABLE 6
Selected performance targets

Indicator	Target
1. Childhood immunization rate	70–80 percent
2. Cholesterol screening	60 percent in past 5 years for people 40–64
3. Mammography	75 percent of women age 45–64
4. Cervical cancer screening	70 percent of women over 19 have a pap smear every 3 years
5. Low birthweight	less than 5 percent
6. Prenatal care	90 percent visit 26–44 weeks prior to delivery
7. Asthma inpatient admission rate	188 per 100,000

Set (HEDIS) developed by the National Committee for Quality Assurance (NCQA) targets or Healthy People 2000 will provide a strong starting point for program planning. HEDIS "represents a core set of performance measures developed to respond to a complex, but simply defined employer need: How to understand what value the healthcare dollar is purchasing and how to hold a health plan accountable for its performance." The information in Table 6, from HEDIS 2.5 and Healthy People 2000, may provide a framework from which to begin building management strategies.

In summary, the outpatient setting may be stratified into three categories: preventive management (where screening and immunization actually prevent illness and its associated costs); outpatient management of chronic disease (e.g., diabetes and congestive heart failure); and aggressive management of acute illness.

Delegation and de-delegation

As NCQA accreditation becomes the standard for health plans, it is important to recognize the standards reveal that health plans need to de-delegate administrative and medical management activities that have been delegated to the independent practice associations (IPAs) and medical groups. For instance, utilization activities, quality management, and credentialling may be the health plan's focus to create a powerful accountability. Because of this shift, it is important for groups to clearly articulate a plan that, depending on the group's performance, lessens the burden of control by the health plan. It is recommended that a series of interventional phases be agreed upon with objective measures that demonstrate a group's improved performance. The goal is to be able to practice without implicit or explicit utilization controls in a manner that delivers a quality product with superior treatment outcomes.

The quality measurement component generates specific indicators that demonstrate efficiency and quality. For example, measurements for a group's diabetic population should be able to predict needed resources (e.g., pharmacy, hospitalization, and education) and establish outcomes of care such as decreased admissions, reduced end-stage renal failure, decreased diabetic retinopathy, and fewer emergency department visits. Dictated guidelines and pathways will not meet this objective because the medical profession does not respond well to external coercion. However, collaborative practice improvements with modest ranges of performance measures will.

The five phases are summarized as

1. Physicians' roles

   This phase begins with significant controls and tightly defined roles exercising these controls. This start-up phase resembles an implicit contract of professional norms. As the roles are defined and principles discussed, the bureaucratic structure is built. This bureaucracy acts as the control and feedback center for the group

2. Transition

   The transition from start-up to developing medical group capacity begins to shift emphasis from control to more feedback on cost effectiveness and cost benefit of practices

3. Growth and development

   This phase addresses the challenges of growth, internalizing services into the group of capitated providers and adding new staff. The medical group easily manages the growth and additions of new physicians and members because the majority of physicians accept appropriate group-based medical practice patterns. It is at this developing phase that many physicians quickly move to an autonomous practice. At this phase, managed care plans in a region begin to eliminate most hospital utilization review (UR) and referral authorization reviews. The feedback of practice effectiveness and efficiency is mostly generated by the individual physician

4. The art of medicine
   The transition from developing to mature practice patterns is where most groups will end after several cycles of growth. To move beyond phase 4 is rare for a large group practice but not impossible. Phase 4 eliminates most explicit controls in favor of self-motivated professional autonomy. This phase is reached when physicians practice medicine based on outcome goals and clinical guidelines adjusted to meet particular practice beliefs—beliefs that have been molded by peers and through a self-realization that medical practice is a blend of art and science. The UR bureaucracy should now be purely a support function that manages data and supplies requested information

5. Pure autonomy
   This occurs when physicians manage their own practice in concert with the patient. There are no microcontrols over inpatient or outpatient care. The physician intuitively practices medicine as an art that is scientifically sound and economically efficient. This idea is difficult to obtain and sustain but can be accomplished through a planned program that builds consensus and raises the level of practice through education

Through aggressive and realistic performance targets, a strong working foundation for practice development can be formed. Within this foundation, strategies for improvement can be planned.

The target staffing ratios cited above open the path for understanding appropriate devolution of care delivery. For example, most physicians may be able to give lower-level practitioners much of their day-to-day practice activities, including taking patient histories, physical examinations, immunization, preventive screening, rechecks, chronic illness management, and even acute illnesses or minor trauma.

Today, groups should evaluate their practice needs to include using more midlevel practitioners because there is a three-to-two financial ratio of nurse practitioners to physicians. This ratio translates into more than doubled performance yield for the medical group. Assuming that orthopedic surgeons earn $300,000 per year, their practices may be halved by decreasing discretionary procedures and delegating musculoskeletal ailments to the primary care physician (PCP). By eliminating two surgeons, at a cost of $600,000, a group can bring on at least three PCPs with an assumed income of $125,000 (minus office overhead). This allows for a savings of $225,000 in salary and a significant reduction in hospital costs. Even further, a group may be able to replace two PCPs with at least three nurse practitioners, thus increasing access and improving key targets such as preventive screening rates. Obviously this causes alarm for the medical community. In fact many groups have realized that the trend is growing and the act of devolution is reducing actual practice costs and improving access while not decreasing the quality of care. Unfortunately, some groups have resorted to eliminating nurse practitioners and are attempting to further limit the latter's professional scope of practice.

The medical community often works without a strategy instead of planning for the future. Managed care was originally viewed by the medical community as a side business that was limited to a few practitioners. As physicians attempted to wait out the emergence of managed care, most health plan boards were discussing managed care contracts, capitated business, costs, market position, sales strategy, reimbursement rates, and quality of care. Many medical groups discuss protecting their turf, remaining autonomous, and increasing the capitation or reimbursed rate. No wonder these two powers often are at odds. This is even more evident as outpatient care becomes the dominant setting for health services delivery and physicians shift their role to the manager of care with specific functions delegated to other professionals. Office practices become more of a piece of the overall continuum of treatment settings that have developed over the past several years. This remarkable shift in points of service and delivery personnel will continue to redefine and potentially eliminate the physician role as it is today.

Developments in infomatics and systems point to a very different future for the practice of medicine. Artificial intelligence coupled with pathway development paint an interesting evolution of medicine from labor-intensive assembly-line-like management to a model that relies on the ancient shaman approach to care. This role is one of a hands-on healer supported by the intelligence of the computer. The future will depend on those who have developed strong assessment and communication skills. Knowledge of medicine may not be the principal currency.

Imagine the rapid growth of the Internet and how it may be potentially used. A 42-year-old female is awakened by sudden sharp abdominal pain. It is 11 P.M. and she would normally place a call to the paging service to contact her physician or go to the emergency department. Instead, she logs on to the Internet directly to a symptomatic database that walks her through typical assessment questions that consider her past history and medications. The result is an increase in one medication and a scheduled office visit the next day. At the visit the caregiver (not necessarily a physician) downloads the information, adds some physical assessment information, and the computer program delivers a diagnosis and treatment plan. This could even be completed at home by the patient while on-line with the caregiver.

While there may be debate about this scenario, the capability exists today. Patient care systems are becoming so advanced in hospitals that diagnostics are programmed into and coupled with guidelines for treatment without physician intervention. Finally, robotics have entered the surgical suite as extensions of the surgeon's hands and are becoming more advanced with each generation of technology. The logical progression of the changes in medical practice suggests that the educational process of medical school will be obsolete.

So, the question is raised about physician knowledge as the currency of measurement for the future. It appears futile for a person to attempt to learn the breadth of knowledge currently available due to the vast and rapid electronic access to information and knowledge. The most sensible direction is to understand patients, their needs, their symptoms, and have the ability to quickly access whatever new knowledge is needed.

The key for medical groups is to understand these trends and to plan for the future in terms of financial requirements, changing practice patterns, and quality management. This will be a prerequisite for adjusting to rapid and ongoing fluctuations in market dynamics.

4

Physician autonomy and provider accountability

William Riley, PhD
Chief Executive Officer

David Yauch, MD
Medical Director
Aspen Medical Group
Minneapolis/St. Paul, Minnesota

MULTIPLE APPROACHES to managed care have emerged as the healthcare industry responds to demands for better care for more people at less cost. There is a range of managed care acceptance by the healthcare providers, patients, and payers. To healthcare providers, the most acceptable form of managed care is one that maintains clinical and economic autonomy.

This article examines an approach to perform managed care successfully in a medical group in a way that preserves clinical autonomy and reasonably maintains economic autonomy. Internal-based managed care will be defined, and components of a successful managed care approach will be examined including group structure, compensation, and provider performance review.

The best medical decision making occurs between the provider and the patients and their families. This approach is usually the most satisfying approach for the patient and the most professionally rewarding for the provider. And though the provider should be in the best position to make clinical decisions and accept responsibility for those decisions, not all managed care approaches empower the provider to do so.

Thus, two managed care paradigms can be identified and distinguished: internal- and external-based managed care. Internal-based managed care is a totally provider-driven approach to care delivery, where all decisions are based on direct medical judgment of the provider to achieve desired outcomes. Internal-based managed care consists of managed care systems inside the organization, under the provider's direction, and offers providers decision making without external interference.

External-based managed care is where providers are directed with external forces to guide their decisions. This type of managed care imposes outside interference in the provider's decision-making process and is characterized by extensive outside review systems including prior authorization, retroactive denial, and inspection-driven protocols. These processes all second-guess provider decision making and treatment recommendations. External-based managed care is usually based outside the provider's organization and relies on micromanagement of patient care by nonproviders. Today, this is a prevalent form of managed care and is defined by the Institute of Medicine as techniques by third parties to "manage healthcare costs by influencing patient care decisions through case-by-case assessment of appropriateness."[1]

External managed care models that incorporate discounted fee-for-service mechanisms can generate quality care but are limited by a reimbursement mechanism that may motivate excessive utilization. Appropriately structured managed care leads to quality and efficiency. Internal-based managed care achieves this as well as greater clinical autonomy and economic autonomy.

The contrast of internal managed care against external managed care places a focus directly on the extent to which the provider has the clinical autonomy to make medical decisions and still be accountable for quality and efficiency outcomes.

An internal-based managed care paradigm, with provider-driven case management, is a preferred approach that can result in better attainment of both quality and efficiency goals. This type of managed care is preferred because it is simple, more effective, more acceptable to patients and providers, and avoids increasingly expensive and intrusive health plan systems.

TABLE 1
Quality and efficiency relationship

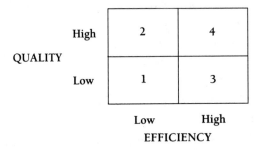

		Low	High
QUALITY	High	2	4
	Low	1	3

Low   High
EFFICIENCY

Conducting internal managed care

The optimal managed care system provides quality and appropriate care through empowerment rather than coercion. The key factors for success include salaried providers, incentives for performance, timely internal communication of performance results, and a provider-driven managed care paradigm. A culture and philosophy with explicit commitment to managed care depends on a working definition of managed care, emphasizing a commitment to both quality and efficiency.

Table 1 shows successful managed care as the outcome of an appropriate relationship between quality and efficiency.

Cells 1, 2, and 3 indicate how managed care performance can fail to meet quality expectations, efficiency expectations, or both. The combination of low quality and low efficiency found in Cell 1 is probably uncommon. Cell 2 shows high quality and low efficiency. It is easy to perform quality care in an inefficient way. For example, the disparity of inpatient utilization rates in various areas of the country, with no apparent difference in outcomes, suggest that quality care can be delivered in a very inefficient manner. Cell 3 reflects low-quality care that is highly efficient. This may occur when a provider is at personal financial risk for utilization by capitated patients and care is withheld because it directly affects provider compensation. Cell 4 reflects both high quality and highly efficient care. This result can best be achieved through a properly aligned managed care system, purposefully structured to accomplish high-performance goals in all areas of patient satisfaction, medical outcomes, and preventive services.

Provider-driven managed care

An internal-based managed care paradigm presupposes a managed care approach led by the primary care provider. Provider-driven managed care means that the provider is in total charge of directing the clinical care coordination for the patient. Provider-driven managed care can be used across the entire spectrum of care delivery. In the ambulatory care setting, provider-led managed care is characterized by

- Primary care focus

- Quality providers committed to managed care

- Flexibility to spend time necessary with patients without pressure of production quotas

- Ability to make referrals as necessary without external oversight

- Knowledge-base of efficient referral providers to facilitate referral decisions

- Emphasis on long-term patient-provider relationships

- Systems for patient education

Managed care initially emerged in part as a response to the inefficiencies of traditional fee-for-service (FFS) medicine, whereas external-based models developed to manage providers who were uncommitted or resistant to the concept of care management.

An internal-based model requires primary care providers (PCPs) who are committed to managed care goals, eliminating the need for external review. Here rigid controls of external managed care are replaced by flexible approaches that allow providers and patients to mutually arrive at treatment decisions. When referral care outside the group is needed, it is important that providers have the freedom to make referrals as well as seek information on specialist consultants. Provider-driven managed care depends on well-established, long-term, patient-provider relationships. Disrupted or short-term relationships will create poor decision making and ultimately higher cost and lower quality. Patient education systems are an important part of this system to avoid the need for layers of rules and guidelines.

Provider-led managed care in the inpatient setting is characterized foremost by a care concept that allows the PCP to make decisions regarding inpatient care without prior approval, conformance to external review, or outside inspection of the patient's treatment. It includes

- Advance planning for discharge prior to admission

- Education of hospital staff and specialist consultants on care management expectations

- Concerted effort to communicate with patient and family

- Ongoing dialogue with peers

- Coordination of care among specialists

- Continual monitoring by provider-directed staff to assist with discharge planning

- Working with nonhospital resources to ensure continuity of care in the appropriate setting after discharge

Efficient inpatient care systems require maximal education and communication among providers, patients, and their families. The process starts prior to admission where possible. All hospital staff and consulting providers must understand what is expected from them as part of the patient care team. Communication with patients and, when appropriate, families avoids unnecessarily prolonged hospitalization, which creates increased costs and suboptimal outcomes.

A provider-directed staff works throughout the hospitalization to assist with all aspects of discharge planning including medical, social, and psychological. The end result is an inpatient process that has the potential to improve medical and patient satisfaction outcomes without the imposition of costly and frustrating external review.

In summary, internal-based managed care is a provider-directed team working to make high-quality yet appropriate decisions regarding care. It also includes forgoing care if it does not affect the outcome or improve quality of life.

Internal-based managed care is simple, not complex. This approach does not need rigid algorithms, pathways, or protocols that may impose added complexity. Inherent in this approach is starting with the patient's needs and determining a treatment course that best meets those needs.

Finally, internal-based managed care is not a benefit-driven approach where the benefit plan design represents a starting point that providers may attempt to manipulate to provide necessary care.

Medical group structure

A provider-driven managed care system requires a compatible organizational structure that incorporates provider direction and control as a central feature. Today there is a tendency in large healthcare organizations to become highly centralized, with systems installed to oversee and control operations at the patient-care level. However, a decentralized structure is the most suitable for internal-based managed care. A highly decentralized clinic operating structure positions patient care as the load-bearing pillar. Centralized functions are avoided and limited to those that do not directly affect patient care and those that can be done more efficiently at the central level such as contracting, MIS, and financial systems.

The closer the locus of responsibility is to the provider, the more responsive the organization will be to patient needs. The most effective and efficient operating unit for managed care is a local clinic that offers personalized care on a decentralized basis. The local clinic is the focal point where care is delivered and rendered. All decisions regarding patient care and clinic operation need to be delegated to the local site, which is managed by a provider. These include

- Provider recruitment and termination

- Provider and support staff scheduling

- Provider call schedules

- Volume expectations

Clinic operating decisions cannot be made in isolation from patient care decisions and should include

- Budget development, implementation, and control

- Clinic operations

- Support staff management

Though all these functions could be performed centrally, they are best performed at the clinic level with central coordination. When healthcare organizations do not delegate budget development and accountability to the local clinic, then the clinic may not assume responsibility for efficient care. Clinic budget accountability is essential for internal managed care when aligned with a provider-compensation system structured to promote quality and efficiency. The financial success ultimately depends on provider acceptance of responsibility for group performance. This accountability starts with understanding of the budget and involvement in its development.

Support staff direction is also better performed at the local site level, rather than from a distance; the further the distance for support staff direction, the longer the time for potential delays and the greater the unresponsiveness to local needs.

Components for successful managed care

PROVIDER-DRIVEN AND PROVIDER AUTONOMY

A provider-driven system implies assigning total responsibility to the provider for patient care, without external review and protocols. This is done free from outside overview and protocols. Provider-driven care, however, does not mean "blank check" medicine or low-quality medicine.

Provider autonomy allows clinical and economic autonomy. The characteristics of clinical autonomy are the ability of the provider to control the terms of practice, including the course of diagnosis and therapy for the patient. Economic autonomy is the ability of the provider to determine the charges and amount of work.[2]

Allowing providers to control the content and terms of their work seems anachronistic with the prevailing dominance of external managed care. It can be argued that providers have tolerated intrusion into clinical autonomy to maintain economic autonomy. However, a recent study of Medicare participation by providers found that some providers forgo economic autonomy to maintain clinical autonomy by refusing to participate as Medicare providers or to balance bill.[3]

It is ironic that internal managed care driven organizations may actually enjoy more clinical autonomy than both traditional FFS providers and providers participating with external managed care approaches.[4] Internal managed care does not require a tradeoff of clinical autonomy for economic autonomy. It may be an erroneous perception that independent FFS providers enjoy greater freedom in decision making.

QUALITY AND APPROPRIATENESS

Outcomes measures represent the intersection of cost and quality factors. The goal of outcomes measures is to achieve desired clinic results at the optimal cost efficiency. Health economists criticize the FFS incentive system because it places the provider in an untenable situation of having a direct economic relationship with the number of tests ordered, examinations recommended, and treatments prescribed. Compensation systems with providers directly at-risk may also be criticized for placing the provider of care in an untenable situation of having a direct economic relationship with the number of tests, exams, and treatments. Numerous studies suggest that delivering greater amounts of care does not necessarily relate to improved care outcomes. Table 2 expresses the relation between quality and appropriateness.

This matrix shows that low-quality care can be care that is either too little or too much. Poorly structured compensation systems could motivate providers to withhold services or provide unneeded services if compensation is connected to the care delivery decision.

TABLE 2
Levels of care

QUALITY				
	High			Patient receives needed care based on condition
	Low	Patient does not receive needed service	Patient receives service that does not affect outcome	
		Care withheld (At-risk compensation)	Excess care (Production compensation)	Care that matches need (Salaried compensation)

TABLE 3
Ancillary utilization
Fee-for-service salaried comparison

	Dr. Smith		Dr. Jones		National average*	
	Per encounter	Total dollars	Per encounter	Total dollars	Per encounter	Total dollars
Lab	$20.44	$76,656	$38.86	$143,734	$31.47	$118,000
X-ray	$10.71	$40,182	$18.42	$ 68,154	$13.71	$ 52,000
Total ancillary	$31.15	$116,838	$57.28	$211,888	$45.18	$170,000
Total clinic visits	3,750		3,700		3,780	

*National average is from the Medical Group Management Association PEER study September 1993.

An analysis of different medical practice approaches based on the economic incentive system is shown in Table 3. The table compares two primary care providers, Dr. Smith, a salaried provider with a managed care practice and Dr. Jones, whose compensation is production based. Both practices are in the Twin Cities and are managed by Aspen Medical Group, a multispecialty medical group. The table compares the number and cost of total patient visits for each provider, as well as the number and cost of ancillary testing associated with the clinic visits. Although the total visits for each provider were nearly identical (3,750 visits for Dr. Smith and 3,700 visits for Dr. Jones), there is a marked difference in the laboratory and x-ray tests ordered for each clinic visit. Dr. Smith, the salaried provider, had lab and x-ray tests of $31.15 per encounter, compared with $57.28 of tests per encounter for the production-based provider. This represents 83 percent greater charges for ancillary tests with no measurable difference in the outcome of the two providers with respect to quality and satisfaction measures.

However, there was a major difference with respect to efficiency measures. The production-based provider ordered more than $95,000 of additional ancillary tests compared to the salaried provider. Although this is a case study example and should not be generalized, it reflects years of accumulated experience, common sense, and basic economic theory that the structure of a financial incentive system for provider compensation will inexorably affect provider practice patterns.

COMPENSATION SYSTEM

This example leads to a discussion of how to develop a compensation system linked to accountability, which results in successful managed care operations. There are two compensation components necessary for successful internal-based managed care: salaried providers and clinic-site accountability.

Any provider compensation system will affect medical decisions if there is a direct economic consequence for compensation based on medical decisions. Thus, the ideal compensation system should motivate providers to deliver appropriate care and quality care, while avoiding care that does not affect the outcome. Appropriate care consists of delivering all care necessary to achieve a desired outcome. The comparison of Dr. Smith and Dr. Jones suggests that Dr. Jones's practice pattern included almost $100,000 of care that did not affect the clinical outcome and could represent inappropriate care. It is a function, in part, of a fee-for-service compensation system.

Another requirement for a compensation system is to promote quality. To summarize, quality consists of delivering the right care, the right way, in the right setting, at the right time. Salaried compensation with incentive is a method that promotes quality without creating inappropriate utilization such as with fee-for-service payments.

Accountability is the second factor in the formula for successful managed care. Accountability implies an obligation to perform a task and evaluate how well the task is accomplished. Accountability is a companion to salaried providers because salaried providers do not have the same "pressure to perform" as production-based providers. Accountability becomes a method to measure performance when production quotas and production-based compensation are absent. Two components of accountability are efficiency and successful operating results.

A salary compensation system promotes quality and appropriateness for individual care, but the clinic must also be accountable for delivering care to an entire enrolled patient population at a competitive market price. Functioning as a team to deliver care to an enrolled patient population, the clinic is accountable to deliver care at a cost that allows sufficient surplus for the group to be successful over time.

Another aspect of accountability is to ensure that each clinic closes each operating cycle with a financial surplus from operations. Cost accountability combined with salaried compensation measures performance and replaces production as the driving financial mechanism.

The equation below relates the two aspects of salary compensation and accountability.

$$\frac{\text{Salary compensation}}{\text{Appropriate care}} + \frac{\text{Clinic accountability}}{\text{Efficiency}} = \frac{\text{Quality and}}{\text{successful results}}$$

SYSTEMS AND ORGANIZATION

A striking feature of internal-based managed care is the complexity of care organization and systems information technology needed to manage populations as well as individuals. Neither traditional FFS or external-based managed care need sophisticated information systems at the medical group level. Internal-based managed care does not need elaborate systems of policy and procedures. It does need real-time information, monitoring of data, and provider-driven management. The nature and structure of internal-based managed care should require less investment in information systems, care management systems, and personnel than external care management delivery models.

Provider performance evaluation

A provider performance evaluation (PPE) system should be a formal, uniform, predictable mechanism to teach and remind providers what must be done by every member for the group to succeed. Proper feedback to each provider that focuses on relevant areas of managed care performance for quality, outcomes, and efficiency is the ultimate goal of a performance evaluation.

An effective PPE should measure performance, communicate the results in a way that reinforces desired performance, and identify opportunities for improvement. Critical factors to a successful PPE include internal development by providers with input from all participating providers; consensus on key areas; information systems developed to support PPE; mixture of subjective and objective elements; input from patients and nonprovider staff; and annual review of process to create PPE evolution in response to internal and external change.

Information systems are an important part of a PPE. Manual data systems can be useful and workable if simple; however, the most useful information, such as patient panel size, requires manipulation of large data sets.

Many data elements critical to the PPE process may not exist in many organizations reflecting the predominantly financial orientation of most early MIS departments. For the PPE to work, the organization must commit to developing useful clinical information systems. The current emphasis on continuous quality improvement is generating large amounts of provider-specific clinical information that is relevant and useful.

Involvement of support staff and patients in the PPE process is extremely important. Their response, gathered in an anonymous survey format, allows very important provider-specific information to be gathered. It also allows patients and staff to feel a part of an organization where their input is valued. This can have many benefits, including improvements in patient satisfaction, office efficiency, and workplace morale.

One of the most important features of the PPE process is that it has the appearance of and can actually be an evolving system. Providers must have the ability to change the entire process if it does not work for them as a group. Just as they must be involved in initial design, they must participate annually in a mechanism that reviews the PPE process.

THE INSTRUMENT

The Aspen PPE is a composite evaluation instrument with 10 pages of provider specific information compared to departmental averages. Table 4 shows the five components in the PPE, measured with 21 items. The measurements have different values assigned and a total of 50 points. The five components are patient satisfaction, interpersonal skills, quality, production, and utilization. Each of these have been identified as important performance areas for each provider to achieve managed care success for the organization.

Patient satisfaction receives high priority in the instrument. This component is measured with five items that total 12 points. Multiple-page questionnaires on satisfaction and service assessment for each provider are distributed to patients, support staff, and peers. The provider is

TABLE 4
Summary of five components for PPE

1. Patient satisfaction	Overall score
A. Patient satisfaction survey	4
B. Support staff assessment of provider	3
C. Peer assessment of provider	3
D. Complaint rate of provider	2
E. Provider/manager comments	0
	12 points

2. Interpersonal skills	
A. Interaction with staff	4
B. Interaction with peers	5
C. Provider/manager comments	0
	9 points

3. Group involvement	
A. Participation in committees	4
B. Peer assessment	5
C. Current CPR certification	1
D. Provider/manager comments	0
	10 points

4. Production	
A. Encounters	4
B. Capitated charges	4
C. FFS charges	4
D. Provider/manager comments	0
	12 points

5. Utilization	
A. Lab utilization	1
B. Radiology utilization	1
C. Peer assessment	3
D. Special efforts	2
E. Provider/manager comments	0
	7 points

Grade total	50 points
Average for specialty	_____

measured on 23 areas from these three sets of respondents. In addition, the provider complaint rate is used as a measure for satisfaction. Provider/ manager comments regarding patient satisfaction are also included as part of the feedback.

In each of the five areas measuring patient satisfaction, the provider is evaluated according to established performance criteria. Table 5 shows how these various five areas are evaluated. For example, a provider who is rated over 95 percent satisfaction by patients is awarded four points,

TABLE 5
Patient satisfaction and service—Internal Medicine

1. Complaint rate—Individual provider   Rate: _____
(Number of complaints per 1,000 encounters)

0 – ≤1/1,000	_____	2 points
>1/1,000 – ≤2/1,000	_____	1 point
>2/1,000	_____	0 points

2. Patient satisfaction survey   Average: _____%
(Average satisfaction for questions 15–20, 22–24, 26, 27, 30)
(Using very satisfied and satisfied response categories)

>95%	_____	3 points
>90 – ≤95%	_____	2 points
>85 – ≤90%	_____	1 point
≤85%	_____	0 points

3. Nursing and ancillary staff assessment of provider
(Patient satisfaction, timeliness, accessibility)
(Attachment A: 1–7 scale, questions 1–4)   _____
Average score: _____

≥6 – ≤7	_____	3 points
≥4.5 – <6	_____	2 points
≥3 – <4.5	_____	1 point
<3	_____	0 points

4. Peer assessment
(Attachments B, C: 1–7 scale, questions B1–2, C1–2)   _____
Average score: _____

≥6 – ≤7	_____	2 points
≥4.5 – <6	_____	1 point
≥3 – <4.5	_____	0 points

5. Total: 0–10 points   _____

6. Provider/manager comments:

while a provider who scores between 90 to 95 percent satisfaction receives three points.

INTERPERSONAL SKILLS

Interpersonal skills consist of three items totaling nine points. Both support staff and peers complete a questionnaire consisting of five measurements to address interpersonal performance in areas of communication, work performance, and extent of cooperation.

GROUP INVOLVEMENT

Group involvement measures the extent to which providers participate in activity that benefits the organization. Various measurements are used to recognize participation on committees, quality improvement, special projects, and other activities that may serve community benefit or affiliated organizations. This component is also used to identify selected areas that may be deemed important for clinical or quality reasons. For example, Table 4 shows that one point is awarded for current CPR certification. There is flexibility to determine each year what areas can be emphasized.

PRODUCTION

Healthcare financing complicates efforts to evaluate production. Increased production may be desirable in a production-based compensation system. However, as discussed in Table 3, increased production can lead to inefficiency while not necessarily affecting care outcomes.

The production component of the PPE analyzes individual provider production for both managed care and FFS payer sources. The analysis extends to all care settings and points are awarded on the basis of comparison to department performance. In recognition of the importance of efficiency, providers are also measured on the size of patient panels and evaluated on the basis of departmental comparisons.

UTILIZATION

Appropriate utilization is a pivotal element to provide efficient quality care. The PPE measures five areas within this component to identify appropriate utilization patterns and evaluate performance. Thus, it is possible for two providers to achieve similar clinical outcomes, yet exhibit a wide range of efficiency. The utilization measurements compare individual provider performance with departmental averages in several selected areas.

THE PPE PROCESS

The PPE process is conducted yearly with the actual review being done by a provider/peer manager. The process has evolved in the group from initial resistance to healthy skepticism to acceptance. The majority of providers value it as a formal mechanism for receiving valuable feedback. It is understood that the PPE tool will continue to evolve.

There are many barriers to creating a PPE. Most providers leave residency or perhaps their final board exam with an expectation that they will not be judged or critiqued in their future career. After years of intense inspection, providers feel relief at finally practicing without someone looking over their shoulder. Older providers, who have practiced for years without an evaluation process, are insulted a "tool" can adequately assess their skills. They may worry that another external system will interfere with the relationships they have developed with their patients over the years. Providers resist performance evaluation systems for a variety of other reasons, including concerns over data reliability, patient severity indexing, subjectivity, confidentiality, perverse financial incentive, and distraction from patient care.

Conclusion

An internal-based model of managed care can be successful. It can create the highest quality care in the most efficient manner. Patients and providers of care can feel empowered to participate together to improve health. This approach requires energetic, committed providers, with a primary care approach. It also requires a compatible structure and significant administrative systems development. Internal managed care depends on a salaried compensation structure with accountability for performance. Mechanisms for provider communication and education are critical.

By respecting provider clinical autonomy and economic autonomy, the long-term success of this approach is enhanced, despite the complex demands of the healthcare industry in the future.

NOTES

1. B. H. Gray and M. J. Fields, *Controlling Costs and Changing Patient Care? The Role of Utilization Management* (Washington, DC: National Academy of Sciences Press, 1989).

2. E. Freidson, *The Profession of Medicine: An Essay in the Sociology of Applied Knowledge* (New York: Dodd Mead, 1970).

3. R. Culbertson, "Physician autonomy: Sociological theory of the professions examined through physician participation and assignment decisions under Medicare" (Unpublished Dissertation, University of California, San Francisco, 1993).

4. U. Reinhardt, "Healers and Bureaucrats in the All-American Health Care Fray," in *Technology, Bureaucracy and Healing in America,* ed. R. Bulger (Iowa City: University of Iowa Press, 1988).

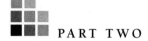

PART TWO

PHYSICIAN COMPENSATION DESIGN

5

Distribution of capitation within physician organizations

John L. Miller
Principal
Integrated Healthcare Development Group
Westlake Village, California

THIS CHAPTER DISCUSSES how capitation is distributed within a physician organization. The concepts presented apply whether physicians are considering a commercial HMO, a senior HMO, or a capitated point-of-service product. Regardless of the product, the various internal income distribution methodologies within a physician organization are essentially the same.

Accepting a capitation payment for professional services can be a complex and emotional process. Countless hours may be spent to negotiate the master capitation agreement and review the actuarial assumptions used to calculate the overall capitation payment to the physician organization.

Capitation transfers the financial risk from a health plan or insurance carrier to a provider organization. In a traditional fee-for-service (FFS) program, providers have no direct financial stake in the insurance company's financial performance or costs of care. The insurer's solvency or premium rates are of little concern to the provider who is delivering care. To control escalating costs, insurance companies have historically used a variety of external control measures (e.g., hospital utilization review and second surgical opinions) to reduce unnecessary utilization. While these interventions have been somewhat successful, they have added complexity and expense to the already overburdened healthcare system.

In a capitated HMO, however, there is more opportunity to restrain costs by making providers financially responsible for their decisions. In these cases, financial risk for the payment of services is transferred to the provider. Typically, this process of transferring risk is called "capitation" because providers are prospectively reimbursed (usually monthly) for the cost of anticipated medical services on a per member basis. Reimbursement is prepaid and received before the services are actually rendered. It is determined based on actuarial calculations that predict the cost of medical services for an enrolled HMO population. If the cost of these claims exceed the available funds, a deficit results. Conversely, if medical services are rendered efficiently and within a budget, there is a surplus. In effect, through the capitation process the provider becomes the insurer.

While capitation provides an incentive for physicians to render only needed services, it is not intended to withhold necessary care. Today, most successful capitated physician organizations realize providing appropriate care is the most cost-effective way to practice in a prepaid environment over the long term.

To most physicians, acting as an insurance company by accepting risk seems mystifying. They are faced with having to quickly understand insurance-related concepts such as premium budgeting, actuarial analysis, and the process of projecting utilization and the cost of medical services based on historical trends and future predictions. However, through sophisticated actuarial calculations, health plans have the ability to predict the utilization and cost of professional (i.e., physician), hospital, and ancillary services with amazing accuracy.

Health plans develop their health insurance premiums based on a budget that includes both the expected cost of medical claims plus the insurance company's own administrative expenses and profit. Generally, the premium budget is based on the development of three financial categories: professional, hospital, and administration. Each component represents an individual financial pool from which appropriate expenses are paid. In the case of professional capitation, all (or some, depending on the services covered) of the financial responsibility for the cost of care is the responsibility of the physician organization under contract with the health plan. However, the actual mechanical activity of paying the claims may be the responsibility of either the health plan or the provider organization.

Insurance pools

FIGURE 1
Insurance pools

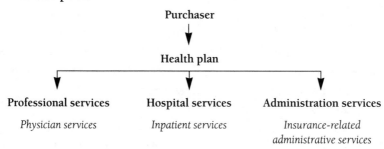

PROFESSIONAL SERVICES POOL

The cost of all professional services included in the benefit plan are mathematically projected by the health plan on a service-by-service basis. In practice, most actuarial projections are expressed based on a population of 1,000 enrollees. As an example, a health plan may state that it expects 2,300 office visits to a primary care physician (PCP) for every 1,000 enrolled members within a year. The array of capitated professional services may be comprehensive and include specific items such as routine office visits, physical examinations, surgeries, radiology, medications, and durable medical equipment (DME). About 40 to 50 percent of the premium is allocated to the professional services pool.

As a physician organization assumes financial responsibility for all professional services, it moves closer to being at "full risk." However, not all services included in the professional services pool are necessarily included in the capitation payment. For example, the responsibility for mental health and chiropractic may be specifically excluded from the physician organization's capitation payment. The exact list of services included are dependent on negotiations between the physician organization and the health plan. Sometimes, these services are determined based only on the services directly available within the group. In other situations, the physician group may be responsible for all services, regardless of what services are offered within the organization. In the latter case, the organization must subcontract with outside providers who offer the services. Subcontracting with providers outside the group in order to offer a wide spectrum of services is common in capitated arrangements.

HOSPITAL SERVICES POOL

Costs for room and board, emergency room, maternity, operating and recovery rooms, in-hospital radiology and pathology, psychiatric, and other specific services are calculated and included in the hospital service portion of the premium. For some outpatient services performed at the hospital (e.g., outpatient surgery, radiology) the hospital may only be financially responsible for the facility charge. However, if a nonhospital affiliated or stand-alone surgery center is used, the professional organization may assume responsibility for the entire cost.

Approximately 35 to 40 percent of the premium is allocated to the hospital services pool. In recent years, however, the size of the hospital pool has decreased as more services have moved to the outpatient setting and become the financial responsibility of the physician organization.

Initially, capitation was thought to apply only to professional services. However, more recently it has also been used to reimburse hospitals as a way to encourage prudent utilization. The basic concepts of hospital capitation are similar to those involved in capitating a professional organization.

HEALTH PLAN ADMINISTRATION SERVICES POOL

The cost of health plan administration may vary depending on a number of factors. For example, health plans perform certain administrative and management tasks such as marketing, managing enrollment and eligibility, paying broker commissions, maintaining the HMO licenses, providing underwriting, and actuarial services. All such services have associated costs that are met through a deduction from the premium. These funds are allocated to the health plan's administrative services pool.

However, in addition to purely administrative services, health plans may decide to retain funds for certain insurance-type risks that can be better managed at the health plan level. Some health plans, for example, will remove certain specific services (such as the cost for the treatment of AIDS or services rendered while the patient is out of the provider's service area) from capitation payments to contracted providers.

The legal status of the health plan (i.e., for profit or not for profit) may also affect how much money the plan retains from the premium. For-profit health plans must often compete for capital in the public equity markets and must generate earnings (i.e., profit) to justify the price of their stock. Total health plan fees for these types of HMOs can exceed 25 percent of the premium. Fees for non-profit plans often range between 10 and 20 percent.

Types of physician organizations

While some physician groups have been around for decades, others are relatively new. Some are large and have a strong central administrative and management structure, others are decentralized. However, there are two basic types of physician organizations: integrated group practices and the contracting organizations.

INTEGRATED GROUP PRACTICE

An integrated group practice is a single legal organization of physicians. The practice usually employs its physicians, has a central governance and management structure, owns its assets, bills under one provider number, and collects all revenue. Physicians are usually full-time employees and may also be partners or stockholders. Income distribution methods for integrated groups vary, but generally physicians are either salaried or have some combination of salary and production incentives.

There are different types of groups that fall under the definition of an integrated group practice. For example, in addition to stand-alone group practices, integrated groups may also include physicians employed by a hospital through a group practice division, a management company, and a staff model HMO. Also, some groups are less centralized or "integrated" than others. For example, hybrid groups (e.g., groups without walls) have been formed that have some characteristics of traditional group practices but lack their full integrative nature in terms of a unified governance structure, common culture, and pooling of accounts receivable.

CONTRACTING PHYSICIAN ORGANIZATION

The second general type of physician structure is a nonintegrated organization of physicians formed for contracting. Unlike the integrated medical group, the contracting physician organization is usually composed of independent providers who maintain their individual offices but join together to secure capitated health plan contracts. This model resembles a provider network rather than a unified medical group. Typical of this model are independent practice associations (IPAs), physicians organizations (POs), and physician-hospital organizations (PHOs). While each model has its own particular characteristics, they may be considered as one general type.

Contracting organizations have several advantages over integrated practices including the ability to form quickly and a lower level of capital investment than integrated groups. However, they may also have more difficulty in achieving economies of scale and suffer from management problems caused by the looser form of organization.

Basic principles in negotiating capitation agreements

Various models are available for distributing capitated funds within a physician organization. The basic principles of designing effective capitated arrangements are very different from how providers are typically accustomed to receiving reimbursement.

Five basic principles of negotiating professional capitated agreements are presented below. These guidelines apply to a physician organization negotiating with a health plan or with a colleague to render subcontracted services.

1. Comprehensive contracted provider network

   At the nucleus of the contracted professional organization is a group of physicians. When a professional organization agrees to accept a capitation payment from a health plan, it may agree to provide (directly or indirectly) all services within the scope of the payment. The scope of contracted professional services in HMO agreements is typically rather large and generally encompasses more than just physician services. For example, the professional organization may need to provide DME, laboratory, and home healthcare in addition to its typical array of physician services that may be offered through a network of outside providers

2. Upside gain, downside loss

   Risk is based on a chance for both gain or loss. In a capitated agreement, physicians must accept the chance that they stand to suffer a loss as well as realize a gain. However, depending on the degree of risk shared by all, physicians may also be "at-risk" based on how their colleagues practice. For example, a physician could be paid less should insufficient funds remain in the professional services pool. This shortfall may be caused by the overutilization of services by other physicians within the organization. Therefore, all individuals who are paid from the pool need to understand and accept responsibility to practice in a cost-effective manner

3. Determining the scope of services
   The amount of the capitation payment is based on the scope of services to be performed. While not designed to be a complete list, the following services are representative of those found in the capitated professional services pool

PCP SERVICES

- Office visits

- Inpatient visits

- Health maintenance

- Immunizations and necessary injections

- Regular physical exams

- Minor office surgical procedures

- Maternity visits

- Related diagnostic and laboratory services

SPECIALIST SERVICES

- Emergency room visits

- Consultations

- Immunizations and necessary injections

- Allergy tests

- Surgical procedures

- Anesthesia

- Obstetrics and family planning including sterilization and termination of pregnancy

- Radiology

- Pathology

ALLIED HEALTH AND ANCILLARY SERVICES

- Mental health

- Physical therapy

- Laboratory

- Radiology

- Home health

- Durable medical equipment

- Miscellaneous other professional and ambulatory services

4. Determining the volume of services
   The volume of services for any particular capitated product depends on the nature of the product sold (e.g., covered benefits, the target market, retained risk, and the underwriting requirements of the health plan). Each of these factors is important and may impact the financial viability of the health plan agreement. Many studies, for example, have shown that even a small patient copayment in an HMO product can significantly lower the level of utilization of primary care services. Also, certain industries are known to have employees with more health problems and risks than other industries (e.g., construction versus office workers). In addition, enrollees in a standard commercial HMO product will have different medical needs than seniors. All of these factors will have some effect on the demand for medical services. Therefore, some type of product and market analysis is critical to project expected utilization of professional services. Usually, the health plan will be able to supply important utilization data to the physician organization

5. The law of large numbers
   Assuming a normal distribution of illness in a covered population, the degree of risk decreases with the number of individuals insured. From an insurance perspective this concept is called the "law of large numbers." Therefore, financial exposure to loss is greater when capitated

enrollment is low. Physician organizations are often advised not to convert to a capitated arrangement until a minimum threshold of covered members is achieved. While there is no magic number associated with this threshold, many physician organizations considering their first capitated agreement want an aggregate minimum of several thousand covered health plan members before converting to a capitated reimbursement model. This requirement may represent a problem for a new HMO without substantial market share. In such cases, some physician organizations have agreed to assist the health plan in getting into the market by accepting a negotiated fee-for-service payment until the minimum threshold of plan members is achieved

Spectrum of contracted professional services

The scope of professional services under capitation is defined by the master agreement between the physician organization and the health plan. From the health plan's perspective, the intent of capitated agreements is to offer the full spectrum of professional services to enrolled members while delegating the financial responsibility for rendering these services in a quality and cost-effective manner to the physician organizations under contract. A list of typical CPT-4 procedure codes found in capitated professional arrangements may be found in Exhibit 1.

Most HMO capitated arrangements require that the PCP act as the entry point to the provider system and take overall responsibility for being the patient's care manager. Therefore, in addition to the role of a direct caregiver, the PCP coordinates and monitors the patient's care as they move through the provider system including care from specialists, the hospital, or allied personnel in the home. A list of typical CPT-4 procedure codes for a PCP is in Exhibit 2.

Models for internal distribution

Once a capitation agreement is properly negotiated, the next step is to determine how the organization will distribute the capitation proceeds to its providers. Primary care, specialist, and ancillary providers must be compensated for rendering services to assigned HMO patients. It is important to note that there is no clear-cut right or wrong model. Seldom is one model perfect. More realistically, internal distribution systems are on a continuum whose success is based on their overall effectiveness in terms of achieving the professional organization's goals.

There are many factors that help to develop a workable internal compensation system, such as making it clear and understandable, simple in operation, and perceived as equitable by physicians. However, the central issues in designing an effective internal reimbursement methodology are to develop a system that is both financially responsible and rewards the behavior the organization wishes to reinforce.

FINANCIALLY RESPONSIBLE

A financially responsible reimbursement system seeks to maintain the financial integrity of the contracted physician organization (e.g., establishing a conservative, yet equitable, reimbursement methodology). Proper monitoring and control of utilization also reduces inappropriate or unnecessary internal expenses and helps to maintain a fiscally solid organization.

REINFORCING POSITIVE BEHAVIOR

Rewarding positive behavior has several elements. First, many physician organizations adopt the policy that a physician member must comply with the organization's policies and procedures if they are to be reimbursed. Stating this in a positive manner, only desired behavior will be reimbursed. Therefore, as an example, a physician who does not follow utilization review procedures may be denied reimbursement for services.

Another factor that influences behavior involves how surplus, or bonus, funds are distributed. There are several sources of bonus payments. However, regardless of the source, surplus funds are usually distributed internally to reward the behavior the organization wishes to reinforce.

The most appropriate internal reimbursement mechanism often depends on the degree of integration and internal control present within the professional organization. For example, highly integrated and centrally managed group practices often pay internal providers a salary. The actual amount of capitation received each month may not directly affect a physician's paycheck. A contracting organization, such as an independent practice association (IPA), may reimburse providers on a subcapitation or modified FFS basis that may be highly sensitive to the monthly flow of income and expenses. In such cases, provider payments may be adjusted frequently as the organization seeks to achieve a financial balance between capitated income and claims expenses.

INTEGRATED GROUP PRACTICE DISTRIBUTION MODELS

There are four primary models that integrated physician groups use to compensate their employed physicians. The common models include production, straight salary, salary and production, and internal capitation.

Production model

Purely production-based reimbursement systems have been used successfully by FFS group practices for years. Here physicians usually receive income based on what they collect minus an allocation for group overhead. Often physicians will be guaranteed a minimum monthly draw to level seasonal fluctuations in income. However, this draw is usually set based on production assumptions from the preceding year.

Physicians under a production system are given income credit for the direct care they render to patients. Because of recent federal regulations (commonly referred to as Stark amendments), income from ancillary procedures is usually pooled and shared equally among physicians within the group, or distributed on a nonproduction formula.

It is often assumed that if a physician organization is capitated its individual physicians are also capitated. This is not necessarily true and some early-stage capitated organizations still compensate physicians on a production basis. However, pure production-based systems can lead to providing unnecessary care that has little benefit to the patient. Such compensation systems may lead to utilization levels far beyond those projected by the health plan's actuary. Most successful capitated integrated group practices recognize the inherent conflicts associated with accepting capitation and paying physicians on a production basis. Therefore, these compensation arrangements are seldom used when the group has more than 20 percent of its revenue generated from capitation agreements.

Straight salary model

Straight salary arrangements are at the opposite end of the continuum from pure production distribution systems. Many integrated medical groups employ physicians and pay them a salary. Employee benefits (e.g., health insurance, life insurance, and retirement plans) are in addition to the salary paid.

Internal salary arrangements vary depending on the group's history, physician makeup, and values. As a general rule, physician salaries are paid based on a competitive salary survey of the immediate market. PCPs are usually paid less than physicians in the specialties. While the difference in pay scales can be quite large (with some specialists making two to three times more than PCPs), the overall level of primary care salaries is generally increasing. In fact, recently the salary for many specialists has been remaining constant or decreasing. The growing importance of primary care physicians is related to the increasing demand for PCPs to be used as the gateway into the managed care system.

Typically, straight salary arrangements do not directly reflect production. In fact, many physician organizations have argued that a salary arrangement is the most conducive system to a successful capitated arrangement since physician compensation is not dependent on rendering a large volume of services. On the other hand, opponents of straight salary systems stress that physicians may not be incented to work hard. Some groups have, in fact, experienced a 20 percent or greater reduction in physician productivity shortly after they converted from a production to a salary system. Generally, to make such a change in compensation systems effective, the group must also clarify physician performance expectations and reward positive physician behavior in merit reviews and incentive payments.

Salary and production model

As many integrated groups convert from FFS to capitation, they attempt to maintain a pure production income distribution methodology within the group. Certainly, such a system can make accepting capitation more politically acceptable within the group. However, the absence of fiscal accountability usually creates a "business as usual" attitude. Many groups who adopt this form of income distribution lose money in terms of their capitated business. To the extent that total practice revenue from fully capitated arrangements remains relatively small (from 5 to

10 percent), the financial loss can usually be accommodated. However, it is increasingly difficult to accommodate such losses when capitation receipts exceed 20 percent of total practice revenue.

While straight salary models are the most typical internal distribution method for integrated groups with large capitated enrollment, some groups also use a modified salary approach. A modified salary system usually begins with a minimum or base salary but adds additional compensation as a physician's production increases. The base salary (usually set at a low level) becomes a floor, and the physician is further compensated based either on the volume of patients seen or the equivalent FFS collections. (Retail charges are seldom used as the benchmark because of the vagueness associated with contractual allowances.) Additional compensation may range between 10 and 20 percent of collections.

This method of distribution also has its advantages and disadvantages. For example, many physicians find this system attractive because it reflects the efforts of a physician who is managing a larger patient load. However, it also has the potential to incent physicians to perform unnecessary services and tests. This, of course, is the exact problem that capitation seeks to resolve, and the medical group adopting this method may find itself in the uncomfortable position of paying out more in physician compensation than is being received in capitation.

Internal capitation

Some integrated groups choose to internally capitate providers. In these cases, PCPs may be capitated for their assigned HMO members while specialists may be paid on a modified FFS basis. However, in some cases one financial pool may also be created for all specialty services, or individual pools may be created on a service-by-service basis. Specialists are then reimbursed from the pool. If insufficient monies remain in the pools, reimbursement is lowered. Conversely, if the pools show a surplus, reimbursement may be increased or bonus payments made at predetermined times.

CONTRACTING PHYSICIAN ORGANIZATION
DISTRIBUTION MODELS

Common contracting models include IPAs, physicians organizations (PO), and physician-hospital organizations (PHO). Typically, these are network-type organizations formed to secure managed care contracts.

Much like an integrated medical group, a nonintegrated organization will also need a management entity to administer its internal managed care affairs (i.e., health plan contracting, provider contracting, capitation processing, data processing, utilization review, and quality assurance). In an integrated group this administrative function is largely internal to the organization and may simply represent the addition of a new operating department that is charged with the responsibility to manage the capitated business (i.e., processing claims, capturing encounter data, and producing utilization reports). A nonintegrated organization will either need to develop its own management capability or contract with an outside organization (i.e., health plan or claims administrator).

Contracting organizations usually do not pay their providers a salary since they are not employed by the organization. Rather, physicians who are members of a contracting organization maintain their own independent offices and overhead structure. Therefore, internal reimbursement is usually limited to FFS, fixed pricing for each service ("case pricing"), and subcapitation models. These three models of reimbursement may also be used by an integrated group model to compensate outside contracted providers who are part of its network.

FFS models

FFS payments may represent the most readily acceptable form of internal reimbursement. This is particularly true when the nonintegrated physician organization is relatively new and physicians are reluctant to accept subcapitation. However, the cost of claims may quickly exceed income. Capitated physician organizations usually withhold some funds from a FFS payment as a financial safeguard. These withholds are usually calculated as a percent of a provider's eligible payment (e.g., 10 to 20 percent of reimbursement). Physicians are at-risk for the amount of funds placed in the withhold pool in the sense that the withhold fund is usually used as the first source of funds to pay for unexpected claims. All or a portion of the withhold fund may be depleted if utilization and/or costs cannot be controlled. Most capitated physician organizations have adopted a withhold arrangement for physician members who are paid on a FFS basis. Assuming that actual claim payments are less than projected expenses, the withholds are returned to each provider on a pro rata basis.

Provider organizations that are relatively inexperienced in capitation contracting are often criticized by their membership for not returning withholds. This may be a valid criticism, but the problems contributing to it may be caused by the actions of the physician membership. For example, deficits in the withhold pool may be caused because the provider organization is unable to secure sufficient discounts from their membership or the provider panel is rendering too many unnecessary services. As a general rule, proper compensation policies and appropriate utilization of services usually result in withholds being returned.

FFS payment arrangements include payment based on billed charges, discount from charges, and fee schedules. Provider withholds are often applied to all models.

Billed charges. Though not typically found in most managed care arrangements, some physician organizations still pay physicians for services based on their charges. In situations where there is strong physician resistance to health plan growth, a capitated physician organization may have little choice other than to adopt this methodology. Unfortunately, it does not usually work well when the physician organization is capitated. For example, while this method may have some initial advantage in securing a larger physician network, it usually does not reward practitioners who are attempting to use resources wisely and practice medicine in a conservative manner. Considering the capitated physician organization has a fixed amount of income—which is usually targeted at less than traditional billed charges—such a reimbursement system may quickly bring financial collapse even if utilization is watched closely. Also, as a practical matter, charges may not be the best yardstick in terms of equitable reimbursement. For example, one physician may charge more to account for a costly and, perhaps, inefficient overhead structure.

Discount from charges. A discount of 10 to 30 percent from a participating provider's billed charges is common. This methodology may help to control claims costs (assuming that general utilization does not increase) simply because fewer dollars are being paid to providers for services. However, experience shows that discounts often bring an offsetting and unwarranted increase in utilization. Thus, contracted physicians may see little difference between a noncapitated preferred provider organization (PPO) and a fully capitated, at-risk HMO—a potentially serious problem.

Fee schedules. Fee schedules apply a relative weight to a given professional service (in terms of units of complexity) multiplied by a conversion factor (dollar amount). The goal of all fee schedules is to reimburse physicians equitably, based on the relative complexity of their activities. This weight can then be multiplied by a common conversion factor that expresses the monetary value for one unit of care. If the relative weights are correct and the conversion factors are set properly, the fee schedule is usually an acceptable method to compensate physicians.

Unfortunately, there is not one fee schedule methodology widely accepted by all physicians. Many physician groups, particularly on the West Coast, use the 1974 California Relative Value Study. Other groups use Medicare's Resource Based Relative Value Schedule (RBRVS). Still others use the fee schedule published by McGraw-Hill. To complicate matters further, many HMOs also develop their own unique fee schedules (e.g., Blue Cross and Blue Shield) that providers may use. While details vary between these schedules, their purpose and general methodologies are similar. The physician organization is usually well advised to decide on one internal fee schedule to be used with all capitated agreements.

One advantage of fee schedules is that they are easy to adjust to meet the competitive conditions of individual marketplaces. To increase fees, a physician organization needs only to increase the conversion factor, thereby injecting a higher multiplier into the financial equation. The relative complexity of one procedure to another remains constant. In addition, conversion factors for cognitive services (such as office visits and counseling patients) may be increased without increasing the factors for procedural services. Such an adjustment may provide a higher level of compensation for PCPs.

Subcapitation models

Many capitated contracting organizations subcapitate individual providers. The methodology is similar to that employed by integrated group practices and may be applied to primary care, specialists, and ancillary services. Actuarial-based cost and utilization data is available for all primary care physicians, every specialty, and all ancillary services. Developing a subcapitation payment for internal providers is the same process that health plans use in developing the total capitation payment. The actuarial process used by the health plan is able to identify expected costs for each service on a per member per month (PMPM) basis. To determine monthly reimbursement the contracting organization simply multiplies this rate times the number of members assigned to each capitated provider on a service-by-service basis. In effect, participating providers are subcapitated based on the actuarial equivalent of their specialty, multiplied by the number of their health plan members.

In addition to individual provider-based capitation and capitated primary care, specialty and ancillary pools may also be created. For example, orthopedics may have its own capitated pool based on the group's budget for orthopedic services. Actual distribution to individual providers may be on a FFS basis. This technique forces all providers to live within a fixed budget.

Primary care subcapitation. One of the most common internal reimbursement arrangements within a nonintegrated risk-bearing physician organization is to subcapitate the PCP. In arrangements that subcapitate PCPs, other providers may still be compensated based on a modified fee-for-service payment or case rate, both of which may be subject to a withhold.

Establishing the dollar value of primary care capitation is closely related to the scope of services represented by the capitation payment. Ideally, the intent of primary care capitation is to bundle all basic PCP services into one monthly payment. The greater the number or the more complex the services that fall under the scope of the PCP, the greater the payment. Not all physicians acting as PCPs, however, feel comfortable with all the primary care services. For example, groups heavily weighted with general internists may find it difficult to incorporate minor operative services into a primary care subcapitation because internists do not usually perform invasive procedures. In such cases, however, the subcapitation payment may be adjusted downward to reflect the necessity of referring minor surgical procedures to another physician.

Approximately 25 to 35 percent of the total professional capitation for commercial enrollees should be set aside for primary care services. For capitated Medicare products, about 18 to 25 percent of the total capitation received by the contracted organization should be allocated to PCP services. The exact percentage varies depending on a number of factors including ability to attract PCPs willing to accept capitated risk, the scope of services performed, and the level of control exercised by specialists within the organization. The remainder of the capitation is allocated for specialty and ancillary services, internal administration, and claims reserve.

Attracting and retaining PCPs is an important factor to consider in designing an internal compensation system. Most health plans and employers will not find a physician organization attractive unless there is an adequate primary care network. There are many practical reasons for such requirements. For example, PCPs are able to triage patients and quickly determine if further specialty care is required. PCPs can also establish a comprehensive view of a patient's health status and manage the overall healthcare process. In addition, PCPs are able to manage most routine health problems in a lower cost setting. PCPs are both direct caregivers as well as patient care managers. Therefore, much of their time is spent communicating with specialists and the hospital, handling patient-related administrative tasks, and coordinating with patients and their families.

Historically, many of these responsibilities have been considered as within the normal scope of a PCP's activities. However, a capitated product often demands that PCPs play a more intensive role in patient management and administration. Therefore, it is not uncommon to find a more generous primary care subcapitation that adequately compensates these physicians for their patient management activities. Some physician organizations have adopted a patient management fee in addition to their regular PCP reimbursement. Such a fee is calculated based on the number of members enrolled with a PCP and is usually expressed as a dollar amount paid on a monthly basis (e.g., one dollar per patient per month).

Some contracting organizations want PCPs to be more accountable for the entire patient care process and make them financially accountable for all claims expense associated with their prepaid patients. These claims expenses include the costs of all covered specialty and other outpatient services. A professional services pool is created for each PCP based on their assigned HMO membership multiplied by the total capitation received on a PMPM basis. All professional claims (including those related to primary care activities) are paid from the pool. A settlement is made at the end of the accounting period, usually each year. If the pool has a surplus, the PCP may receive all, or most, of the funds available as additional compensation for a job well done. If a deficit results, the PCP may need to make up the shortfall either through direct capital contribution or lower personal reimbursement in the following years. This model of reimbursement has created mixed reviews. Some physicians feel that it truly places the PCP in charge of the patient's care. Others, however, believe that it may place financial considerations above the practice of appropriate patient care.

Specialty, allied, and ancillary subcapitation. The intent of paying all providers within the system on a subcapitated basis is to encourage the appropriate use of healthcare services throughout the delivery network. Certainly, an effective utilization review program helps to control unnecessary specialty referrals. However, as a practical matter, placing a specialist or ancillary provider at-risk through a subcapitation arrangement provides a further financial inducement to minimize the number of unnecessary procedures and encourage the most efficient mode of practice.

Table 1 depicts sample actuarial data by service for a commercial HMO population on a PMPM basis.

It is usually not advisable to subcapitate these services when capi-tated enrollment is low. Sufficient patient volume is necessary to properly amortize financial exposure across the patient base. For this reason, most physician organizations do not begin to subcapitate specialty, allied, or ancillary services until the entire organization achieves a minimum capi-tated enrollment of at least 7,500 members. Also, because of varying volumes, not all specialty care providers should be capitated at the same time. For example, higher volume services (e.g., laboratory, radiology, orthopedics, and cardiology) are usually first to be capitated. Specialists and other medical services that are used infrequently (e.g., neonatologists, neurosurgeons) or "high ticket" specialists (e.g., open heart surgeons) are usually capitated last, if at all. The cost of their services is relatively high and a miscalculation in projected membership or actual utilization can have a large financial impact.

Subcapitation of specialists may also create a problem of patient "dumping" whereby the PCP simply refers everything to a specialist. The logic of the argument is that since specialists are capitated, there is no financial downside for the PCP to make indiscriminate referrals. While many physicians believe that the likelihood of such a problem is remote, it is important to place safeguards to ensure that inappropriate referrals do not take place. In response to the potential for abuse, many contracting

TABLE 1
Examples of specialty subcapitation payments for a commercial HMO product

Service	Dollar value of capitation
Allergy	$ .18
Anesthesiology	1.80
Cardiology	.84
Dermatology	.18
Emergency (MD)	.60
Endocrinology	.07
Gastroenterology	.50
Hematology/oncology	.95
Infectious disease	.04
Lab/pathology	1.35
Neonatology	.28
Nephrology	.18
Neurology	.15
OB/GYN	4.08
Ophthalmology	.85
Otolaryngology	.60
Orthopedics	1.44
Physical therapy	.07
Psychiatry/psychology	.34
Pulmonary	.12
Radiology	4.08
Rheumatology	.05
Surgery, cardiology	.55
Surgery, colon/rectal	.10
Surgery, general	.75
Surgery, neuro	.20
Surgery, oral	.03
Surgery, pediatric	.12
Surgery, plastic	.15
Surgery, thoracic	.08
Surgery, vascular	.05
Urology	.42

organizations have established patient referral guidelines and maintained a tight utilization management process.

Actuarial costs for services vary significantly, and there is no accepted average. However, health plans often have historical cost data by service for their enrolled population. Professional organizations should rely on data specific to their contracted health plan partner and local marketplace since utilization patterns vary widely based on geography, individual market demographic characteristics, level of managed care experience, and available benefit packages.

There are two basic forms of internal distribution of specialty subcapitation, single provider subcapitation and service specific specialty pools.

SINGLE PROVIDER SUBCAPITATION. Not all physician networks have a large and diverse group of specialists. Rather, some networks are able to centralize certain specialty services, such as orthopedics or radiology, with one provider group willing to accept subcapitation for their services. Also, capitating one exclusive provider for a group of services is administratively easier and offers the specialists assurance that their volume will grow as network membership increases. It is important to note that the political fallout from nonparticipating providers to this narrow approach may be significant.

SERVICE SPECIFIC SPECIALTY POOLS. Service specific subcapitation attempts to capitate a specific specialty service but, unlike the model above, does not require an exclusive relationship with any individual provider (e.g., surgery may be capitated and all qualified surgeons may participate). Because the arrangement is not exclusive to any particular provider group, service specific subcapitation usually requires the development of a financial pool on a specialty-by-specialty basis. Largely, this is an accounting procedure rather than the costly development of a new formal organization for each group of specialists. Typically, individual providers within the subcapitated pool are paid in one of two ways, regular billing or fixed price.

REGULAR BILLING. First, subcapitated providers may send a regular bill (usually a HCFA 1500) to the provider organization for payment. The provider organization pays the bill on a modified FFS basis, usually subject to a withhold.

FIXED PRICE. Providers may also be reimbursed from a subcapitated pool on the basis of a fixed price or case rate for their services.

Regardless of the method used, if sufficient funds are present in the pool to cover payments, all physicians who participate in the pool will receive their expected level of contracted reimbursement. If, however, sufficient funds are not available, providers will receive less than contracted reimbursement until the financial shortfall within the pool is corrected. Conversely, if a financial surplus accrues at the end of the accounting period, all participants receive a bonus payment in addition to their contracted reimbursement and return of all withholds. Usually the intent of the professional organization is to distribute most monies available after retention of a prudent financial reserve. Common reserve levels are 60 to 75 days of claims expenses.

Case pricing

Case pricing attempts to fix the cost of specified procedures by paying an agreed upon rate for a specific service. Case prices are common for services that lend themselves to a standard and discrete procedure. Case pricing is appropriate for procedures where the level of intensity and resource consumption is relatively predictable. Surgical procedures, for example, are often reimbursed on a fixed case basis regardless of the surgeon performing the operation. The case price usually includes all care rendered by the provider such as preoperative and postoperative care. Case pricing may also involve the use of hospital services, such as where the technical and professional component are closely related. Much like capitation, case pricing rewards internal efficiency because the final level of provider reimbursement is fixed. Unlike capitation, however, there is no barrier to unwarranted utilization.

Bonus arrangements

Generally, capitation income equals about 65 to 70 percent of FFS charges. Some providers may do better while others may do worse depending on several factors such as the level of reimbursement, utilization of services, and overhead.

Bonus income, however, is an additional reimbursement available to individual physicians. Bonus income represents revenue in addition to the money physicians receive from any regular payments. Bonus arrangements may have a substantial bearing on the adequacy of physician compensation and may even bring the overall level of reimbursement to well over 100 percent of billed charges. In fact, many experienced physician organizations seek only capitated contracts because of the significant opportunity for financial gain from assuming risk and carefully managing utilization and the cost of care. Such rewards are not available in traditional FFS or preferred provider arrangements.

SOURCES OF BONUS PAYMENTS

Typically, bonus income is generated from financial surplus from one or more of the following sources.

Capitation bonus surplus

Capitation bonus surplus is achieved when the cost of all claims paid by the contracting professional organization (minus any operating costs) is less than the amount of capitation received by the organization. To achieve such a surplus, the physician organization must ensure that utilization patterns and internal payments to providers are fiscally conservative. It is important to note that the internal payment amount may be adjusted upward for PCPs who are also charged with the additional responsibility of acting as "case managers" and downward for procedural (e.g., surgery, ophthalmology) and diagnostic (e.g., radiology, pathology) specialties.

Operational bonus surplus

Operational surplus results when administrative costs (e.g., provider and health plan contracting, processing claims and encounters, producing data reports, provider services, and insurance) are less than the amount budgeted and reserved by the physician organization. In an integrated group practice, operational surplus is usually calculated from income produced from all lines of business, not just capitation. In a contracting organization such as an IPA or PO, operational surplus is usually only produced from the direct cost of administrative support required to operate the contracting organization. Depending on the services provided, the cost of administering a capitated agreement by an outside management company is usually between 8 and 14 percent of gross capitation.

Hospital bonus (shared risk)

Significant additional revenue may be gained by a bonus payment from the surplus in the hospital pool as a reward to the physician organization for the appropriate use of hospital services. This bonus pool reflects the surplus of funds remaining in the hospital pool after payments for hospital-related services. Generally, the potential surplus of funds in this pool is significant (often between 2 and 4 percent of the total premium) if utilization or costs of hospital services is lower than that budgeted. Usually, the accounting for the bonus pool is administered by the health plan that is responsible for paying the hospital claims. An audit by the physician organization is advised of at least a portion of hospital claim payments against the final health plan settlement to ensure proper accounting.

Commonly, the hospital bonus pool is split on an equal basis between the health plan and the physician organization. Hospitals often question why they are not included in the bonus pool. The answer is that most health plans reimburse hospitals on a per diem or discount-from-charges basis. As such, the hospital is not technically at-risk for their services since they are paid the negotiated amount regardless of utilization. Compare this with the at-risk physician organization that receives a fixed amount of money monthly and must pay all claims from the funds available. However, in some recent health plan agreements, the hospital is also capitated. When a hospital is capitated the surplus from the hospital services pool is usually shared between the hospital and the physician organization, and the health plan seldom participates.

TYPES OF BONUS ARRANGEMENTS

The opportunity to share in bonus income is highly dependent on the nature of the contractual arrangement between the provider and the health plan. Consider, for example, the two general types of health plan capitation methods discussed below.

Direct capitation arrangements

These arrangements involve direct contracts between the health plan and the individual providers. PCPs may be directly capitated by the health plan for specified services while specialists and ancillary services are paid on a modified FFS basis. In direct capitation arrangements, the health plan usually administers the capitation pool, the payment of claims, and the utilization review program. Physicians receive payments directly from the health plan. Therefore, the physician organization may often be relegated to the minor position of being the contracting conduit for its individual members. It may also retain some limited level of oversight of the credentialing, utilization review, and quality assurance functions. This arrangement is particularly prevalent in nonintegrated physician organizations that lack a strong central governance structure or the ability to provide for their own internal administration. It is also more common where the providers are not fully at-risk because the assumption of total financial risk demands that providers assert more direct clinical and management control over the activities of their organization.

Assuming sufficient funds in the professional services pool, withholds are always returned. The health plan may also distribute any additional funds remaining in the pool. However, physicians may also be held financially accountable if the professional services pools show a loss. Financial losses in these pools are often made up by the health plan through lower reimbursement or higher withholds in following years. As a general rule, physicians operating under direct capitation arrangements seldom participate in surplus from the hosptial pool. Depending on the terms of contract, they may participate in any surplus funds in the professional pool. This is largely because of the health plan's dominant role in the overall management of the provider network and the lack of a strong professional organization to negotiate on behalf of members. Of course, direct capitation arrangements will vary greatly between health plans.

Capitation plus bonus

The second type of health plan reimbursement system relies on a capitation payment plus the opportunity to share in surplus from both the professional services and hospital services pools. Bonus dollars in the hospital bonus pool are accrued when actual hospital expenses (either through lower-than-budgeted utilization or hospital payments or both) are less than expected. Often these arrangements are present where the physician organization is strong, has demonstrated to the health plan that it can manage its own affairs, and has strong internal administration (e.g., claims processing, data reporting) and management capability in place. These arrangements are most common in situations where the physician organization is fully at-risk for the professional services pool and is able to help the health plan negotiate a favorable level of reimbursement with the hospital.

Considering its ability to manage its own risk pools, any surplus from the professional services pool will immediately accrue to the physician organization. Any surplus in the hospital services pool is usually shared between the health plan and the physician organization. Depending on the relationship with the partner hospital, some physician organizations also share their bonus with the hospital as a return for lower negotiated institutional rates.

ACCUMULATION AND DISTRIBUTION OF BONUS FUNDS

Bonus dollars from hospital, capitation, and operational sources can be combined into one bonus pool. Some physician organizations believe that all bonus funds should be distributed in the same manner regardless of the source. Others believe that behaviors that result in a capitation surplus from the professional services pool are very different from those that result in a surplus from the hospital services pool. The later types of organizations usually have one distribution methodology to distribute capitation surplus and another to distribute hospital bonus funds. One method tends to reward individual members for the organization's overall performance while the other method tends to reward individual physicians for their performance in specific areas. The methodology for rewarding overall and specific performance is different.

Rewarding overall performance

There are several methods to reward overall performance, including simple allocation, equal distribution, distribution based on billing and payments, and distribution based on members.

Equal distribution. Here, physicians are distributed the same amount regardless of their specialty, the number of patients seen, or amount of reimbursement received. This is a very egalitarian method and rewards physicians equally for being members of the organization.

Simple allocation between PCPs and specialists. In a simple allocation formula, the physician organization needs to determine what percent of the total surplus will be distributed to PCPs and what percent to specialists. Often 50 percent or more of the surplus is distributed to PCPs even though they may represent less than half of the organization's total physicians.

Distribution based on billings and payments. This method is more common where physician reimbursement is based on FFS payments rather than subcapitation. Using this method, physicians are rewarded based on the relative proportion of payments received from the organization. This method favors more highly compensated services, such as surgery, and may actually provide a disincentive for the higher volume but lower reimbursed cognitive specialties, such as primary care.

Distribution based on capitated members. In direct contrast to the method above, distribution based on capitated members is used in situations where the provider is subcapitated. Since primary care may be the only subcapitated specialty, it is most commonly used to reward family practitioners, general internists, and pediatricians. Using this method, PCPs are rewarded based on the percentage of their enrolled members to the entire enrolled population times the surplus available for distribution.

As a practical matter, physician organizations may use a combination of these methods. For example, the PCP distribution formula may be calculated based on 60 percent of the total surplus times the relative percent of the PCP's membership to the total. Specialists may be entitled to a surplus distribution of the remaining 40 percent based on their pro rata share of their payments to the total payments to all specialists.

REWARDING SPECIFIC PERFORMANCE

There are also two common methods to reward specific performance such as participation in incentive funds and rewards based on a point system.

Incentive fund arrangements

Surplus may be accumulated by the use of incentive pools. These are financial pools whereby certain amounts from incoming health plan capitation payments are set aside for specific purposes. For example, a primary care incentive fund is often used to induce PCPs to manage their enrolled patients in a cost-effective manner and not unnecessarily referring to specialists. Each month the physician organization accrues an amount of an individual PCP's monthly reimbursement into a fund. At the end of the year the organization will compare the PMPM referral expenses for each PCP against a predetermined PMPM referral expense. If a PCP's performance is equal to or better than the PMPM referral budget, the organization may provide an incentive payment as a reward.

Similar incentive fund arrangements also may be designed to reward specialists for controlling costs. As a general rule, however, all incentive funds are developed based on budgets or some type of financial target.

Accumulated point method

Surplus can be distributed based on factors that attempt to directly measure a physician's contribution to the organization. Consider, for example, the formula in Table 2 and Table 3.

The categories may be changed to reward any specific performance that the organization deems is important. For example, sophisticated organizations may be able to measure patient outcomes. The relative points can be changed to place more weight in one area versus another. While specific performance systems focus attention on areas that the organization feels are important, they may also take time to manage. Some information, such as data on average length of stay, may be readily available from a data processing system. However, tabulating patient satisfaction responses may involve a great deal of time-consuming manual activity.

TABLE 2
Sample PCP accumulated point method

Factor	Maximum points
Inpatient utilization	
Admissions per 1,000 members	15
Length of stay per 1,000 members	15
Professional cost per member	
Referral cost	15
PCP cost	15
Patient satisfaction survey	15
Compliance with procedures (e.g., UR, QA)	15
Other (e.g., open practice)	10
Total	*100*

TABLE 3
Sample specialist accumulated point method

Factor	Maximum points
Average length of stay	25
Compliance with procedures	25
Patient satisfaction	15
Compliance with medical management guidelines and protocols	35
Total	*100*

Use of utilization data in negotiation

Complete and accurate utilization data is necessary to negotiate a workable capitated arrangement with a health plan. Without such data, professional organizations either ask for unrealistically high or settle for unrealistically low capitation payments. Both can be harmful to the professional organization. Seeking to achieve an unrealistically high level of capitation may inhibit the negotiation process with the health plan, and the contract may be signed with a competing provider group. Settling for a low capitation payment may quickly place the professional organization in financial jeopardy.

Initial experience data, often generated by the health plan, should have detailed information about utilization by specialty and associated costs. In the absence of any direct experience with capitation, the professional organization may need to rely heavily on such data. Information can be supplemented by capitation data from professional periodicals, experience of other groups, actuaries, and consultants.

During the negotiation process, the physician organization should consider the possibility of requiring the health plan to supply necessary data on a timely and regular basis. If the health plan is providing administration (i.e., paying claims, processing referral authorizations, and accounting for withhold pools), the professional organization will have little choice but to rely extensively on the information presented by the HMO. Timely data allows the physician organization to take quick and responsive correction action. Therefore, most successful capitated organizations strive for prospective and concurrent review of performance. Unfortunately, however, health plan data is often presented after the fact, and the physician organization's only remaining recourse is retrospective review. However, if the professional organization is managing its own administrative function, data should be readily available.

The importance of accurate and timely data presented in an understandable format is vital. Information about utilization is essential to ascertain the financial condition of the professional organization on an immediate and ongoing basis. The more risk the professional organization assumes, the more critical meaningful and timely data becomes.

Data typically collected and evaluated on a regular basis includes

- Inpatient hospital utilization (days per 1,000 enrollees)

- Total costs (ambulatory and inpatient) PMPM versus cost PMPM

- Incurred but not reported claims

- Appropriateness of referrals and use of ancillary medical resources (e.g., lab, MRI)

- Physician productivity (usually more appropriate in staff model groups)

Such data is of obvious importance to the general management of the group and also provides feedback on the appropriateness of the internal distribution system. If the group is not achieving an acceptable level of reserve, either utilization levels are excessive or provider compensation is too high or both. Likewise, if too much surplus is being retained, utilization or reimbursement may be too low. The internal reimbursement system may need to be fine-tuned until the correct balance is achieved. Professional organizations should view compensation and reimbursement systems as having the capability to change to meet different circumstances. The professional organization should prepare and review the financial statement of the group monthly. Modifications to the internal distribution system may need to be made quickly.

Conclusion

Effective internal reimbursement systems must be designed around solid financial and utilization principles. The aim of capitation is to change provider behavior toward the more efficient use of healthcare resources. Therefore, the "business as usual" approach has generally met with devastating financial results.

Methods to reimburse providers for services rendered within a capitated professional organization vary widely depending on a number of factors. The financial risks and potential rewards can be great. However, new models for effective practice must be quickly developed once a professional organization accepts the challenge to manage under a fixed dollar reimbursement system. These models should consider a variety of factors including care maps, critical paths, and emphasis on less costly forms of quality patient care.

The movement to managed care has also created an emphasis on efficiency in practice. Changes in the reimbursement system have altered the way physicians view their practice. Managed care forces competition within the provider community. Competition requires a need for greater capital investment for better office systems and more cost-efficient modes of practice. However, competition and changes in the reimbursement system may also lead to decreased reimbursement. Such forces have encouraged many physicians to search for more effective ways to practice. Some successful physician organizations also have found that an important key to their survival is to move from solo practice into the group practice setting where resources are shared.

Many hospitals have assisted physicians to secure capital and have sought to develop practice management relationships to better position them for the future. Typical of these relationships are management service organizations (MSOs) that allow physicians and hospitals to work together toward common goals. In states that have banned the corporate practice of medicine, MSOs and nonprofit medical practice foundations particularly have found favor with providers. In these models, physicians and hospitals move from separate entities toward an integrated healthcare delivery system. Publicly traded practice management companies also are an option for enterprising physicians searching for more equity-driven models. However, in response to managed care, other models have also developed across the country, such as large physician-led multispecialty or single-specialty medical groups. HMOs are also becoming more aggressive in purchasing physician practices.

Each of these models of affiliation has advantages and disadvantages. What is important to remember is that changes in the reimbursement system will eventually cause physicians to rethink their practice modes as well as their clinical style. It is premature to assert the end of solo practice. Indeed, IPA models continue to demonstrate that solo physicians can continue to be successful in traditional practice settings. However, continuing pressures caused by capitated reimbursement will likely force different linkages between physicians and among physicians and hospitals in the future.

EXHIBIT 1
Typical capitated professional CPT-4 procedures codes and other services

Physician services	CPT-4 procedure codes
Surgery	10000–58999, 59525, 60000–69979
Anesthesia	00100–01999, 99100–99140
Inpatient visits	99221–99223, 99231–99233, 99238, 99431, 99433, 99301–99313, 99199, 99160–99174, 99291–99292
Office visits	99201–99215
Physical exams	99382–99387, 99392–99397, 99178, 99401–99429
Well baby	99381, 99432, 99438, 99391
Emergency room	99062, 99065, 99281–99285, 99288
Home visits	99341–99353, 99321–99333
Consultations	99241–99255, 99261–99263, 99271–99275
Immunizations and injections	90708–90799, 90701–90749
Obstetrics:	
Nondeliveries	59000–59350, 59812–59899
Deliveries	59400–59430, 59510–59515
Radiology	70010–79999
Pathology	80002–89399
Outpatient psychiatric and chemical dependency	90801–90899
Physical therapy	97010–97799
Allergy testing and injections	95000–95105, 95115–95199
Vision, speech, and hearing exams	92002–92371, 92499, 92506–92508, 92551–92559
Miscellaneous	92950–93799, 90935–90999, 90900–90915, 91000–91299, 92502–92504, 92511–92520, 92531–92547, 93875–93979, 94010–94799, 95805–95999, 96400–96549, 96500–96599, 99499, 99000–99058, 99070, 99150–99151, 99175–99199, 00440

Other services	
Home health	Approved noncustodial private duty nursing and home health visits if ordered by the attending physician.
Laboratory	In-office and reference laboratory services.
Ambulance	Professional ambulance service as determined by the attending physician.
Extended care	All facility charges including room and board and ancillary charges for individuals who are patients at an extended care facility. Confinements must be medically necessary.
Durable medical	Needed appliances and equipment to restore normal functioning. Prosthetics are usually included.

EXHIBIT 2
Typical capitated PCP CPT-4 procedures codes

Medicine	90782, 90784, 90788, 90798, 92002, 92012, 92551, 93000, 93005, 93010, 95115, 95117, 99000–99090, 99150–99151, 99195, 99201–99215, 99221–99223, 99231–99233, 99238, 99281–99285, 99301–99303, 99311–99313, 99321–99323, 99331–99333, 99341–99343, 99351–99353, 99381–99387, 99391–99397, 99401–99404, 99411–99412, 99420, 99431–99433, 99438
Surgery	10040, 10060, 10080, 10120, 10140, 10160, 11040, 11050–11401, 11420–11421, 11700–11701, 11730–11732, 11740, 12001, 12011, 16000, 16020, 17000–17002, 17100–17104, 17110–17201, 19000, 21800, 21920, 23500, 30300, 30901, 36400–36410, 36415, 42970, 45300, 45330, 46220, 46600, 49080–49081, 55000, 57150–57170, 58300–58301, 65205–65220, 69000, 69200, 69210

6

Refining reimbursement methods for physician services

Peter R. Kongstvedt, MD
Partner
Ernst & Young LLP
Washington, DC

MANAGED CARE ORGANIZATIONS (MCOs), primarily health maintenance organizations (HMOs), frequently use some form of risk-based reimbursement for some physicians, especially primary care physicians (PCPs).[1] Specialty care physicians (SCPs) may also be paid under some form of risk-based reimbursement, although with less frequency than with PCPs. This chapter provides an overview of the most common risk-based methods.

All risk-based reimbursement systems require a change in attitude from "unmanaged" fee for service (FFS)—economic rewards come from lowering total healthcare costs. Depending on the reimbursement system design, this financial reward may be directly or indirectly related to total healthcare costs. Financial reward may be only partially related to utilization and may be affected by member satisfaction and quality of care delivered. Reimbursement systems may be perceived as primarily punitive, primarily reward based, or as a system that shares with providers savings accrued from good medical utilization. Those perceptions are partially driven by the reimbursement system design and partially by how the HMOs manage the reimbursement system. A reimbursement system, one of the many tools available in managed care, has limited ability to achieve desired goals without other tools such as utilization and quality management.

Neither the divisions by provider type nor the reimbursement mechanisms discussed are found in a pure state in the field. Managed care is marked by a high degree of continual change and variation.

PCP reimbursement

Approximately 40 percent of open panel HMOs use FFS to reimburse PCPs while the remaining 60 percent use capitation (see Figure 1). While this distribution of reimbursement methods has been relatively stable for the past several years, there is no guarantee it will remain stable.

The reasons for this level of FFS reimbursement are varied and have not been systematically studied. One hypothesis is that since FFS is more frequently acceptable to physicians, many HMOs use FFS to get more physicians to sign up, at least during an HMO's initial development period. This is especially true in markets where managed care penetration is low. HMOs also may try to capitate individual practice associations (IPAs), which pay FFS to the physicians. Certain products, such as point of service (POS), are also difficult to capitate and lead many HMOs with a large POS enrollment to use FFS. Lastly, some HMOs, which have reimbursed PCPs under FFS for more than 20 years, believe it is a sound reimbursement methodology.

FEE FOR SERVICE

There are two broad FFS categories: straight FFS and performance-based FFS. The straight FFS is less common in HMOs, although nearly universal in preferred provider organizations (PPOs) and Blue Cross Blue Shield (BCBS) plans. In Pennsylvania, for example, an HMO may not even be allowed to use straight FFS, since the PCPs are required to be at some level of financial risk in order for the HMO to qualify for state HMO licensure.

Performance-based FFS refers to the fact the PCP's fees will be influenced to some degree by performance. Whether performance refers to overall plan performance, performance of one segment of medical costs, or individual PCP performance is variable. How performance is defined and how it affects the fees is also variable. Figure 2 illustrates the relative percentages of MCOs using straight FFS versus performance-based FFS.

FIGURE 1
Reimbursement of primary care physicians

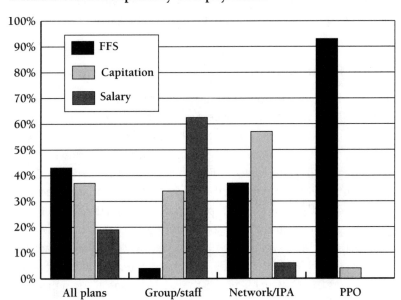

Source: Mathematica Policy Research, Inc. and The Medical College of Virginia, 1994.

Straight FFS

In straight FFS, the fees are unaffected by performance. Like fee structures in a PPO or BCBS plan, fees are constrained but do not have a direct relationship to utilization or any other performance measure.

Fees, however, are slightly constrained through maximum fee allowances. The physicians simply submit their claims using a standard claim form and code their fees using current procedural terminology (CPT) codes. The MCO maps these codes against a maximum fee allowance for that code and then pays the claim. The physician agrees to accept that fee as the maximum to be collected and not "balance bill" the member for any difference between the maximum allowance and the submitted claim. For example, if the physician submits a claim for $100 and the maximum allowance is $75, then the physician cannot bill the member for the $25 difference. The physician is free to bill for any deductible, coinsurance, or copayment the member pays directly but cannot collect more than $75.

The MCO usually uses some form of relative value scale (RVS), which assigns a value to each CPT code. To adjust fees, the plan simply changes the multiplier (i.e., a value that the relative value is multiplied by) to

FIGURE 2

Fee-for-service reimbursement of primary care physicians

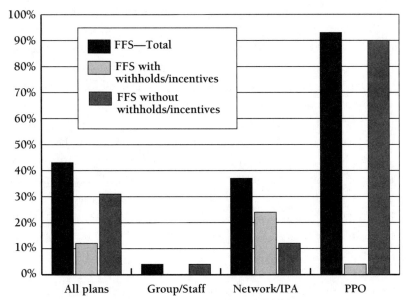

Source: Mathematica Policy Research, Inc. and The Medical College of Virginia, 1994.

obtain new fees for each CPT code. Several years ago the Health Care Financing Administration developed a new resource-based relative value scale (RBRVS), which many private plans have subsequently adopted. The RBRVS tries to correct the historical imbalance between high fees paid to surgeons and low fees paid to PCPs.

Performance-based FFS

Performance-based FFS is relatively common in those HMOs that use FFS to reimburse PCPs. Within performance-based FFS, there are three forms of adjustments—withholds on fees, fee adjustments, and global fees. Global fees, however, are not commonly used.

Withhold on fees. In a withhold, the plan withholds a portion of the fee for a predetermined period of time, usually one year. At the end of that period, the plan determines how medical costs compare to an established budget. If costs are equal to or better than the budget, the withhold is paid to the PCPs. If costs are higher than the budget, the withhold is used to offset cost overruns. If it does not take the entire withhold to satisfy the excess cost, the remainder is returned to the PCPs. However, if the withhold is insufficient to make up the cost overrun, the plan may look to other sources to make up the deficit, such as increasing the level of withhold the next year, or it may simply absorb the deficit.

There are numerous types of costs that a plan may measure in order to determine if the withhold will be paid out to the physicians or used to cover excess costs. The withhold may be applied to overall medical costs or may be applied to only one portion of costs such as hospital expenses. Plans that use this form of reimbursement always apply it to PCPs, but some apply it to SCPs as well.

Performance against which the withhold is applied may be by individual physician, by physician group, or over the entire network. For example, in an individual performance model, a PCP's use of specialty services is the primary measure, and cost overruns for that PCP's referrals are what the withhold is used to cover. At the other end of the spectrum, an entire network of PCPs is measured as a single entity, regardless of how each PCP performed.

It is rare for a plan to hold an individual PCP accountable for hospital expenses. Even in those plans that hold a PCP accountable for referral expenses, hospital costs are applied across a larger group of PCPs, frequently the entire network. How a plan uses the withhold if there is a cost overrun in hospital costs is variable. Many plans use the withholds of all PCPs, regardless of whether or not the PCP had a surplus, to cover hospital cost overruns. In other words, a PCP can have low referral costs and expect to receive a withhold but not receive it because hospital costs in the entire network were too high.

Many experienced medical directors believe withholds are generally not useful, since many PCPs have little expectation of receiving the money and simply consider the withhold another discount. Other medical directors, who feel that withholds are seen by physicians as punitive, prefer to use positive incentive-type reimbursement systems (i.e., physicians receive incentives to control utilization rather than relying on a withhold). While many view an incentive program as the flip side of a withhold, an incentive program shares savings while a punitive-type program takes money away in the event of overutilization.

Fee adjustments. Fee adjustments, prospectively based on past performance, are the other common form of performance-based FFS. They are often used simultaneously with withholds. A relative value scale is used to set fees. If performance is better than budget for the year (or period), the fees are raised using the RVS multiplier. If performance is worse, then fees are cut or not increased.

The method used to adjust fees is similar to how withholds are constructed. Fees are adjusted in one of the following ways: for all physicians in the network (PCPs and SCPs), for all PCPs only, or for subsets of PCPs.

Global fee approach. In this uncommonly used approach, the plan rebundles CPT fees into a single global fee. Regardless of what the PCP bills the plan, the plan pays the same fee. The level of the global fee is tied to performance, similar to fee adjustments, and may be used by groups of physicians or across the entire network. This approach can prevent the problems of "upcoding" (i.e., using CPT codes that inflate the value of the service to receive more money) and "unbundling" (i.e., billing for multiple services that used to be billed as a single service). This approach, however, does not prevent the problem of "churning" (i.e., seeing patients more often than necessary in order to increase income).

CAPITATION

Capitation refers to a fixed payment to a provider on a per member per month (PMPM) basis. The payment may vary, usually based on age and sex, and can vary by product (e.g., different copay levels). It does not vary by use or intensity of service or by the degree of patient illness. The capitation payment is all-inclusive, although a plan may occasionally carve out specifically defined services. These carve outs are confined to services that have highly variable costs and are not subject to abuse, such as immunizations. Under capitation, the plan pays the PCP FFS for those services.

Service risk

In service risk, the PCP receives a fixed payment but is not at financial risk. If service volume is high, then the PCP receives relatively lower income per encounter, and if service volume is low, the PCP receives higher income per encounter. While the PCP may not be at obvious financial risk, if volume is high the PCP loses the ability to sell services to someone else under FFS.

Financial risk

Financial risk refers to actual income placed at-risk, regardless if the PCP has a service risk as well. There are two common forms of financial risk: withholds and capitated pools for nonprimary care services. Figure 3 illustrates relative percentages of MCOs that use withholds and incentives as part of their capitation of PCPs.

Withhold. As with performance-based FFS, the withhold is a common form of financial risk. A portion of the capitation payment, usually 20 percent, is withheld by the plan. For example, if the PCP's capitation payment is $12.00 PMPM (based on the age and sex of that PCP's enrolled membership base), the plan will pay the PCP $9.60 PMPM and hold on to the remaining $2.40. If utilization is equal to or better than the budget, then the withhold is paid to the PCP. If utilization is higher than the budget, the withhold is used to cover overages. The issues regarding measurement (and whether PCPs are measured individually or as part of a larger unit) are similar to those described under FFS.

PCP risk pool capitation for nonprimary care services. PCP risk pool capitation for nonprimary care professional services (i.e., specialty services) is a form of financial risk where capitation money for spec-

FIGURE 3
Capitation to primary care physicians

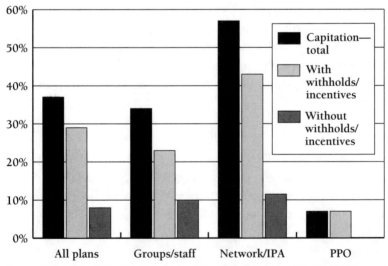

Source: Mathematica Policy Research, Inc. and The Medical College of Virginia, 1994.

ialty services is not paid to the PCP but rather is accrued into a pool and held by the HMO. Any claims for relevant specialty services are paid by the HMO and the risk pool is debited. There are various ways that HMOs handle these types of risk. Figure 4 illustrates schematically how some of these risk pools operate.

There are three broad classes of nonprimary care risk pools: referral (or specialty care), hospital (i.e., institutional care, regardless of whether or not it is inpatient, outpatient, or emergency department), and ancillary services (e.g., laboratory, radiology, and pharmacy). Many HMOs also use a fourth pool, usually called "other," where they accrue liabilities for such things as stop-loss or malpractice. In these cases, the physicians have no stake. It is not uncommon for these risk pools to be handled differently regarding the flow of funds and levels of risk and reward for the physicians and the plan.

REFERRAL POOL. In a referral pool, the plan tracks funds and costs for nonprimary care professional services. Plans often elect to include non-physician professional services such as mental health, optometry, and rehabilitation into an ancillary services pool. Some plans may elect to include hospital-based physicians (pathology, inpatient radiology, and anesthesia) in the hospital pool, although there is no current standardization. The referral pool is often PCP specific—the referral pool is tracked solely on each individual PCP's enrolled members. Although not necessarily a requirement, many plans combine referral pools of groups of PCPs or even the entire network of PCPs.

FIGURE 4
Capitation risk pools

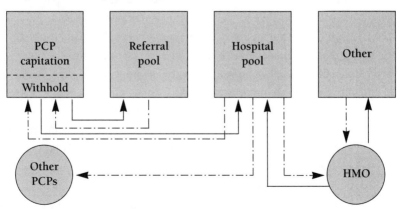

Plans add funds to the referral pool each month on a PMPM basis, adjusted for age and sex (and perhaps product design) and calculate the pool's debits for any claims from SCPs. Any deficits or surpluses in the referral pool are carried over from month to month.

Funds left in the risk pool at year-end are paid to the PCP while deficits are handled in a variety of ways. If there is a deficit, it may be covered by the withhold or covered by a positive balance by a hospital risk pool. In some cases, the plan also may make an adjustment to capitation for the next year. Occasionally, a plan carries over a deficit from year to year, but this is not common since it sends a negative message. It also tends to demotivate the PCPs. Usually, if a deficit cannot be covered by withholds or surpluses in other areas, the plan will absorb the deficit and wipe the slate clean.

HOSPITAL AND INSTITUTIONAL POOL. In a hospital pool, the plan tracks funds and costs for institutional services, including inpatient care, outpatient care, emergency department care, after-hours care, extended and skilled nursing care, home health, and any other services either part of or in lieu of hospital care. Mental health and substance abuse are commonly not included, since HMOs often subcapitate those services in their entirety.

As with the referral pool, the hospital pool is not paid directly to the PCPs but is accrued by the plan on a PMPM basis (again, adjusted for age and sex and possibly product design). Any claims for relevant institutional services are paid by the HMO and the risk pool is debited. Surpluses and deficits are carried over from month to month.

Funds left in the hospital risk pool at the end of the year are paid out to the PCPs. Surpluses are frequently shared with the HMO, often on a 50/50 basis. The reason for surplus sharing is that positive results in hospital utilization are due not only to the efforts of the PCPs but also to the HMO's utilization management function and discounts or other financial arrangements the plan negotiates with the hospitals.

Surplus payouts are used rarely by individual PCPs, since no PCP has a large enough panel of members to reduce the effects of chance. In other words, one or two severe patient cases (or conversely, having no hospital cases) may be as much due to luck as to good patient management. Therefore, the plan usually pays out surpluses based on some level of PCP aggregation, either into segments or over the entire PCP network.

Some plans may only pay hospital pool surpluses to those PCPs with positive referral pool balances, using the theory that low specialty service use is a good proxy for hospital use (since specialists hospitalize patients at a far higher rate than do PCPs). Other plans simply pay out the surplus on a prorated basis to all PCPs. In most cases, the payout is related to the size of the PCP member panel.

Deficits in the hospital pool at the end of the year are covered by the withhold if there is one and may be covered by the positive balances of PCPs in the referral pools. In plans that do not use withholds or referral pools, the plan may simply absorb the deficit. Some plans that use nonutilization-based incentive compensation do not pay that incentive unless there is a positive balance in the hospital pool.

Individual versus pooled risk. All forms of financial risk are affected by how the HMO handles individual risk versus pooled risk. In other words, to what degree are individual physicians at-risk for their performance, versus the degree to which that risk is shared with some or all other PCPs? It is human nature to wish to share the downside risk (and pain) with others but keep the upside (profit) for oneself.

While many HMOs contract directly with PCPs, there are many that contract through IPAs. In the true IPA model, the HMO capitates the IPA, but the IPA may or may not capitate the PCPs. In fact, many IPAs pay the PCPs on a FFS basis, using one or more of the performance-based FFS reimbursement methods described above. The use of IPAs to manage and reimburse physicians was in decline for many years, but the increase in vertical integration between hospitals and physicians has renewed interest in this model.

Yet in the absence of an IPA, the question remains: Who actually is being capitated and for what? The individual PCP? A subset of the total network of PCPs (i.e., pools of doctors—PODs)? The entire network of PCPs? The answers may not be the same for each category or risk. For example, a plan may wish to capitate PCPs individually for their own services, combine them into PODs for purposes of referral services, and use the performance of the entire network for purposes of hospital services. A plan can also choose to use different categories for risk and for reward. For example, a plan may spread risk across the entire network but only reward a subset of PCPs.

There are common and predictable problems with individual risk. The majority of those problems relate to the issue of small numbers. As noted earlier, luck can have as much or more of an impact on utilization as does good management, at least in small member panels. As a PCP's panel grows to more than 500 members, this problem starts to lessen but still persists. When PCPs have good utilization results, they generally desire to keep the reward of their hard labor; when results are poor, they frequently feel that they have been dealt an abnormally sick population of members and should not be held accountable for the high medical costs.

The more money at stake, the more dangerous the problem of small numbers becomes to an individual PCP. While stop-loss and reinsurance somewhat ameliorate the problem, it still remains. Thus, many plans use individual pools for referral services but will not do so for hospital services, where the dollars are substantially higher.

The other major problem with individual risk is the ability of some PCPs to "game the system." In other words, to enhance income, PCPs manage to transfer their sickest patients out of the practice, with a resulting improvement in individual PCP's medical costs. While all plans prohibit PCPs from moving members out of their practice due to medical condition, a wily and unethical PCP can find a way to do so yet remain undetected.

There is also another concern that individual risk incents a PCP to withhold necessary medical care. While this charge has been leveled at the HMO industry for many years, it has never been proven.

Lastly, there have been cases of HMOs requiring an individual PCP (or small group) to write a check to the plan to cover cost overruns in medical expenses (as opposed to simple reconciliation of accidental overpayments). This has usually occurred when the plan agreed to not actually keep the withhold (in response to the PCP's plea to improve cash flow) but nonetheless track it. Whenever a PCP is required to pay money back to the plan, a problem in provider relations is likely to occur.

If the plan chooses to pool risk across the entire network, then the flip side of individual risk may occur: the impact of any individual PCP's actions are diluted so much as to be undetectable. If PCPs are having good results, then they may resent having to cover for their colleagues' poor results. If the plan does not track individual results, then it will have little capability of providing meaningful data to individual physicians to help them better manage medical resources.

Because of these two extremes, many plans have chosen to use PODs for at least some financial risk management. Although there is no standard size, PODs are a subset of the entire network. PODs may be made up of a large medical group, an aggregation of 10 to 15 physicians, or all participating PCPs in an entire geographic area. A POD could also be made up of the physicians in a physician-hospital organization (PHO) that accepts risk. The common denominator is that there are sufficient members enrolled in practices in the POD for statistical integrity, but a small enough population to allow the POD to make changes seen in utilization results. The chief risk is that PODs require support from the plan in the form of data and utilization management.

While many have chosen PODs to share financial risk, they are not a panacea. If a POD fails, the repercussions are greater than if an individual physician fails—more members are affected and costs are greater. There are times when individual risk and reward is best, times when the entire network should be treated as a single organization, and times when PODs will make sense.

Full risk capitation

Full risk capitation is when the PCP receives money for all professional services, primary and specialty but not hospital services—although the group may still be on a hospital utilization management incentive program. The PCP not only authorizes the referral but actually reimburses the SCP. This type of reimbursement was once marginally popular, but today is rare; some PCPs did not have sufficient funds to cover specialty costs, and members were exposed to balance billing. However, there has been a recent resurgence of interest in this form of capitation as PCPs band together into large groups or other forms of collective activity such as integrated delivery systems.

A large group or organized system of PCPs can best support full risk capitation. To the degree that the primary care group can capitate specialists for services, the risk of having insufficient funds is lessened. However, many state insurance departments will only allow a licensed HMO, not a provider, to subcapitate.

Any medical group accepting full risk capitation needs strong financial management skills and good management information systems (MIS). In the absence of such sophistication, many HMOs will be reluctant to enter into such arrangements because they do not wish to be exposed to the risk of failure. This form of full risk capitation is similar but not identical to total capitation where an integrated delivery system (IDS) accepts capitation for medical services, both institutional and professional.

Specialty physicians

As illustrated in Figure 5, approximately 20 to 30 percent of specialty care physicians (SCPs) in HMOs are paid through capitation. The majority of SCPs are paid through FFS, with others reimbursed through salary, retainer, or hourly rates.

FFS AND SCPS

Fee for service as applied to SCPs is generally a straightforward proposition. It is not commonly performance based but rather is usually straight FFS, based on a fee allowance schedule. SCPs must accept the fee as payment in full (except for collectible deductibles, copayments, or coinsurance) and may not balance bill the member at all. The SCP must also agree not to balance bill the member in the event the plan fails or refuses to pay at all, unless the service is clearly for a benefit not covered under the plan's schedule of benefits.

While relatively uncommon, there are plans that use performance-based FFS for the SCPs in the network. The most common examples are through withholds and fee adjustments in an IPA where all—both PCPs and SCPs—are treated the same.

FIGURE 5
Reimbursement of specialty physicians

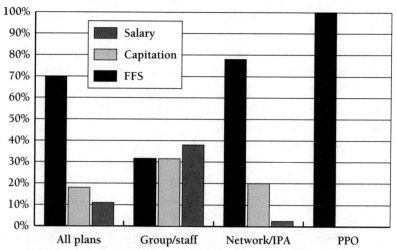

Source: Mathematica Policy Research, Inc. and The Medical College of Virginia, 1994.

A few IPAs have tried to adjust fees based on each specialty, so-called "budgeted fee for service." In this approach, each specialty has a PMPM budget (e.g., $2.50 PMPM for cardiology), and actual costs are measured against that budget. If costs exceed budget, then fees are lowered for that specialty; if budget exceeds costs, fees are raised. This arrangement requires a highly sophisticated management information system, sound actuarial analysis, and a large membership base to ensure statistical integrity to ensure that utilization patterns are based on provider performance.

Global fees, however, are more common for certain specialties than for PCPs. Obstetrics and surgery are two examples in which MCOs apply global fees to cover the preadmission period, admission, and postadmission care. Unfortunately, global fees are relatively easy to "game" in that if SCPs choose to, they can find ways to bill for services outside of the global fee to enhance revenue. Nonetheless, global fees are useful for routine procedures to provide some protection against gross upcoding and unbundling.

CAPITATION AND SPCS

SCP capitation is generally simpler than PCP capitation. In theory the same utilization issues apply to specialty care and to primary care—the numbers in SCP capitation are often significantly smaller for a given specialty (even though specialty PMPM costs as a whole are usually one and a half to two times higher than primary care). For example, PCP capitation may average $14 PMPM, while neurology capitation may be $0.55. Thus, adjustments can become small and may not be worth the effort.

Capitation for specialty services is usually provided through a simple payment, although it may be performance based, which may employ a withhold or use an incentive pool to control utilization. In each case, the plan sets targets for utilization, using a combination of professional and institutional PMPM costs. As with PCP incentives, the withhold or incentive is paid based on performance against those targets.

How to capitate specialty services

Capitating specialty services can be more problematic than PCP capitation. When capitating PCPs, a member must choose a PCP—then it becomes a straightforward issue for the MCO to track that membership. Specialty capitation is different. Any given SCP will provide care to patients of multiple PCPs with no requirement on the part of a member to choose a SCP.[2] Because of these issues, HMOs must use alternate methods to determine how to capitate SCPs. Some of these methods are described as follows.

Organized groups. The easiest form of SCP capitation is through organized medical groups. In some cases, the group is a multispecialty group, inclusive of primary and specialty care. In these cases, it is assumed that a member assigned to a PCP in that group will also be assigned to the SCPs in the group.

Organized single-specialty groups are also good candidates for capitation. If the group is large enough, then it may be capitated for the entire network. If it is not large enough to cover the entire medical service area, then it may be capitated for that portion of the geographic medical service area that it can cover.

A new variation on this type of capitation is for single-specialty services to a specialty corporation (e.g., a vendor that specializes in cancer services). The corporation employs physicians and support staff and provides facilities and ancillary services and is then responsible for providing all of that specialty's services within the HMO's medical service area.

Geographic distribution. Geographic distribution is somewhat similar to the way an organized medical group is capitated. In essence, a small (i.e., two or three) physician specialty group accepts capitation for all specialty services, but in a specific geographic area rather than for the entire service area. For example, a group of general surgeons might be capitated to cover all services rendered at a single hospital or in an urban area. A capitated SCP might cover all PCP practices located in a particular set of zip codes. Since it is not uncommon for PCP (or SCP for that matter) practices to have multiple locations, assignment is based on whatever office is considered the physician's principal office.

Specialty IPAs. Specialty specific IPAs are uncommon, but the recent increase in vertical integration activities (such as PHOs) has led to increased interest in this form of specialty capitation. The specialty IPA operates similarly to a standard IPA. It accepts a capitation from the HMO but usually pays FFS to the participating specialists. Capitation of individual SCPs within the specialty IPA is certainly possible but rare because specialty IPAs are often created to preserve the opportunity for multiple, unrelated SCPs to participate with aggressive HMOs. Whether or not specialty IPAs will remain viable is unknown.

Single-specialty management. Single-specialty management and its two approaches are uncommon but may increase as managed care experiments with different capitating specialty service methods. Here, the HMO contracts with one single entity to provide all services within a single specialty, although that entity does not provide all the services.

In one approach, an HMO capitates a single specialist (i.e., an individual physician) to manage all services in that specialty for all HMO members, even though the SCP cannot provide the services. The contracted SCP must then subcontract with other specialists to provide services throughout the medical service area. The primary contract holder (i.e., the SCP with the overall capitation contract with the HMO) either makes or loses money depending on how efficiently specialty services are managed. The primary SCP may subcapitate with other SCPs if allowed by the state insurance department (many states will not allow a provider to capitate another provider) or may pay FFS. In all events, the primary SCP acts like a second "gatekeeper" in that the PCPs work through the primary SCP to access specialty care for members. Sometimes, the primary SCP receives the full capitation payment and must pay the other SCPs directly, or the HMO may administer the claims payments and provide accounting and reporting for the primary contract holder. The HMO may often wish to manage payments and other administrative tasks in order to track performance on a real-time basis and to protect members from possible nonpayment of claims by the primary contract holder.

In the other approach, an HMO contracts with a single institution for single specialty services (e.g., the HMO contracts with a local university faculty practice plan for all cardiology services). The contracted institution is then responsible for arranging specialty services it cannot provide itself. The primary specialty contract holder receives the capitation payment and must then administer payment to subcontractors. In some cases, the administrative cost to the primary contractor is often a manual process, and it may be greater than the total capitation payment.

By PCP choice. Another capitation method is through the mechanism of "PCP choice." Although seldom used, this model requires each PCP to choose a SCP to be used on an exclusive basis. The presence of choice means that multiple SCPs have agreed to a capitation rate, but no single SCP has exclusive rights. The plan is then required to track the members assigned to those SCPs by virtue of being on the PCP's panels and pay the SCP capitation based on that. While this approach is interesting, most HMO management information systems are not capable of handling it, and the administrative headache would be great.

Specialty capitation and cost control

Capitation, especially SCP capitation, requires clear delineation of the services covered. There are times when a SCP will be unable or unwilling to provide all relevant specialty services (e.g., an ophthalmologist may not perform laser retinal surgery). When this occurs, the plan pays FFS for these services known as carve outs (i.e., those services not covered under the capitation are "carved out" of the capitation payment).

Carve outs can create utilization problems if the same SCP who has the capitation provides the carved-out service under FFS. The reason is obvious: the SCP is being paid capitation to determine if he or she should also be paid FFS to provide additional services. Seasoned medical directors will almost never allow a capitated SCP to bill FFS for any services. If the SCP is unable to provide the service, then the utilization problem is much diminished—there is no financial incentive for the SCP to recommend the carved-out service.

Usually a carved-out service is simply not included in the capitation rate. Occasionally, a plan will use a capitation rate that includes the carved-out services and then deduct the FFS cost of those services from the capitation payment as services are rendered. In this way, the SCP has more financial stake in monitoring the use and cost of the carved-out services.

An HMO needs to ensure that all capitated specialty services will be rendered by the capitated providers, or else the HMO will pay twice— once through capitation and once through FFS. Often, inexperienced managers assume that since the care is now capitated, then costs are predictable and fixed. This may be true in a mature plan with years of experience and a stable membership but is unlikely in a plan that has recently capitated specialty services.

There are several challenges to capitated specialty services including out-of-area emergencies, which are clear examples of costs outside the capitation. In the early periods of changing to a more limited, capitated SCP panel, both members and PCPs will be less than completely efficient in changing referral patterns. Thus, there will be considerable use of noncapitated SCPs. Another major problem is that capitated specialty services are sometimes perceived as "free" by both PCPs and the medical director. If specialty utilization rises dramatically because of this, the capitated SCP will demand a substantial increase in the capitation payment, leading to difficult negotiations by both parties.

Total or global capitation

Total or global capitation applies to a vertical IDS that is capable of accepting full or nearly full risk for medical expenses, including all professional, institutional, and many ancillary services. This differs from the full capitation described earlier that applied to primary care groups. Total capitation includes institutional as well as professional services, and the party accepting the capitation payment is a large, vertically integrated organization with greater resources. Even though the IDS accepts total capitation, it often purchases reinsurance to protect against catastrophic cases. That reinsurance is either provided by the HMO or purchased by the IDS from a reinsurer.

Although the HMO may have capitated the IDS, the IDS still faces the issue of how to divide up the revenue and risk. In a sense, total capitation simply transfers the burden of payment and management from the HMO to the IDS, but the fundamental issues remain. If the IDS employs the physicians, then it is relatively easier to distribute income.

Most IDSs, however, are combinations of private and employed physicians. Even hospitals that employ physicians usually still rely on private physicians for at least some services, even though the genesis of the IDS was to allow the hospital and private physicians to remain competitive in a managed care environment.

Therefore, the IDS that accepts total capitation must determine how to allocate risk and reward. IDS managers must be realistic and recognize that individual physicians will be unable and unwilling to bear a high level of financial risk (e.g., how many individual physicians could afford to pay $200,000 as their share of overutilization?) but will usually demand a disproportionate share of financial reward. While risk and reward are always related, IDS management must be careful to properly incent the physicians as well as avoid the legal problems of private inurment and fraud and abuse regulations.

The last major issue in total capitation is to determine who is the licensed health plan. If an IDS accepts total capitation, then a state's insurance department may require the IDS to become licensed as an HMO. One state's insurance commissioner has dubbed totally capitated IDSs "stealth HMOs." This is even more complicated if the IDS accepts capitation from a self-funded employer under ERISA, without any licensed health plan involved. Regulation of IDS accepting full risk capitation is undergoing considerable scrutiny by state insurance departments.

To capitate or not to capitate

While capitation is a powerful and useful method of reimbursement, there are reasons to capitate and reasons why capitation is not preferable. Likewise, there are times when capitation would be desirable but cannot be implemented. A number of such reasons are discussed below.

Reasons to capitate. The first and most powerful reason for an HMO to capitate providers is that capitation puts the provider at-risk for medical expenses and utilization. Capitation eliminates the FFS incentive to overutilize medical services and brings the financial incentives of the capitated provider in line with the financial incentives. Under capitation, costs are more easily predicted by the health plan, although not absolutely predictable. Capitation is also easier and less costly to administer than FFS, resulting in lower administrative costs in the HMO and potentially lower premium rates to the member.

The strongest incentive for a provider to accept capitation is financial. Capitation ensures positive cash flow, allowing the provider to receive prepayment at a predictable rate, regardless of services rendered. Also, for effective medical case managers, physicians, and cost-effective providers, the profit margins can exceed those found in FFS today and in the future. Capitation also eliminates any disagreements over the level of provider fees charged to a patient, thus providing some level of financial insulation to the physician-patient relationship.

Reasons not to capitate. There are several reasons why an HMO might not wish to capitate. Theoretically, capitation may lead to inappropriate underutilization. While capitation methods have been accused of withholding necessary care, it has never been systematically demonstrated in actual practice. In fact, most studies of quality of care and member satisfaction in HMOs demonstrate equal or superior results, making the capitation appear to be harmless.

Since capitation is statistically based, it is not sensitive to small enrollment and may not accurately represent the actual health status of a single physician's panel of members. This becomes a more important issue if an individual physician is at considerable financial risk for a small number of members or less of an issue if risk is spread over a large base of members and physicians.

Although capitation is commonly adjusted for age and sex, it must be adjusted if benefits are not uniform, at least if there are large differences in benefits an HMO offers to its members. Similarly, certain product lines such as Medicare and Medicaid pose similar problems in that substantial adjustments in capitation must be made due to varied utilization. Adjusting copayments is easy, while adjusting for different benefits may not be so simple. For example, a plan may offer different levels of coverage for obstetrics or may offer benefit riders to cover unusual cancer treatments and transplants.

A physician may not want to capitate because of fear of the unknown. Although most physicians have experience with FFS, they may have concerns about the way capitation affects their income. Physicians tend to be risk averse and capitation clearly has an element of risk. Some physicians hold an unwarranted but firm belief that capitation will incent them to inappropriately withhold services. It is unlikely, however, that these physicians would admit that they would deliberately provide inferior-quality care to receive money (and in fact they would not knowingly practice bad medicine).[3]

POINT OF SERVICE

Point of service (POS) is especially difficult to combine with capitation, particularly with individual physicians. It is possible to capitate IDS under POS, with the IDS responsible for both in-network and out-of-network costs. This only works with large IDSs with reasonably large enrollments.

The problem with POS and individual provider capitation is in determining the levels of in-network versus out-of-network use. While actuaries may predict that the typical POS plan design is expected to yield, for example, 30 percent out-of-network use, that percentage is applied to the entire membership, not to an individual physician's member panel. Any individual panel may have 10 percent or 50 percent out-of-network use. If the plan applies a uniform capitation payment, then some providers will be underpaid while others are overpaid. This problem applies to primary care capitation as well as risk pools for nonprimary services.

Two rather useless approaches to individual capitation in POS are to adjust the capitation prospectively or retrospectively. In the former, the plan lowers the capitation payment by the expected out-of-network utilization (e.g., lowers the capitation payment by 30 percent if that is what the actuaries conclude out-of-network utilization will be). Because it is unlikely that the individual provider will have exactly that same level of out-of-network utilization, the provider will either be overpaid (and clearly incented to encourage out-of-network use by members, since it will result in higher relative payments for services) or underpaid. The other approach, retrospectively adjusting the capitation payment, requires the provider to refund the plan a percentage of money that equates to the out-of-network utilization. That quickly becomes a difficult exercise for provider relations when the plan demands an individual physician write a check (e.g., a PCP with a $12.00 PMPM rate on 500 members with 30 percent out-of-network utilization would be required to pay nearly $20,000).

A number of HMOs have resorted to using capitation to reimburse providers for their "pure" HMO members but use FFS for POS members. This can create problems, however, due to the different reimbursement systems, and results in what psychologists call "cognitive dissonance." Many HMOs with high levels of POS membership simply do not capitate at all and use FFS exclusively. Applying performance-based FFS in a POS plan is more difficult than in a "pure" HMO, but it is not impossible. It is important to continue to incent the physicians properly, even in a POS plan, so as not to encourage out-of-network utilization. Figure 6 illustrates relative percentages of MCOs that use different reimbursement systems for different product types.

NONUTILIZATION-BASED INCENTIVE PROGRAMS

Capitated incentive programs for providers may not be based solely on utilization targets; there are nonutilization-based incentive compen-

FIGURE 6
Variation in reimbursement by product

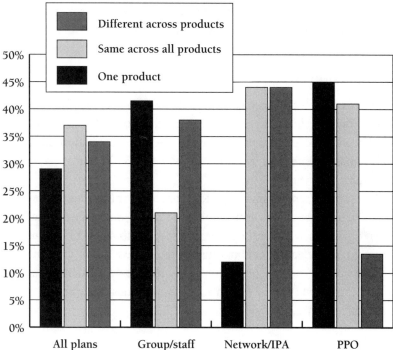

Source: Mathematica Policy Research, Inc. and The Medical College of Virginia, 1994.

sation programs for PCPs in some HMOs as well. Funding of the incentive pool may be from utilization-based withholds or risk pools or may separate line-item capitation in the cost budget.

To determine how incentives are paid, PCP performance is measured most commonly in areas of quality of medical care, member satisfaction, and compliance with administrative requirements (or business quality). Incentive payments are made to those PCPs who qualify. A few HMOs use these programs as their predominant method of incentive payments (e.g., one large plan pays PCPs incentives based 40 percent on utilization and 60 percent on quality and member satisfaction).

Quality of medical care is determined through clinical quality measures from the plan's quality management or assurance program. Member satisfaction is measured through member surveys, complaints or grievances, and transfer rates (i.e., the rate at which members leave one

PCP in order to change to another PCP). Business quality is measured using data from interactions with the health plan such as compliance with the referral panel, compliance with utilization policies and procedures, and submission of encounter forms.

Conclusion

To be effective, a managed care organization, whether an HMO or IDS, must align the financial incentives and goals of all the parties—the health plan and providers who deliver the care. Capitation, and to a somewhat lesser extent performance-based FFS, do this in ways that traditional FFS cannot.

The reimbursement system is a tool and, like any tool, has limitations. Just as a hammer is the correct tool for pounding and removing nails, it fails for cutting wood and drilling holes. A reimbursement system is a powerful and effective tool but can only be effective in conjunction with other managed care functions: utilization management, quality management, provider relations, and many other activities of a well-run managed care organization.

NOTES

1. Primary care physicians are assumed to be in the specialties of Family Practice, Internal Medicine, and Pediatrics; General Practice (i.e., nonboard certified general practitioners) are also considered primary care in those plans that contract with GPs. Obstetrics and Gynecology, while sharing some attributes of primary care, are generally treated as specialty physicians by HMOs. Physician extenders, such as Physicians' Assistants and Clinical Nurse Practitioners, are generally treated as being associated with primary care physicians and so are not discussed separately.

2. The common exception to this last point is obstetrics and gynecology (OB/Gyn). Some plans do require all female members over the age of 12 to choose an OB/Gyn, and the plan in turn capitates that OB/Gyn in a fashion similar to that used for PCPs (although the capitation rate is less frequently varied by age or sex).

3. In most cases, physicians are not worried about their own behavior, "it's those other guys that can't be trusted."

7

Balancing physician financial and nonfinancial incentives

Henry E. Golembesky, MD
Principal

Michael K. Kaplan
Senior Associate
APM Incorporated
San Francisco, California

I N T H E M A N A G E D C A R E W O R L D , California is often viewed as an indicator of where the rest of the nation is headed. In California, capitation rates are as much as 50 to 100 percent lower than those in other states. Many integrated delivery systems (IDSs) experienced a 3 to 5 percent decline in per member per month (PMPM) capitation rates in 1995.[1] It is no surprise, then, that only two of the seven leading California IDSs achieved a return on sales equal to or above the average rate for all U.S. hospitals in 1994, while the remaining five had returns ranging from -2.7 percent to 0.9 percent.[2] The increasing financial pressure on physicians (particularly specialists) and hospitals caused by such reduced managed care payments and compounded by government budget cuts will cause many providers to fail over the next five years.

In response, physicians and hospitals across the country are scrambling to find partners to help protect their patient base against better-integrated competitors. While developing integrated delivery systems, the physicians and hospitals are aggressively seeking more managed care business. They are trying to negotiate capitated reimbursement from managed care health plans and to bear and share the risk of providing all healthcare services to an enrolled population.

But many of these integrated systems will not succeed because the physicians do not have the appropriate financial incentives to make the arrangements work.

Physician incentives are perhaps the least developed yet most necessary component of managed care, especially for bearing risk as an IDS. There is much agreement from both health policy experts and the popular press that the alignment of incentives among all providers is a key success factor in an IDS. Effective incentives and medical management can reduce PMPM healthcare costs by 15 to 33 percent, increase patient satisfaction, and improve the quality of care. But most newly formed or forming networks pay far more attention to which hospitals and physicians are included in the system than they do to making sure those physicians and hospitals are working toward the common goals of access, cost, and quality.

The "hassle factor" approach to incentives

To date, few healthcare organizations have designed an incentive program that actively encourages physicians to assure seamless patient access and high-quality, cost-effective care. Those few that have created incentive programs most often use the proverbial stick rather than the carrot to reduce utilization and cost. The most common program is often referred to by physicians as the "hassle factor" approach, with a new utilization review (UR) system based on penalties, negative reinforcement, and burdensome administrative review of individual physician decisions. The general premise here is that the more difficult it is for a physician to do anything, the less the physician will do.

Physician incentives are not as simple as throwing a new UR system into place and converting to capitation. Nor do these incentives need to be based on hassling physicians. There are many variables to consider, and it is possible to succeed by treating physicians as well-trained, professional care managers who will achieve desirable outcomes if given good data and positive incentives. Creating such an incentive program requires starting with the point of view of the physician.

What do the physicians want?

Surprisingly few health plans or IDSs actually take the time to ask participating physicians what they want or need. When physicians are asked what they would like to see in an integrated delivery system, the answers they give are consistent nationwide. In general, physicians would like

- *Access to patients and the opportunity for new ones.* For their professional and financial growth, physicians need their patients to have access to them, supporting the prime reason that most physicians consider joining an IDS or health plan. An organization that can deliver a stable flow of patients over the long term will be highly attractive to physicians

- *Practice autonomy, especially in clinical decision making.* Lack of autonomy in practice and referrals is a large concern physicians have about integrated arrangements. Physicians want to practice in a collegial and professional environment, not one with many hassles or problems. Furthermore, they would like to see utilization review and medical management designed to work as a positive rather than a negative physician incentive

- *A role in governance and decision making.* Physicians want to have a voice in the decisions that affect them. It is a rare, and perhaps unwise, physician who is willing to delegate all decisions to some IDS or hospital administrator. Physicians need to believe the organization they are joining recognizes their value and importance, not just in attracting contracts but in governance. The importance to physicians of being involved in decision making and forging their own destiny should not be underestimated

- *Participation in plans with high-quality panels and reasonable payment levels.* Top-notch physicians who have invested many years in becoming highly skilled, well-respected professionals often believe that becoming part of an IDS means that their individual reputation will be affected by the group. They want to join groups with highly skilled physicians who are reimbursed appropriately. Although change is inevitable, some physicians will balk at participating in groups not considered to have the best physicians or reimbursement commensurate with their training and skill

- *Help with managed care contracting and cost control.* The basic premise behind an IDS is that costs can be better controlled in an integrated network, enhancing the ability to get additional contracts and patients. But most physicians have not received any education in clinical or administrative cost control and do not have the funding for clinical information systems or protocol development. Thus physicians are looking for a source of education about and capital to support concepts like negotiating managed care contracts, creating clinical practice guidelines, controlling per member per month costs, and developing new reimbursement mechanisms

- *A fair means of dividing capitated revenues.* Under capitation, physicians' incomes become less tied to their individual effort than under fee-for-service medicine. This also means that a larger payment for one physician can mean a smaller one for another—and payments are generally smaller than they used to be. Physicians require that an equitable method be used to allocate capitated funds and determine their income

These factors serve as a realistic backdrop for designing a physician incentive system.

Principles for risk sharing and financial arrangements

As described above, there are a myriad of nonfinancial concerns related to physician desires and incentives. But while the vast majority of physicians do not make individual clinical decisions with an eye toward the bottom line, the overall effects of financial incentives are hard to ignore. After all, this is the primary reason capitation has spread so rapidly. The following set of guidelines can be used to design effective financial incentives that balance patient satisfaction, quality of care, and financial viability.

- Financial arrangements must be designed to motivate the management and delivery of high-quality patient care. Delivering high-quality care and keeping members healthy is critical; compromising on quality today will lead to higher costs tomorrow. The best investment an IDS can make is high-quality healthcare

- The IDS should strive to align the incentives among primary care physicians, specialists, hospitals, and other providers by encouraging shared financial risk and reward. Sharing one capitated bank account will not achieve desired outcomes if individuals are motivated to write themselves checks until the balance is zero. The incentive system should be structured so that all providers who help to achieve a surplus benefit economically if there is money left in the account at the end of the year

- The IDS should attempt to gain control of as much of the premium dollar as possible. Gaining control of the premium dollar should strike a balance between aggressively entering a risk contract (to build market position and force learning) and ensuring fiscal integrity (by not assuming risk until the capability to manage the IDS is successfully developed). In the long term, the only healthcare services excluded from capitation should be those few with the following characteristics: low expected frequency of occurrence; high risk of high-cost and/or low-quality outcomes; and factors that influence cost/quality outcomes that are not well defined or controlled by the IDS

- The contracting model and financial structure should be attractive to payers as well as providers and should be flexible enough to accommodate changes in product design as market conditions require. Different payers will want different arrangements with the IDS—some will want full capitation, some partial capitation, some case rates, and some something different altogether. A few may be willing to develop multiyear relationships that include joint investments in system development. The model that is set up must be able to handle the wide variety of potential contracts that may become available to the IDS over time

- The IDS must learn to manage risk and be prepared. Thorough risk assessment, actuarial analysis, and sufficient stop-loss protections must be part of any and all risk contracts. Comprehensive utilization management and quality improvement programs that include clinical protocols must be established to monitor performance and change behaviors. Patient education, triage, and urgent care systems must support the medical management strategy. Information systems must be available to support the analysis, communication, and risk/reward mechanisms. Continuous financial monitoring and timely reporting are essential

- The distribution of risk and potential financial reward within the IDS must be clearly defined and understood in advance. The distribution should be based on a defined scope of services for each category of provider: actuarial expectations and target utilization levels, volume (e.g., panel size or productivity), quality of care and patient satisfaction measures, and actual control over and the ability to influence performance outcomes

- Incentives should be significant enough to motivate physicians to ensure high-quality and efficient utilization of resources. The potential distributions from incentives such as bonus pools and withholds must be substantial enough to impact practice patterns. A potential year-end payout of $200 is not as powerful as a potential bonus of $10,000 for achieving utilization targets. A recent report by the Advisory Board suggests that these incentives must be between 30 and 50 percent of total compensation to be effective. While this may represent the high end of the spectrum, incentives below 10 to 15 percent of compensation may well be insignificant

- The IDS financial arrangements should minimize administrative burdens on physicians. Adequate funds must be allocated for investments in management information systems (MIS) and support staff for the IDS to operate effectively and physicians to be appropriately leveraged. Population-based MIS will be absolutely critical to manage and monitor utilization patterns and to provide physicians with the data and information needed. Patient outreach and education programs to assist in managing healthcare for the members also must be part of IDS operations and budgets

To capitate or not to capitate or how to pay physicians

Capitated reimbursement changes the financial incentives inherent under fee for service. Under capitation, physicians should have a direct financial incentive to perform only medically appropriate diagnostics, to deliver clinically efficient and effective care, and to keep patients as healthy as possible. But an IDS that receives capitation from a payer does not necessarily have to pay each individual physician or specialty on a capitated basis.

There are benefits and drawbacks both to fee schedule reimbursement and capitation of individual physicians, and these vary between the primary care physician (PCP) and the specialist. Table 1 discusses some physician compensation approaches and issues.

In the end, the right answer for an IDS will depend on its enrollment, its physician panel, and scope of services. It may include a mixture of fee schedules and capitation. One common approach is for PCPs to be reimbursed via capitation and for individual specialists to be paid on a fee schedule as services are rendered. The assumption is that specialist utilization is reduced because the PCPs serve as gatekeepers, reducing unnecessary specialist referrals. But do the PCPs actually have the incentive to do this? Not unless there are other incentives involved. With the PCP capitated, there is a built-in incentive to refer any potential specialist issue because the PCP will not be paid more for seeing that patient or treating that complaint. The specialist, on the other hand, has the incentive to see all these cases. From a purely economic perspective, primary care capitation coupled with a fee schedule for specialists is not optimal. Some health plans and IDSs that have taken this approach have seen a

TABLE 1
Trade-offs between fee schedules and capitation

Primary care	Fee schedule	Capitation
Pro	Incentive to "keep" specialty care and thereby reduce referrals	Incentive to control primary care use
	"Small numbers" problem (patients per PCP) would make capitation difficult	More predictable funds flow Easier way to redistribute funds to PCPs
Con	May result in higher number of visits per member per PCP	May result in higher referrals rates to specialists
	Higher risk of funds shortfall at year-end	Can result in limited patient access
Specialists		
Pro	"Small numbers" problem (utilization per specialty) would make capitation difficult	Incentive for specialists to return cases to PCPs and control utilization
	Utilization still to be wrung out; why give specialists the windfall	Incentive for primaries to over-refer to specialists
Con	Maintains high utilization incentive	Data may not be sufficient to support rate development
	Risk of funds shortfall and need for withhold	Can result in limited patient access

dramatic increase in the number of minor health concerns referred to specialists, (e.g., coughs referred to pulmonologists or sprains referred to orthopedists).

If their enrollment is large enough, IDSs should consider the opposite. By reimbursing the PCPs on a fee schedule within a global budget, these physicians are encouraged to take on as much "specialty" care as they can. And the capitated specialists have the incentive to teach PCPs to manage more of the routine specialty care. This combination can be very effective to reduce specialist referrals, and then specialty capitation rates can be reduced over time to reflect the reduced utilization. The most frequently capitated specialties are psychiatry, ophthalmology, radiology, cardiology, urology, allergy, orthopedics, general surgery, otolaryngology and dermatology.[3] This approach, however, can only be implemented in an IDS with enough enrollment and utilization data to set statistically valid specialty capitation rates. It also must be accompanied by protocols that ensure the PCPs do not underutilize specialists for conditions that warrant a referral.

WHAT ABOUT RISK POOLS AND WITHHOLDS?

Beyond the primary method of reimbursement, two common approaches to physician financial incentives are to create risk pools or to employ withholds.

A risk pool is a percentage of capitation or fund allocation that is set aside for year-end distribution. The basic premise is that superior medical management will generate financial surpluses, which are shared among participating physicians. If at year-end there is a shortage due to overutilization, the risk pool can be used to settle claims, and if there is a surplus, it is distributed among providers according to objective performance measures. Payouts can be linked to a number of individual physician and group variables, some based on utilization statistics (e.g., days per 1,000, referrals per 1,000, or specialist costs PMPM) and some on other factors (e.g., outcomes, patient satisfaction, or physician productivity). In a nonintegrated or noncapitated organization, similar arrangements can be created whenever there is prospective reimbursement (e.g., case rates or package prices), which may lead to surpluses if costs are well managed. Risk pools, particularly when physicians share in the benefits of reduced hospital utilization, can be very effective physician incentives.

TABLE 2
Example criteria for distributing surpluses

Criteria	Relative value	Pool or individual
Volume measures:		
For PCPs: percent of expected (adjusted) panel size	.25	Individual
For specialists: referrals rates, actual to targets		Pool
Productivity measures:		
Visits per member per year compared to targets	.25	Pool
Referral wait times, actual compared to targets		Individual
Resource utilization measures:		
Referral rates, actual compared to targets	.20	Pool
Dollars per patient per year, actual compared to targets		Pool
Patient satisfaction measures:		
Survey results	.10	Individual
Disenrollment or switching rates		Pool
Program compliance measures:		
Notifications	.10	Individual
Process management		Individual
Outcomes measures:		
Morbidity, mortality, redos/recidivism, health status	.10	Pool

Withholds are collected as a percentage of each fee paid to providers. (If all providers are capitated, there is no need for a withhold.) The withholds are used to cover a shortage of funds if there is overutilization, serving as a kind of self-insurance. If the withheld funds are not needed to pay new claims, they are returned to the providers from whom they were retained.

Some believe the incentive value of withholds is questionable. Many physicians assume they will never see the withheld money again, so there is no meaningful effect on practice patterns. Thus, it may be more effective to reduce the fee schedule by the amount of the withhold and set this money aside as a reserve to fund deficits or pay bonuses.

Medical management as a physician incentive

As discussed above, physicians maintain a strong desire for autonomy in clinical decision making even when they join integrated systems. At first glance, this can seem in conflict with the need to tighten medical management and utilization to achieve cost savings. It is possible, however, to design a medical management plan that accomplishes both and to use this plan as a positive physician incentive.

Most new IDSs take an approach to medical management, often called the first stage, where a utilization management (UM) committee is formed, representing all major specialties. The UM committee meets weekly and reviews prospective, concurrent, and retrospective cases. Administrative staff support the UM committee; the full-time RN staff compiles case reviews and round daily on inpatient units. The RNs review requests for services and have authority to authorize them; cases that cannot be resolved by the RN reviewer are brought to the UM committee. Enforcement is left to the medical director, who speaks to noncompliant physicians individually and may impose financial penalties or send out a newsletter highlighting issues of noncompliance.

Before long, the UM committee rarely denies physicians' requests for services, making the use of committee time for individual case review no longer justified. The physicians become disgruntled. Utilization, which improved initially, reaches a plateau with minimal ongoing improvement. In some cases, this first stage approach can deteriorate into the type of hassle factor plan described above. But in an effective IDS, a better approach can develop using this insight.

In the second stage, each physician in the group becomes the utilization manager for his or her patients. Treatment decisions for individual patients are based on providing appropriate treatment for the patient's condition as determined by the treating physician without regard to increasing revenue or saving money. The physicians collectively develop condition-specific treatment protocols, guidelines, and critical pathways and examine new methods to improve the overall health status of members. The goal is to provide appropriate care to each individual promptly, cost-effectively, and without duplicated or unnecessary services. In this stage, the physicians take a continuous quality improvement approach to medical management.

The second stage also requires infrastructure other than a staff of UR nurses. The backbone of second stage infrastructure is the management information systems. All encounters must be captured by the MIS and tracked by patient, by clinical condition, by physician, and by department. Departments meet to develop guidelines, starting first with the most common and most expensive clinical conditions. For example, pediatricians, allergists, and pulmonologists can work together to define the treatment protocol for pediatric asthma, including how the PCP should manage care, under what conditions the patient should be referred to a specialist, what workup the PCP should do, and what services should be included in the initial visit to the specialist.

Data is analyzed to determine where large expenditures occur, then departments review patterns of care using a continuous quality improvement approach. After guidelines are developed, practice pattern data is fed back monthly to departments and individual physicians to assess progress and the need for guideline modification. Here, the UM committee becomes an administrative function overseeing protocol development rather than a decision-making body acting on requests for authorization.

The results of this approach can be impressive. Individual physicians modify behavior with little outside pressure when presented with compelling data on their practice patterns and those of their peers. Resource consumption also declines below the first stage plateau, in terms of PMPM costs, referral rates, days per 1,000, and cost per incidence of care. Physicians regain clinical control of practice, face less administrative frustration, and have improved satisfaction.

Can a new IDS skip the first stage of medical management and pass directly to a second stage approach? Unfortunately not. Several prerequisites are required for the second stage to be effective. These include aligned financial incentives among the PCPs, the specialists, and the hospitals; experience as a group in learning how to manage utilization effectively; and a willingness on the part of the physicians to critically examine their own and their peers' practice patterns. The goal for a new IDS should not be to jump to the second stage of medical management but to gain experience in the first stage and move forward, rather than add more and more constraints. When successful, an IDS can build an effective second-stage medical management plan and use it as a positive physician incentive to complement financial incentives.

Conclusion

While many integrated delivery systems have been formed (with an even larger number in the planning stage), few will be able to achieve the goals they set forth. Some will benignly fade from existence after being unable to obtain the types of risk contracts they were designed to manage. Some will fail financially after getting risk contracts but not managing care and risk effectively. The appropriate alignment of incentives, especially physician incentives, will be one of the key distinguishing variable between those IDSs that succeed and those that fail. By tackling physician incentives actively and effectively, networks can ensure that physicians, hospitals, and payers are working toward the common goals of access, cost, and quality.

NOTES

1. Statistical Abstract of the United States, 1994.
2. Dun & Bradstreet and HCIA annual reports.
3. Warren Surveys, InterStudy.

8

Aligning performance and payment criteria

James Wm. Hager
Director of National Business Development
Blue Shield of California
San Francisco, California

FOR THE HEALTHCARE INDUSTRY to be successful in the next decade, efforts must be made to create value by demonstrating a high standard of quality at a highly competitive price.

$$\text{Value} = \frac{\text{Quality}}{\text{Cost}}$$

Healthcare quality can take on many forms:

- Clinical outcomes that include indicators of care, such as cancer survival rates, surgical outcomes, and complication rates, as well as other measures including pediatric immunization rates and cholesterol screening rates

- Accessibility, routine or urgent appointment waiting times, choice of primary care physicians (PCPs), or after-hour availability

- Service orientation, such as quality of service offered by providers and staff and waiting times in the physician's office, pharmacy, or laboratory

- Provider qualifications, training, privileges, and interpersonal communications skills—bedside manner

Managed care organizations have shown that integrating the healthcare delivery system—such as aligning physicians, hospitals, ancillary providers, and payers behind a common set of goals and strategies—can position providers to deliver quality services.

This chapter identifies areas to consider in designing a compensation structure that aligns provider incentives to deliver value to healthcare consumers.

Compensation design

Inherent in the traditional method of reimbursing providers on a fee-for-service (FFS) basis is a financial incentive to provide services and reward productivity, not efficiency of health service utilization. Financial pressures have pushed payers to move away from FFS reimbursement to a structure that places incentives on providers to control service utilization and length of stay.

Capitation, or paying a provider a fixed amount per patient per month to cover necessary services, shifts the financial responsibility for managing patient care to the provider. While often seen as the ultimate form of provider reimbursement, capitation is no panacea.

When structuring a provider compensation design, the move from FFS compensation to capitation should not be made without

- Considering financial incentives that compensation design places on provider behavior

- Matching financial incentives with provider or group performance objectives

- Developing specific performance incentives into a provider compensation system to identify critical performance variables and data required and to select variables within a provider's control

- Considering the data required to monitor performance

- Assuring that rewards are closely linked to individual provider performance

- Verifying that financial incentives of providers in the entire delivery system are in sync

Given these considerations, compensation design, including capitation, can be an effective tool to create an integrated delivery system (IDS) with a focus on delivering value. In this environment

- Primary care and specialty physicians are encouraged to collaborate on patient care decision making

- Medical outcomes and quality of care are foremost in providers' minds, not competing financial incentives

- Efforts to continually improve the delivery system, streamline use of medical services, and reduce healthcare costs are supported by all involved

The following discussion will explore capitation payment to contract providers.

Incentives and performance objectives

While FFS reimbursement has encouraged waste and overuse of healthcare services, moving to full capitation can miss the opportunities of intermediate levels of risk sharing. Compensation design should consider performance objectives. For example, if an important objective in building a delivery system is to encourage PCPs to expand their scope of practice, referring to specialists only when their knowledge is insufficient, then FFS reimbursement may be the best payment method. Thus, combining FFS payment with opportunities to receive additional training and financial support to establish a clinic to manage lower back pain may make a PCP's practice more diverse and rewarding, while providing a more cost-effective and medically appropriate means of managing lower back pain. In other situations, per diem, case rate, or modified FFS forms of compensation may be the most appropriate.

Capitation, providing an opportunity to create incentives that discourage service utilization, can help address situations where a more conservative use of surgical services, for example, may be desired.

Table 1 shows a wide variation in the incidence rate of surgical procedures using an age/sex adjusted sample of patient populations in managed care organizations in four states. For each of these procedures there

TABLE 1
Procedure rates per 100,000 members in 1992

Procedures	State A	State B	State C	State D
Laminectomy	35	131	35	101
Hysterectomy	156	247	172	221
CABG	63	117	72	99

is a "gray area," where different providers may question the validity of performing surgery on a given patient. "Community standards," whereby common medical practices in one region may be uncommon in another, may play a significant role in explaining practice variation.

To establish payments on a capitation basis, there are two fundamental requirements to consider. First, services to be provided under the fixed payment must be defined. Listing CPT-4 codes in a provider agreement is one way to clearly identify what is to be included in the capitation payment. Second, the patient population to be served by the agreement must be clearly defined. This is more easily done when, for example, a single urology group is under contract to provide services to a health plan's entire membership in a particular city. The situation, however, becomes more complex when a population is divided among provider groups. In these situations, a mechanism (such as dividing patients by zip code) must be put in place to identify members as belonging to the appropriate provider group.

Capitation offers financial simplicity because payment made on a per member per month (PMPM) basis is easier to administer than payment made on a FFS case rate or per diem basis that requires billing information to process payment.

One benefit to the provider is predictable cash flow. Since payment can be calculated without traditional itemized billing information, there is a tendency to simplify things even further by allowing providers to discontinue developing itemized bills altogether. The information on standard billing forms (UB-92, HCFA 1500) is critical to obtain utilization information. Since bill generation is typically a routine automated office activity, discontinuing the billings for a patient group seen as part of a capitation contract may create more, not less, work for the provider. Only when capitation becomes a significant component of a provider's practice can savings from not generating bills offset the costs of establishing a report to capture the utilization "encounter" data required.

There are some risks to be considered when establishing a capitation payment arrangement. For example, a PCP signing a new capitation contract should be concerned about the condition of the patients selecting their practice. A disproportionate share of chronic or high-risk patients could mean a lot of work with little payment, not sufficient to cover the costs of maintaining the practice. There is some actuarial analysis required to determine the minimum number of patients necessary to average the risk of high-cost cases. For example, 500 members may be a minimum required before the risk of high-cost patients is off-set by healthier patients. Outlier protection can be used to limit financial exposure for the provider where volume does not meet such a mini-mum. A payer may offer to pay for all of a physician's charges above $5,000 per year for a patient, until the point where that physician has 500 assigned members.

Another way for providers to protect themselves against this risk is to purchase reinsurance, usually on a PMPM basis, to cover the cost of the outliers.

When calculating capitation payments for certain categories of ser-vices, age/sex or other population adjustments may be necessary. Table 2 indicates some age/sex adjusted capitation payments for primary care services. As expected, predictable age/sex variation also occurs in spe-cialty physician practices (e.g., obstetrics, with practice directed toward women of childbearing age, and urology services, focusing on men over 50 with prostate complications). In these cases, an analysis of the patient population for payment calculation is critical.

Another source of data for risk adjustment is prescription pharmacy data of a given patient population. It can be used to identify the inci-dence of diabetes in a population or the number of patients on heart medications and provide a detailed review of an extensive database used to predict admission rates for a group of patients with chronic illnesses.

Compensation system and incentives

If an incentive bonus system is applicable to an executive staff or sales team, why not to providers? Incentives can be very broad (e.g., placing a group of primary care providers at-risk for hospital costs of their

TABLE 2
PMPM payment example
All physician services

Age	Male	Female
<1 year	$50	$50
1–19	$15	$15
20–39	$25	$55
40–49	$40	$50
50–59	$55	$70
60–69	$80	$90
70+	$110	$100

assigned patient group or for the cost of all specialty referrals). Another approach is to review specific indicators of performance driving quality and cost. For example,

- *Hospitalization*
  Are physicians adhering to critical pathways and clinical guidelines?

  Are they participating in utilization management programs or on committees?

- *Specialty referrals*
  Do PCPs comply with guidelines related to the appropriateness of referrals?

- *Pharmacy*
  Are they adhering to a formulary?

  Are they participating in educational activities on alternative pharmaceutical interventions?

- *Accessibility*
  What is wait time for appointments?

  Are there rewards for offering extended office hours?

- *Service*
  How do they score on patient satisfaction surveys and interviews?

- *Quality of care*
  How is their performance on outcomes measures such as infection rates or complication rates such as cesarean section rates that are specifically tailored to individual specialist categories?

- *Administration*
  Are physicians providing timely encounter data?

  Is this data accurate?

When developing performance indicators, designers should keep things simple and not lose the financial simplicity of a capitation arrangement to elaborate performance incentives. There should be a focus on three or four key variables, verifying that data exist or can be easily collected to measure performance and provide information to providers.

Critical performance variables

Table 3 illustrates a performance incentive structure (i.e., indicator data required and received) for a capitated group of eight PCPs practicing in one clinic.

Incentives should address specific issues encountered by groups in general or tailored to individual groups or groups by specialty. For example, orthopedists may have a separate set of incentives that include adherence to a critical pathway for hip replacement, while neurosurgeons concentrate on laminectomy rates. If accessibility, complication, or surgical rates are not concerns, focus on appropriateness of referral,

TABLE 3
Sample incentive structure

1. Indicator: Pharmacy, adherence to a formulary
   Data required: Complete prescription records for health plan members, by
                       physician, compared against the plan's formulary
   Reward: 0–90% formulary adherence $.00 PMPM bonus
                       90–98% formulary adherence $.25 PMPM bonus
                       98–100% formulary adherence $.50 PMPM bonus

2. Indicator: Accessibility, extended office hours
   Data required: Documentation of extended office hours
   Reward: 3 to 5 evenings per week open until 9 P.M. $.25 PMPM bonus
                       or open 12 to 20 hours beyond 8–5 Mon–Fri $.25 PMPM bonus
                       5 evenings per week, 8–5 Sat–Sun $.50 PMPM bonus
                       or open 36-plus hours beyond 8–5 Mon–Fri $.50 PMPM bonus

3. Indicator: Service during visit, patient satisfaction with provider and staff
   Data required: Patient identification following an office visit
                       Patient satisfaction survey completed and returned by a sample
                       of patients
   Reward: 0–90% overall satisfaction score $.00 PMPM
                       90–95% overall satisfaction score $.25 PMPM
                       95–100% overall satisfaction score $.50 PMPM

4. Indicator: Quality of care, cholesterol screening and winter flu vaccination
   Data required: Percent of patients assigned to the group receiving annual cho-
                       lesterol screening and winter flu vaccination, verified by sam-
                       ple chart review or special data collection tool completed by
                       the provider group
   Reward: 0–70% screened $.00 PMPM
                       0–60% vaccinated $.00 PMPM
                       70–80% screened $.125 PMPM
                       60–75% vaccinated $.125 PMPM
                       80–100% screened $.25 PMPM
                       75–100% vaccinated $.25 PMPM

service, or pharmacy. This information should be provided in an easy-to-read (preferably in graphic) format and distributed on a regular basis so that providers can monitor and improve their performance.

It is also helpful to provide benchmark data where available. For example, sample quarterly reports for a capitated primary care group (Group A) could indicate adherence to a pharmacy formulary. This report could benchmark Group A to other groups as displayed in Figure 1. It could also list providers individually (Figure 2) so that Group A can work with members within the group (PCP 3 and PCP 4) to take corrective action to improve fomulary adherence.

In the 1980s, a common practice for compensating independent practice associations (IPAs) was to pay providers on a fee-for-service basis, withholding 15 or 20 percent to be paid at the end of a period

FIGURE 1
Percent adherence to formulary

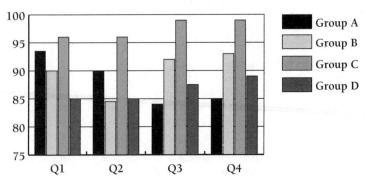

FIGURE 2
Percent adherence to formulary (Group A detail)

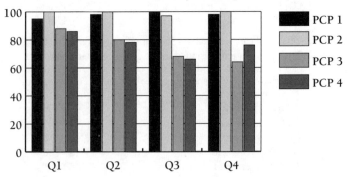

based on performance to budget (or other such indicator). To their surprise, providers commonly discovered that year-end medical costs (associated with their patients) had exceeded budget and the withhold was never realized. The use of withholds was often regarded by providers as another discount in their reimbursement. Subsequently, performance reports went ignored and targets were missed.

A more positive way to improve performance, however, is to use a bonus system. Here, compensation can take the form of a fixed payment amount, such as offering providers $.50 PMPM for keeping evening office hours four days per month or for obtaining a 90 percent satisfaction rating from patients surveyed. Although $.50 PMPM does not seem like a lot, if the eight-member physician group had about 10 percent of their practice with this health plan (1,600 patients) and met the target on all four indicators ($2.00 PMPM), there would be a quarterly bonus of $9,600 for the physicians to divide. Fixed-dollar payments, however, such as $1,000 for meeting performance goals, may be less equitable since it may not vary by patient load.

Caution should be exercised when designing performance indicators. Be sure the rewards cannot be legally interpreted as a kickback or self-referral. Providers should not be receiving financial rewards for withholding services or for referring services to where they have a financial interest (i.e., to a surgery center in which the provider is an owner). Recent legislation has targeted questionable practices in this area. Indicators such as hospital days per 1,000 patients, admission rates, referral rates, dollar amounts under budget—all used as a means to calculate bonus payment—are coming under fire. Legal counsel should be sought when in doubt.

Scope of control

Understanding the services and treatments within a provider's scope of control or practice is critical to designing performance measures. For example, obstetricians may not control hospital admission rates but they do control cesarean section rates. More specifically, transplant surgeons have more control over primary graft failure than do transplant physicians, whereas transplant physicians will take the lead in monitoring graft survival throughout a patient's lifetime. Therefore, when designing performance measures, be sure that the indicators are appropriate for the providers. Do not adopt generic indicators that are not relevant for specific categories of providers.

Rewards and performance

Another variable in designing a performance-based compensation structure is whether an individual or a group is held accountable for the indicators selected. Depending on the indicator used, it is often valuable to hold a small group accountable for performance targets. This practice has some distinct advantages. It encourages collaboration and discussion among the group and allows risk to be spread out over the wider patient population of the group rather than the smaller patient base of an individual provider.

Alternatively, holding a large group of providers accountable for meeting performance objectives can have significant disadvantages. As the group size increases, the influence an individual has on meeting the overall target diminishes. The actions of one high-performance provider in a large group can be diluted in reviewing the group's overall performance. This has become a growing concern among large group or staff model HMOs that have salaried physicians with a bonus structure based on overall group performance. Since individual performance can have little or no effect on a bonus amount paid to an individual, physicians are not directly rewarded for patient immunization rates, patient satisfaction, or productivity. All of these factors have a direct impact on the value equation and the group's competitive edge in the ever-demanding marketplace.

Provider incentives

Determine how financial incentives of one provider align with the incentives of others in the delivery system, making sure there is no conflict among providers. The following case study illustrates.

A group model HMO has a panel of PCPs serving 50,000 enrollees in a midsized city. This group is salaried but shares a small year-end bonus for providing services under budget. They have FFS contracts with two orthopedic surgery groups in town. Although referrals are tightly controlled by the group, there is concern that one group has a higher laminectomy rate and surgical complication rate than the other.

The PCP group made a decision to establish a capitation contract with the preferred orthopedic group to serve the entire population. Since their population of patients is easily counted, a PMPM arrangement is easy to administer. Also, since performance of the group is known and quality of care exceptional, the PCP group decided to have no withhold or bonus structure.

Once the contract was established, however, things began to fall apart. Since the orthopedists were now capitated, the group's primary care providers became less concerned with the financial impact of referring to the specialists. Managing lower back pain was difficult anyway, and patients often wanted a quick surgical remedy to their problem. Referring them to the specialists was an easier way to go. Over time, the orthopedic group found demand for their services increasing, while losses under the contract were mounting. The incentives in the delivery system were not in sync.

To better manage this scenario, the PCP group might have continued to pay the orthopedists on a FFS or case rate basis to keep the incentive on the PCPs to manage lower back pain as they had done in the past. A more cumbersome alternative would have been to develop a performance incentive for the primary care group to manage lower back pain within the group. Since productivity can be an issue with the group, they may want to focus their efforts on designing an incentive plan that rewards individual or subgroup performance.

Conclusion

Capitation can be an effective tool to control healthcare cost but should not be considered in isolation. As payers and providers position themselves to deliver value to the healthcare consumer, they should consider compensation design in its broader form; understand how financial incentives may influence provider behavior; and match financial incentives with the performance objectives of individual providers, of providers within groups, of groups of providers, and of all the various stockholders making up the healthcare delivery system.

Then, providers should develop specific performance incentives to create the greatest return on investment. Specific provider behavior should be targeted to create high-quality, low-cost value for the customer. Performance incentives must be within the provider's control to achieve desired results and be easily measured. Providers should have data available on a regular basis to monitor and improve their performance. Rewards must be tangible and linked to individual performance.

Compensation design can be a very effective tool to incorporate providers into an IDS, poised to deliver value to patients and purchasers of healthcare services in this highly competitive marketplace.

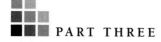

PART THREE

TRANSITION MANAGEMENT TECHNIQUES

9

Managing the transition from fee for service to prepaid incentives

Robert A. Dickinson
Director
BDC Advisors
San Francisco, California

Two patients sit in the waiting room of a physician's office. One is a Medicare beneficiary who recently joined an HMO where she will pay a $10 copayment upon completion of her visit. The physician, who receives $105 each month to provide for the Medicare HMO member's primary care, specialty, and emergency services, wants to keep the senior as healthy as possible. The other patient in the waiting room is a recent college graduate whose insurance company will reimburse his physician on a discounted fee-for-service (FFS) basis for any covered services performed. Besides their sex, age, and appearance, can the patients sitting in the waiting room be differentiated? Is it reasonable or even practical to expect a physician to know how each patient's insurer will pay? Is it moral or ethical?

For physician organizations adding a managed care contract, there is an inherent conflict between productivity-based incentives under FFS reimbursement and appropriate utilization under capitated reimbursement. One alternative is to segregate patients—and the way care is rendered—on the basis of reimbursement, creating a two-tiered system of care. Another alternative is to manage a medically equal system.

This chapter outlines several methodologies for designing physician compensation and work-effort programs in increasingly capitated markets. It is organized into four sections: strategic goals highlight the importance of physician recruitment, performance, and retention;

conflicting messages describe inherent conflicts among physicians about reimbursement incentives and their responses; case examples outline compensation alternatives; and lessons learned offer pitfalls to avoid.

Strategic goals

It is imperative that physician group practices, staff models, and other physician organizations achieve and sustain a growing base of marketable, efficient providers. Three key factors will affect how well a group can achieve its goal: physician recruitment, performance, and retention.

An effective recruitment process can enhance a physician organization's ability to attract high-quality physicians, expand its network geographically, and increase enrollment. For one medical group in San Jose, California, for example, successful recruitment of between 6 and 19 primary care physicians (PCPs) per year since 1990 is largely due to its attractive benefits package, which gives physicians an average starting salary $10,000 higher than adjusted national averages by specialty as well as five additional vacation days.

Performance represents a physician organization's ability to increase revenues while managing costs during and after the transition from FFS to prepaid business. Performance can be damaged without a strong relationship between compensation and physician productivity. For example, the same group practice in San Jose measured its encounters per year and found the average physician productivity and work effort up to 15 percent below national standards by specialty. Low physician productivity increases the group's recruiting requirements and its cost to provide sufficient access to patients.

Retention is a physician organization's ability to keep efficient providers over time. Although the medical group in San Jose can attract PCPs, its current compensation program fails to retain newer members. Average attrition has been 21 percent in each of the past three years; 13 of the 17 departing physicians had less than two years of tenure with the group. In effect, the group provides a source of recruitment for local competitors. Two factors may be driving poor retention of newer physicians at the medical group: poor incentives for cash bonuses and deferred compensation (i.e., bonuses and deferred compensation

FIGURE 1
Compensation and productivity life cycle

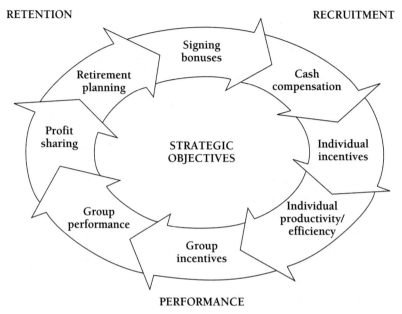

Source: BDC Advisors.

represent 14 percent of total compensation compared to an average of 32 percent among leading integrated delivery systems), and a career path with few distinguishing benefits for partners (e.g., partners receive an additional five vacation days a year, plus participation in a small profit-sharing plan).

As Figure 1 illustrates, physician compensation and work-effort formulas represent an important means by which an organization can successfully recruit, maintain strong performance of, and retain physicians. To be effective, every physician compensation and productivity plan must satisfy a minimum number of requirements, including an ability to

- Support strategic objectives

- Maintain a simple formula that physicians can understand

- Promote fairness

- Predict physician behavior (i.e., anticipate cause and effect from changes to compensation)

- Recognize key values (e.g., preserve quality of care and patient satisfaction)

- Facilitate PCP recruitment

- Retain physicians

- Compensate for appropriate levels of productivity

Compensation plans often follow an evolution that accounts for the inherent conflict between productivity-based incentives under FFS reimbursement and appropriate utilization under capitated reimbursement. As a group increases its capitated business, it may more frequently consider qualitative factors (e.g., patient satisfaction, outcomes, or stewardship) with incentives focusing on group rather than individual incentives. An effective compensation and work-effort system will influence physician behavior by aligning individual and group incentives with long-term strategic objectives.

Conflicting messages

As managed care accounts for an increasing share of physician revenues, physician organizations are tailoring their compensation plans. In a FFS environment, financial performance is based on revenue-generating charges. Higher charges equate with higher profits and more patient visits generate more revenue. Compensation plans, therefore, tend to reward productivity.

Today, most compensation plans still reflect a FFS mentality. For example, five physician shareholders in a family practice group in Chicago reimburse themselves on the basis of net revenues from combined FFS and capitated business. Covering only 200 commercial-risk lives, the family practice group maintains a FFS mentality; physicians providing more services and accepting more enrollees will earn a larger share of group income.

Like traditional FFS, discounted FFS payments from preferred provider organizations (PPOs) and other noncapitated revenue sources reward productivity as well. Providers are rewarded for maximizing patient visits and procedures. Reimbursement discounts under PPO plans may even encourage providers to increase their number of patient visits or services per visit to offset the reduction in reimbursement per service.

For example, a PCP receiving 80 percent of historical charges may want to provide 25 percent more visits or services per visit to account for decreased compensation. Consider that a PCP performing 1,000 visits at $75 per visit earns $75,000. If the physician's reimbursement per visit is reduced to 80 percent of charges, or $60 per visit, then 1,250 visits would have to be performed to earn the same $75,000.

Initially, most group practices and physician organizations attempt to incorporate HMO patients into their existing compensation and productivity program. The conflicting goals of production versus efficiency and cost savings, however, compel groups over time to move away from purely production-based compensation. According to a Leadership Institute survey of integrated delivery systems with group practices, compensation begins shifting from purely productivity-based incentives to salaries with group bonuses or profit sharing when 25 to 35 percent of a group's revenues are derived from capitation.[1] This equates to approximately 450 to 600 commercial risk or Medicaid risk members per PCP, about 200 to 300 Medicare risk members per PCP, or some combination of these ratios.

After a physician organization attracts a significant amount of capitated revenues, compensation systems tend to focus more on the group's goals and performance rather than on the individual physician. Goals may include increased revenues, higher margins, a service line niche (e.g., worker's compensation), full-service capabilities, or simply improved quality of care.

Under capitation, charges represent a use of funds (i.e., any healthcare service rendered to a patient reduces the prepaid funds remaining in the physician organization). Higher charges and more patient visits lead to individual and group losses, resulting in lower profits for the group.

For example, a PCP receiving $15 per member per month (PMPM) for a commercial enrollee earns $180 annualized for this patient. If the physician's average cost per visit is $50 and the enrollee receives three office visits throughout the year, the physician earns $30 for that covered life (i.e., $180 in revenues less $150 in expenses). Correspondingly, if the enrollee receives four office visits throughout the year, the physician loses $20 for that covered life. Groups with significant capitation (i.e., approximately 25 percent or more) find they must adjust the definition of productivity to reflect an optimal use of healthcare resources (i.e., lower average cost per visit or service), maximize incentives for high workloads (i.e., accept a high number of enrollees), and use patient satisfaction and quality (i.e., patient survey results) as a basis for income distribution.

Reimbursement incentives

Groups in increasingly competitive markets strive to increase market share (i.e., number of covered lives served), manage volume (i.e., number of visits and services per visit), minimize cost (i.e., cost per service), and maximize quality and outcomes. As Table 1 illustrates, various reimbursement methods can create different incentives for physicians.

Case examples

At any one time, a group or individual physicians within a physician organization may have some combination of reimbursement methodologies. For example, a group may use a mixed production and capitation formula. Whereas the physician's FFS income can be based on

TABLE 1
Reimbursement incentives

	Units			
Reimbursement method	*Number of visits*	*Services per visit*	*Cost per service*	*Quality or outcomes*
Managed care goals	Decrease	Decrease	Decrease	Increase
Fee schedule				
Without bonus	Increase	Increase	Increase	Variable
With bonus	Increase	Increase	Increase	Increase
Global fees*				
Without bonus	Increase	Variable	Decrease	Variable
With bonus	Increase	Variable	Decrease	Increase
Capitation or salary				
Without bonus	Decrease	Decrease	Decrease	Variable
With bonus	Decrease	Decrease	Decrease	Increase

*Global fees represent fixed payments per episode of care (i.e., case rates for psychiatry, maternity, cardiac surgery).

charges, collections, or visits for FFS patients, capitated income can be based on the number of enrollees assigned. Several alternatives exist for managing this transition from productivity-based incentives to prepaid business, including a prepaid budget, transitional formulas, capitation, and salary plus bonus.

PREPAID BUDGET

A prepaid budget can be used to optimize group income and reimbursement to providers under capitation. The prepaid budget is typically used in physician organizations that separate FFS revenues from capitated revenues, like an independent practice association (IPA) or a group practice without walls.

An overall budget is set equal to the total number of capitated patients under contract with the physician organization and then multiplied by the PMPM reimbursement over the budgeting period, typically one year. An equivalent FFS "super bill" is generated for each prepaid patient seen. Physicians are credited with their hypothetical billings.

The amount of the capitated budget allocated among physicians will be based on the amount of services rendered to prepaid patients and the budgeted cost for each service. The more services individual physicians perform, the greater their individual pro rata share of the budgets will be. But the more services all physicians in the group perform for prepaid patients, the lower the reimbursement amount per unit of service.

As the example in Table 2 illustrates, hypothetical billings are used to allocate capitated revenues among participating physicians in a northern California IPA. An adjustment factor or multiple is calculated by dividing what the IPA is prepaid for capitated enrollees by the total charges billed by participating physicians. As a result, physician charges can be discounted by the adjustment factor so that the IPA never exceeds its budget.

The prepaid budget offers a number of advantages. First, it marries FFS productivity with cost controls by establishing a prepaid budget. Unlike capitating individual physicians, a prepaid budget creates a reduced FFS type of reimbursement. For example, Physician A who billed $20,000 in charges received $18,759 in net revenues, or approximately 94 percent of charges. A physician organization's finance or utilization management committee can also quickly review financial performance with such a prepaid budget.

TABLE 2
Prepaid budget example

Group compensation:

Physician component PMPM	$ 35
HMO membership	× 2,000
Prepaid budget	$70,000
Emergency out-of-network services	−200
Capitation and case rate specialty/ancillary	1,800
	$68,000

Individual compensation:
Primary care and specialty billings

Physician A	$20,000
Physician B	$22,500
Physician C	$30,000
Total	$72,500

Adjustment factor

$$\frac{\text{Adjusted network budget}}{\text{Total billings}} = \frac{68,000}{72,500} = .937931$$

Physician compensation (net revenues)

Physician A	20,000 × .937931	$18,759
Physician B	22,500 × .937931	$21,103
Physician C	30,000 × .937931	$28,138
		$68,000

Second, the adjustment factor is designed to contain overall physician costs within the constraints established by the prepaid budget. This payment mechanism encourages PCPs to provide preventive healthcare services to patients by allowing physicians to bill for services, while limiting total expenditures to the size of the group's prepaid budget. While the prepaid budget is set independent of individual physician treatment and referral patterns, the adjustment factor controls treatment, testing, and billing by limiting physician reimbursement to the budget itself.

Finally, the prepaid budget uses similar incentives found in a large risk pool. If a group participates in capitated plans, members will share the burden and risk equally. The shared incentive of belonging to a common budget or pool assists to motivate all physicians to adopt a common set of practice patterns that promote high-quality, cost-effective care.

A major drawback to the prepaid budget, however, is that it does nothing to encourage physicians to reduce services and referrals. Using physician-specific cost and referral data, however, a physician organization can exert peer pressure, utilization review, and performance reviews on physicians with excessive billings and uncommon practice patterns. Conversely, a prepaid budget minimizes the concern that capitation might encourage nonutilization of necessary services. With no direct relationship between a physician's income and individual patient decisions, physicians can remain patient advocates.

TRANSITIONAL FORMULAS

Rather than segregate capitated revenues from FFS revenues as in the prepaid budget, many integrated physician organizations combine revenues under a single compensation program. There are a number of alternatives to reimburse providers under a system of combined FFS and capitated revenues. These alternatives fall into two major categories: those in which prepaid revenues are allocated directly, and those in which prepaid revenues and work effort are shared equally.

Table 3 provides background information about three physicians in a northern California group practice that serves to illustrate some of these transitional formulas.

Allocating prepaid dollars directly to participating physicians involves calculating individual workloads. Basing physician compensation on hypothetical FFS billings for HMO patients is a simple and effective approach to allocate prepaid revenues directly. The allocation

TABLE 3
Transitional formula example

Fee-for-service receipts	$500,000
Capitation revenues	$150,000
Total revenues	*$650,000*
Physician A FFS receipts	$250,000 (50%)
Physician B FFS receipts	$150,000 (30%)
Physician C FFS receipts	$100,000 (20%)
Total FFS receipts	*$500,000*
Physician A capitated revenues	$ 25,500 (17%)
Physician B capitated revenues	$ 49,500 (33%)
Physician C capitated revenues	$ 75,000 (50%)
Total capitated revenues	*$150,000*
Physician A total visits	3,800 (36%)
Physician B total visits	3,500 (33%)
Physician C total visits	3,200 (31%)
Total visits	*10,500 (100%)*

can be based on number of patients, member months, member visits, an equal split of capitated revenues, or some combination of these criteria. For example, if a physician accepts half of a group's prepaid patients, then 50 percent of capitated revenues should be received.

Since capitated dollars are pooled and distributed according to productivity, the source of revenues (whether primary care visits or subspecialty visits) does not matter. Physicians continue to receive a proportion of the practice's income either based on how much work they do or based on productivity for FFS and an equal split of capitated revenues (see Table 4).

Sharing the responsibility for prepaid patients can be based on an allocation of total receipts based on productivity. It can also be derived from a 50 percent split of revenues divided equally with 50 percent allocated based on productivity (see Table 5).

Whether prepaid dollars are allocated directly or shared equally, a number of transitional combinations can be designed. Among the four examples above, Physician A earns $225,333, $234,000, $275,500, or $300,000 in revenues. For this physician, compensation varies by as much as $74,000 from one scenario to another. Clearly, an appropriate transitional formula will need to be designed with group goals in mind

TABLE 4
Allocating prepaid revenues directly

Physician A	50% of $500,000	$250,000
	17% of $150,000	$ 25,500
	Total	$275,500
Physician A	50% of $500,000	$250,000
	33% of $150,000	$ 50,000
	Total	$300,000

TABLE 5
Sharing revenues

Physician A	36% of $650,000	$234,000
Physician B	33% of $650,000	$214,500
Physician C	31% of $650,000	$201,500
Physician A	$ 108,333 + 36% of $325,000	$225,333
Physician B	$ 108,333 + 33% of $325,000	$215,583
Physician C	$ 108,333 + 31% of $325,000	$209,083

and input among participating physicians. Compensation proposals typically use the previous year's financial data to pilot the impact on the group and individual physicians.

The main advantage of transitional formulas is flexibility, as evidenced by their ability to account for cross-coverage (i.e., when one physician sees another physician's patient after hours or while that physician is on vacation) and differences in physician practices. Cross-coverage of patients can be addressed by allocating prepaid revenues directly to those physicians who see patients or by dividing prepaid revenues equally among all physicians. Dividing prepaid revenues equally among physicians rewards those physicians with practices that attract and direct patients to other providers in the group. Thus, if a capitated patient selects a physician whose practice or appointment schedule is full, the patient may be referred within the group to another physician. While the revenues stay within the group, the original physician should get some credit for attracting additional patients. Dividing prepaid revenues equally also accounts for patients representing a disproportionate risk of care.

To design a transitional formula, many things should be taken into account, such as developing management information systems (MIS) and avoiding a two-tiered system of patient care. MIS will need to process patient claims and encounters, treatment authorizations, and physician and hospital billings; calculate capitation payments; write checks; and produce compensation reports. Furthermore, a physician organization may need patient eligibility, use specific payment rates, adjudicate claims, and assure the accurate processing and payment of claims. Transitional compensation formulas require developing a comprehensive MIS to track visits, collections, and patients and to develop an effective utilization review system to manage capitated revenues.

Transitional models may also result in a two-tiered system where physicians treat FFS patients differently than capitated patients. This not only creates confusion among physicians and tremendous administrative hassles but also leads to poor member satisfaction.

For these reasons, groups often manage all members under the same practice guidelines, utilization review protocols, and standards for quality. In particular, groups often find that as capitation exceeds 25 to 35 percent of total revenue, a decision must be made to become a managed care group as opposed to a fee-for-service group.

CAPITATION

A pure capitation formula has advantages for groups with significant capitated revenue. Physicians are at financial risk for prepaid services and
commit to develop strong utilization management and quality assurance.

One integrated group in southern California followed a number of
steps to determine capitation arrangements among their physicians, as
the following example indicates:

1. Define responsibilities on a menu of services by specialty by CPT
   code. Defining these responsibilities mitigates "dumping" of patient
   responsibilities from primary care to subspecialties under capitation

2. Use actuarial data from the local market and historical utilization
   data to allocate the professional component of capitated dollars by
   specialty. This allocation by specialty should total 100 percent of dollars for physician services, as is seen in this example from the southern California group (see Table 6)

3. Determine in-practice and in-group work versus out-of-group activities (i.e., specialties or services not provided within the group) to
   identify gaps in service for which the group will otherwise be at-risk.
   For example

	In-group
Internal medicine	98 percent
Pediatrics	98 percent
Urgent care	100 percent
Emergency medicine	0 percent

A group should designate services for which it will be at-risk under
a contract, rather than sign a contract requiring many services that the
group does not provide or for which it does not have appropriate specialty relationships

TABLE 6
Allocation by specialty

	Commercial HMO		Medicare HMO	
Internal medicine	$ 7.69	(17.75%)	$ 23.99	(22.85%)
Pediatrics	$ 3.29	(7.59%)	$ 00.00	(0.00%)
Urgent care	$ 2.81	(6.49%)	$ 00.79	(0.75%)
Emergency room	$ 0.28	(0.65%)	$ 00.79	(0.75%)
	⋮	⋮	⋮	⋮
Total	$43.32	(100%)	$105.00	(100%)

4. Compute total revenues by specialty based on budgeted utilization, as in the following example

Internal Medicine:

Commercial member months	12,000
Commercial PMPM	× $ 7.69
Commercial revenues	$ 92,280
Medicare member months	6,000
Medicare PMPM	× $ 23.99
Medicare revenues	$ 143,940
Total Internal Medicine revenues	$ 236,220
In-group coverage	× 98%
Net Internal Medicine revenues	$ 231,495

5. Deduct group operating and physician expenses from the in-group revenue allocation to calculate physician compensation by specialty

Operating expense	54 percent
Physician compensation	+ 46 percent
Total expense	100 percent

6. Identify and deduct a benefit reserve to cover the cost of physician benefits, including malpractice, continuing medical education, medical and dental insurance, and other benefits. The southern California group's benefit reserve totaled 16 percent of physician compensation, as follows

Physician compensation	46 percent
Benefit reserve	× 16 percent
Benefit expense	7 percent

7. Determine how departments will allocate dollars among themselves. Departments or physicians in individual specialties can be creative with the allocation within a specialty. The southern California group applied the following percentages in several specialty departments as a basis for allocating group bonus pools

50%   productivity, as measured by net collections based on relative value units (RVUs)

20%   utilization management, as measured by an equal combina-
        tion of length of stay, days per 1,000, use of generic drugs,
        referral patterns, and in-group versus out-of-group activity

12%   patient satisfaction, tabulating a survey instrument at year-
        end

10%   citizenship, as measured by meeting attendance, coverage,
        and communication individually scored on a scale of 1 to
        5 and administered by a compensation committee (i.e., 4 =
        everything expected, 5 = outstanding)

8%   efficiency, as measured by cost per visit

For a physician organization with approximately 60 percent FFS and 40 percent capitated revenues, the customized allocation criteria are consistent with the group's emphasis on managed care.

Capitation establishes budgetable income for allocating dollars among physicians, rewarding efficiency, and giving physicians control over compensation and bonuses. Audits, however, must be incorporated with any capitation system to mitigate underutilization of services to maximize income, lack of coordination, and adverse selection. Capitation also assumes that insurance risk will be well managed to minimize adverse selection and outlier cases. Insurance risk can be managed financially through prudent subcontracting, risk-sharing incentives, stop-loss coverage, aggregate reinsurance, and self-funded reserves. Finally, for groups just beginning capitation, specialties with one physician will receive all the capitated dollars for that specialty, regardless of how many patients are seen.

SALARY AND BONUS

Salary and bonus or profit-sharing plans provide a guaranteed compensation base and incentive for individual productivity and group profitability. Physician organizations with salary and bonus compensation programs integrate revenues and expenses among physicians. Thus, these arrangements require clearly defined basic values and principles, stable and educated physician leadership, consistent management, an identifiable group culture, and an organization to administer the plan. Physician organizations in both Hawaii and northern California use "guiding principles" that physician members carry around on wallet-sized cards to remind them of important values and to recenter their thoughts when difficult compensation issues surface. Once physicians are comfortable sharing all overhead expenses, a group practice can modify or add bonus criteria as managed care revenues become an increasing part of group business. The group overhead percentage is assigned to each dollar earned by the group, and bonus criteria may change from productivity only to criteria based on utilization, outcomes, and patient satisfaction.

First, all group revenues (i.e., FFS, discounted, and capitated) are pooled together. Next, a base salary for each specialty in the group is determined. Salaries and work-effort requirements are linked in a compensation system, with requirements developed for each specialty. Work effort may be defined by weeks worked per year, hours worked per week, encounters per day, week or year, or time spent performing extracurricular activities that support group efforts (i.e., utilization review and quality assurance meetings). For example, one group practice defined the following work-effort requirements for its internal medicine physicians:

Availability: 45 weeks per year, 36 hours per week, 1,620 hours per year

Productivity: 19 office visits per day (10 on a half day), 2.4 office visits per hour, 86 office visits per week, 8.5 hospital or skilled nursing facility visits per week, 32 hospital or skilled nursing facility visits per month

Once salaries and work-effort requirements are defined, group expenses such as nonphysician wages, rent, professional and office supplies, and equipment leases should be totaled. The difference between group revenues and group expenses equals group income. At this point, group income can be pooled for allocation among physicians, or a group can segregate group income into two bonus pools: a FFS pool based on its FFS receipts as a percentage of total revenues and a capitated pool based on capitated revenues as a percentage of total revenues (see Figure 2).

Regardless of whether there are one or two income pools, income can be allocated based on criteria defined by participating physicians. For a group practice starting out with a salary and bonus approach, the FFS

FIGURE 2
Salary and bonus formulas

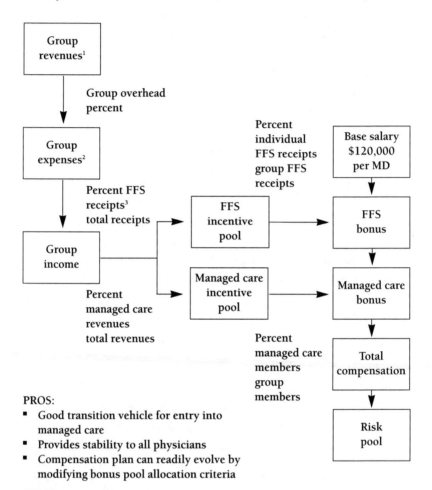

PROS:
- Good transition vehicle for entry into managed care
- Provides stability to all physicians
- Compensation plan can readily evolve by modifying bonus pool allocation criteria

CONS:
- May not adequately reward highly productive/efficient practices
- May be difficult to administer specific allocation criteria

1. Group revenues include risk pool income.
2. Group expenses include base salary of $120,000 per MD.
3. FFS receipts include ancillary revenues and other group income.

NOTE: Statistics represent base-year figures.

Source: BDC Advisors.

bonus after salary can be based on each individual physician's pro rata share of total FFS receipts. Likewise, the capitation bonus can be allocated based on each individual physician's pro rata share of total group HMO enrollees.

As groups become more advanced, more sophisticated criteria can be applied. Bonus criteria may include physician productivity (i.e., FFS) or capacity to see patients (i.e., capitation), financial results (i.e., group profitability), utilization management (i.e., bed days per 1,000), referral patterns, outcomes (i.e., lower readmission rates by ICD-9 code), patient satisfaction, community service, and group participation among others. Table 7 depicts examples of bonus criteria applied in highly integrated, highly managed group practices.

Groups can change incentive criteria or the weighting of such criteria to achieve desired physician behavior and goals as capitation represents a greater proportion of total revenues. A group is always well advised to align compensation incentives with strategic objectives.

Bonuses for cash incentives and profit sharing should comprise at least 20 to 30 percent of total compensation. Bonuses, however, should only be paid when there is money left in a shared pool after reimbursing physician, ancillary, and hospital covered charges. The criteria used to distribute incentive pay should at least reflect a group's mix of revenues.

TABLE 7
Selected bonus criteria

Outcomes indicators:	Percent of hospital readmissions
	Percent of repeat surgeries
	Percent of cases with adverse reactions
	Percent of poisonings
	Percent of deaths following care
	Percent of patients with full functioning
Appropriateness of care:	Percent of care performed in a questionable setting
	Percent of admits with preoperative days
	Percent of questionable care in a short-stay setting
	Percent of cesarean sections (OB/Gyn)
	Percent of expense for lack of self-care
	Percent of expense for preventable conditions
	Percent of expense for experimental treatments
Patient satisfaction:	Overall satisfaction
	Travel time
	Waiting time to schedule an appointment
	Waiting time while in the office
	Time spent per visit

For example, if 50 percent of a group's revenues are derived from FFS business, then it makes sense that not more than 50 percent of the incentive pool be based on productivity.

Lessons learned

Each of the different approaches above relates to the revenue sources and goals of a group practice. Compensation plans can help carry out the goals of a group practice, motivate physicians, and influence behavior. There are compelling relationships between compensation and productivity, productivity and motivation, motivation and behavior, and behavior and group success in a competitive marketplace.

There is no perfect plan to develop or restructure compensation for a group practice. Group compensation plans often start out simple (i.e., productivity based), become more complex (i.e., transitional), and finally end up being easier to understand and administer again (i.e., salary plus bonus). Nevertheless, the following should be considered by group practices in developing their compensation methodologies:

- Identify strategic goals before designing or restructuring the compensation system

- Achieve a coherent culture and build trust to focus on group incentives

- Avoid segregating FFS from capitated patients based on compensation and incentives

- Design the compensation plan and formulas for ease of understanding

- Vary each physician's prospective capitation by prior year's performance

- Link salaried or fixed compensation formulas with explicit productivity requirements

- Create incentives that amount to at least 20 to 30 percent of total compensation

- Base bonuses on outcomes, patient satisfaction, and financial performance

- Provide physicians with guidelines and protocols to use in meeting performance incentives

- Provide physicians with timely feedback

As healthcare markets increasingly integrate and consolidate, appropriate physician compensation programs and their incentives to providers will be drivers of market leadership. Whether it is an HMO looking for profitability among its staff model physicians, physicians looking to increase revenues and profitability, hospital systems striving to align incentives with physicians, or outside investors looking for an appropriate return on investment for their physician organizations, physician compensation will need to be carefully designed throughout the transition from FFS to capitation.

NOTES

1. B. Harrington, "Trends in Physician and Executive Compensation" (The Leadership Institute, San Francisco, March 23, 1994).

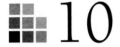 10

Physician compensation models for phasing in capitation

Kevin M. Kennedy
Manager

Daniel J. Merlino
Vice President
ECG Management Consultants
Seattle, Washington

INCREASING MANAGED CARE PENETRATION has radically altered the flow of revenue for many medical groups. This fundamental change in business should cause groups to consider altering their current compensation arrangements to reflect the new economic realities. A major concern of many groups is the desire to retain the successful parts of their old compensation plan while making the transition from fee-for-service (FFS) to capitated reimbursement.

Compensation plans in this mixed FFS/capitated environment are especially difficult due to the contrary incentives of the models. To address this complexity, groups can develop phased compensation plans that change funds-flow characteristics in step with increased managed care penetration. This chapter describes the goals of a compensation plan in a mixed FFS/capitated environment and suggests appropriate payment methodologies tied to the level of capitated business.

Compensation objectives

The three primary objectives of any compensation plan are to gain physician support, maintain proper incentives, and contribute to group success.

GAIN PHYSICIAN SUPPORT

It is not possible to make every physician happy with a compensation plan. However, maximizing three attributes—fairness, simplicity, and flexibility—will tend to minimize problems.

Fairness

Fairness is basic to the success of any compensation plan. Physicians must believe compensation is roughly proportionate to effort expended in patient care and other work activities. This does not mean that compensation must be related directly to the number of patient visits or office hours, but that physicians will want less-productive physicians to "pull their weight" in other areas (such as administration) or to accept reduced compensation. If the plan is not perceived as fair in this respect, the physicians will resent it, which will contribute to group malaise.

Simplicity

A compensation plan should be simple enough for a physician to explain it to a spouse or prospective group member. Physician compensation is an extremely complex issue, with calculations involving a large number of variables. While it may be possible to design a theoretically correct plan that incorporates all relevant variables, such an elaborate plan is likely to confuse physicians and be difficult to administer. Any "improvements" to a compensation plan need to be carefully weighed against corresponding increases in complexity.

Flexibility

Although a compensation plan's purpose is to define rules and expectations, an inflexible plan has the potential to cause unnecessary conflict. Does the plan accommodate the physician who wants to work extra hours to support children in college or the partner who wants to reduce office hours to three days per week? Plans should have a mechanism for addressing unforeseen circumstances, with a designated governing body (such as the board or the compensation committee) having authority to modify the plan.

MAINTAIN PROPER INCENTIVES

A physician compensation plan's success often hinges on the appropriateness of the behavior the system encourages. Physicians, like others, will show remarkable ingenuity to exploit the incentives in a compensation plan. Therefore, once incentives are set, the group should be prepared to accept the consequences that result from unanticipated behavior.

Physicians also will deny they respond to economic incentives and may provide examples of occasions when incentives were ignored. In designing a compensation system, care should be taken to avoid offending a physician's sense of propriety. In the early days of managed care, physicians were often offended by suggestions that capitation incentives could affect their resource utilization; but for most physicians, the effect was dramatic.

Some of the proper incentives include

- *Hard work.* In general, physicians prefer compensation systems that provide additional rewards for increased effort and time devoted to the practice

- *Appropriate utilization.* Under capitation, the group will benefit financially from reduced utilization. Physicians should have incentives that encourage utilization that is economical, yet does not compromise patient care

- *Patient satisfaction.* Satisfied patients will refer other patients to the group. In addition, patient satisfaction data can be used in negotiations with payers. Providing a satisfaction incentive to physicians can help physicians stay focused on consumers

- *Service to the group.* Physicians who devote time and effort to nonclinical activities that benefit the group should be rewarded. As managed care penetration increases, physician input into contracts and utilization review will become increasingly valuable, and physicians should have an incentive to make these contributions

CONTRIBUTE TO GROUP SUCCESS

A compensation plan can be a powerful tool to develop a stronger group culture and to orient physicians toward group success. Because every group will define success differently, it is important to recognize explicitly the organization's goals as part of the compensation planning process. For example, does the group need to increase its market power through growth? Will the group need to replace retiring physicians? How important will capitation be to the group's future? Does the group need to attract additional primary care physicians (PCPs), and if so, how many? The answers to these questions should influence the structure of the group's compensation plan.

Compensation model

The following examples propose compensation models that correspond to increasing levels of capitation:

- Low capitation (0 to 15 percent of total revenues)

- Medium capitation (16 to 35 percent of total revenues)

- High capitation (above 35 percent of total revenues)

LOW-CAPITATION ENVIRONMENT (0 TO 15 PERCENT OF REVENUE)

Retain status quo; FFS-oriented system

In a low-capitation environment, it may be advisable to retain an existing compensation plan if it has been successful. The small shift in incentives and payments at this level will rarely justify the expense and effort required to develop a completely new plan.

However, if a significant portion of reimbursement under a capitated contract depends on risk pools, the corresponding proceeds may be distributed based on incentives that mirror those used to calculate the pool distribution. For example, many primary care capitation contracts provide an incentive payment (or a return of withholds) based upon inpatient utilization. The group may elect to distribute risk pool funds (or a portion of them) based upon each physician's performance under this criteria.

In the example provided in Figure 1 and Table 1, the four-physician group considers capitated revenue in the same manner as FFS receipts. Per member per month (PMPM) payments are added to the production pool and distributed based on preexisting methods such as production or relative value units (RVUs). In this case, risk pool revenues are distributed based partly on inpatient days per 1,000 enrollees and partly on the number of covered lives. Total overhead is allocated using two concurrent methods: half is distributed evenly among the physicians, and half is divided according to each physician's production.

FIGURE 1
Example 1: Low capitation

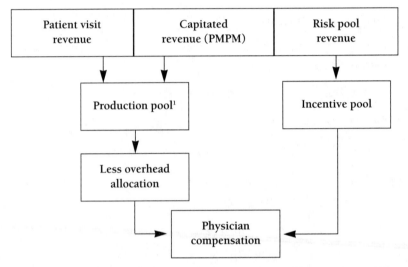

1. To comply with "Stark II" regulations, it may be necessary to establish a separate pool for ancillary revenues, such as laboratory and x-ray services. This pool would be allocated using criteria not related to ancillary volumes. Legal counsel should be consulted before making this determination.

TABLE 1
Example 1: Low capitation—calculations

1. Summary: revenue and overhead allocation

	Allocation, production pool (A)	Incentive pool allocation (B)	Total revenue allocation (C) = (A + B)	Total overhead (D)	Physician compensation (C − D)
Physician A	$324,000	$7,168	$331,168	$199,665	$131,503
Physician B	$351,000	$7,551	$358,551	$207,495	$151,056
Physician C	$378,000	$9,557	$387,557	$215,325	$172,232
Physician D	$405,000	$7,724	$412,724	$223,155	$189,569
	$1,458,000	$32,000	$1,490,000	$845,640	$644,360

TABLE 1 (CONTINUED)

2. Production allocation

	FFS production (assumption)	Capitation revenue (750 lives at $12 PMPM)	Total pro- duction (A)	Percentage of total based on FFS pro- duction (B)	Production pool allocation (A × B)
Physician A	$300,000			22.2%	$324,000
Physician B	$325,000			24.1%	$351,000
Physician C	$350,000			25.9%	$378,000
Physician D	$375,000			27.8%	$405,000
	$1,350,000	*$108,000*	*$1,458,000*	*100.0%*	*$1,458,000*

3. Incentive distribution
Total risk pool revenue (assumption): $32,000 (A)

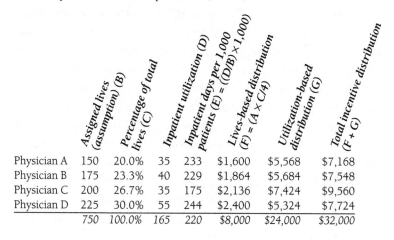

	Assigned lives (assumption) (B)	Percentage of total lives (C)	Inpatient utilization (D)	Inpatient days per 1,000 patients (E) = ((D/B) × 1,000)	Lives-based distribution (F) = (A × C/4)	Utilization-based distribution (G)	Total incentive distribution (F + G)
Physician A	150	20.0%	35	233	$1,600	$5,568	$7,168
Physician B	175	23.3%	40	229	$1,864	$5,684	$7,548
Physician C	200	26.7%	35	175	$2,136	$7,424	$9,560
Physician D	225	30.0%	55	244	$2,400	$5,324	$7,724
	750	*100.0%*	*165*	*220*	*$8,000*	*$24,000*	*$32,000*

4. Overhead allocation
Total group overhead (58 percent of revenue): $845,640 (A)

	Shared overhead (B)	Physician's percentage of total production (C)	Overhead based on production (D) = (A × C)/2	Total overhead (B + D)
Physician A	$105,705	22.2%	$93,867	$199,572
Physician B	$105,705	24.1%	$101,900	$207,605
Physician C	$105,705	25.9%	$109,510	$215,215
Physician D	$105,705	27.8	$117,543	$223,248
	$422,820	*100.0%*	*$422,820*	*$845,640*

MEDIUM-CAPITATION ENVIRONMENT (APPROXIMATELY 16 TO 35 PERCENT OF REVENUE)

Retain production orientation with significant bonuses
for performance under capitated contracts

Developing or adjusting a compensation plan is not a decision to be taken lightly. Nevertheless, when a group's capitation revenue approaches 15 to 20 percent of the total, the benefits of adjusting the compensation system to the new environment will begin to exceed the time and expense of developing a new plan. Effective management of capitated patients is now critical, as the traditional utilization patterns (e.g., referrals, tests, and procedures) may be unprofitable under capitated reimbursement schemes. Therefore, failure to readjust incentives that encourage traditional utilization may negatively impact group income. Allocation of capitated revenue becomes an increasingly important issue as the simplifying assumptions of the past are questioned and discarded. Some of these invalidated assumptions may include equal distribution of capitated patients among physicians, approximately equal utilization patterns and behavior, and equality of efforts directed toward building a practice.

To cope more effectively with the new prepaid environment, two new pools may be created: capitation and incentive. The capitation pool consists of all PMPM revenue received from a capitated plan. The incentive pool is created from other revenue available to the group and may include risk pool revenue, ancillary revenue, and a portion of FFS revenue. These pools are allocated based upon factors related to success in the medium-capitation environment.

The capitation pool is allocated among physicians based on the need to develop fair allocation of capitated revenue, shield physicians from the risk of adverse selection, and provide compensation for patients whose revenue is assigned to one physician but who may receive care provided from another.

While physicians who are new to capitation will often believe that adverse selection and seeing another physician's patient may distort their earnings, those with more experience realize these issues will tend to affect physicians equally over time.

Establishing compensation criteria contrary to the FFS mindset is a crucial step in the evolution of a compensation plan, and one of the most

TABLE 2
Methods of allocating PMPM revenue

Method	Issues
Assigned patients	Simplest approach
	Rewards physicians for attracting patient enrollees
	Provides the most direct incentive to develop capi tated business
Capitated patient office visits	Compensates for unassigned patient care
	May encourage physicians to schedule multiple office visits when a single visit or telephone inquiry would suffice (churning)
FFS-equivalent charges on capitated patients	Compensates for adverse selection and unassigned patient care
	May encourage overutilization
Even split among physicians	Income spread may reduce concerns regarding adverse selection and unassigned patient care
	May fail to reward the hardest-working physicians
A weighted combination of these methods	Potential to combine the advantages of other methods
	May become too complex to easily understand and administer

difficult. There are, however, a number of ways to allocate revenue from the PMPM portion of a capitated contract (Table 2).

These factors should be chosen based upon the relative importance of each issue to the physicians, but caution should be used when considering formulas that take more than two factors into account. The simplest approach is to allocate capitated revenue based upon the number of patients assigned to each physician under each capitated plan. Although this approach does not address a number of the issues raised above, a strong case can be made that adverse selection and providing care to nonassigned patients will tend to be equally distributed among physicians over the long run. Physicians may need to be persuaded to take a long-term perspective on this issue; it is a part of the normal process of accepting and managing risk.

The incentive pool also can be allocated using a number of criteria. Several measures are typically weighted to arrive at the ultimate distribution (Table 3).

Availability of credible data may pose a significant hurdle to crafting an appropriate distribution of this pool. Hospitals and payers may be good sources for utilization data, but the physicians need to be confident that the data accurately measure performance. If possible, physicians

TABLE 3
Methods of allocating incentive pool funds

- Office activity,[1] possibly including
  RVUs
  Office visits
  Patient contact hours
- Performance under risk pool criteria (usually inpatient or referral utilization)
- Performance under UM and quality improvement criteria
- Patient satisfaction
- Equal distribution
- Assigned lives
- Governance and administrative activities
- Community activities
- A weighted combination of these methods

1. To preserve the activity-based incentive and move from the FFS indicators, measures that depend on cash collections or charges should be avoided.

FIGURE 2
Example 2: Medium capitation

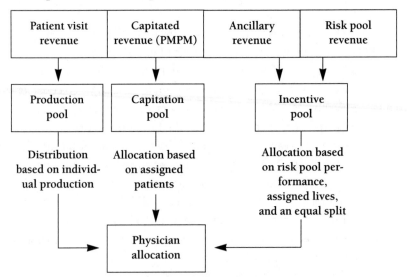

should receive several months' worth of performance data in advance to allow them to become familiar with the data and gain assurances they can affect the data through conscious efforts to change their utilization behavior. This data will be most meaningful when shown in comparison to the data of other physicians.

In Figure 2 and Table 4, the four-physician group allocates capitated PMPM revenue strictly on the basis of assigned patients. The incentive

TABLE 4
Example 2: Medium capitation—calculations

1. Summary: revenue and overhead allocation

	Patient visit FFS revenue (A)	Capitation pool distribution (B)	Incentive pool distribution (C)	Total revenue allocation (D) = (A + B + C)	Total overhead (E)	Total compensation (D – E)
Physician A	$225,000	$43,200	$45,473	$313,673	$199,665	$114,008
Physician B	$250,000	$50,400	$48,017	$348,417	$207,495	$140,922
Physician C	$275,000	$57,600	$55,074	$387,674	$215,325	$172,349
Physician D	$325,000	$64,800	$51,436	$441,236	$223,155	$218,081
	$1,075,000	$216,000	$200,000	$1,491,000	$845,640	$645,360

2. Capitation pool distribution

	Assigned lives	Percentage of total lives (A)	Capitation revenue (1,500 lives at $12 PMPM) (B)	Capitation distribution (A × B)
Physician A	300	20.0%		$43,200
Physician B	350	23.3%		$50,400
Physician C	400	26.7%		$57,600
Physician D	450	30.0%		$64,800
	1,500	100.0%	$216,000	$216,000

3. Incentive pool distribution

Risk pool revenue (assumption):	$100,000
Ancillary revenue (assumption):	100,000
Total incentive pool	$200,000 (A)

	Assigned lives (B)	Percentage of total lives (C)	Lives-based distribution (D) = (A × C)/3	Inpatient days (E)	Inpatient days per 1,000 patients (F) = ($1,000 ÷ B) × E
Physician A	300	20.0%	$13,333	70	233
Physician B	350	23.3%	$15,556	80	229
Physician C	400	26.7%	$17,778	70	175
Physician D	450	30.0%	$20,000	110	244
	1,500	100.0%	$66,667	330	220

	Utilization-based distribution (G)	Equal distribution portion (H) = (A/4)/3	Incentive pool compensation (D + G + H)
Physician A (cont.)	$15,473	$16,667	$45,473
Physician B (cont.)	$15,795	$16,667	$48,018
Physician C (cont.)	$20,630	$16,667	$55,075
Physician D (cont.)	$14,769	$16,667	$51,436
	$66,667	$66,667	$200,000

pool, which consists of revenue from group ancillaries and risk pools, is allocated based on assigned lives, inpatient utilization (related to risk pool measures), and an equal split. Overhead remains allocated on a 50 percent fixed/50 percent variable split, with risk pool revenue excluded from the calculation. Table 4 provides the calculation detail.

HIGH-CAPITATION ENVIRONMENT (MORE THAN 35 PERCENT)

Select a salary or productivity orientation

Among the successful highly capitated medical groups and integrated delivery systems, two distinct schools of thought have emerged regarding appropriate compensation plans. The more common is salary-oriented and provides a high level of base compensation with managed care-compatible incentives. The other is productivity-oriented, retaining many of the incentives of FFS medicine. This relies on strong utilization management (UM) to ensure physicians practice cost-effective medicine.

The salary-oriented model tends to equalize physician incomes since a relatively small portion of income is at-risk. This model relies less on individual productivity incentives and more on group performance. It offers individual physicians more compensation security but less economic potential to maximize income.

Under this model, a budget is developed that projects group revenue from all sources (except risk pools) and deducts projected overhead expenses. The remaining amount is budgeted physician compensation, typically based on a percentage of a standard measure of compensation, by specialty (e.g., 60 percent of the average compensation of family practitioners in the South). This may be calculated based upon readily available data or from a specific salary and compensation survey. Modifications to this base amount may be made to adjust for tenure with the group (such as a higher percentage of the standard base salary). This budgeted compensation amount is paid to the physicians as their monthly salary. Remaining funds are allocated to an incentive pool that includes risk pool proceeds. The incentive pool is then allocated based upon the factors described in Table 2.

The productivity-oriented approach will tend to have larger disparities in physician incomes since a greater piece of income is performance based. This model retains a strong incentive orientation, but to be successful in a managed care environment, it requires a group culture commitment to efficient utilization, backed up by a very focused group UM orientation.

This model begins with estimates of revenue and expenses to calculate a projected amount for total physician compensation and is allocated based upon measures of physician productivity. These measures may include RVUs, patient visits, and patient contact hours. Relatively small monthly draws are paid to physicians based upon their expected performance, with bonuses and other adjustments paid out quarterly or semi-annually.

This model provides simple and direct incentives that physicians appreciate. Physicians who work hard and see more patients will tend to make more money. However, it also encourages behavior, such as overutilization, that can bankrupt a group with significant managed care exposure. To guard against this, potential groups must have a sophisticated and experienced UM program. The group's entire culture must reflect a clinically cost-efficient orientation. Since these programs often require years of planning, the UM program should have an extensive track record prior to implementation of this type of compensation plan.

Physicians focused on stability and a strong group culture will tend to favor the salary-based model, while more entrepreneurial physicians will tend to gravitate toward the productivity-oriented model. The productivity approach will not necessarily result in a fragmented group and an economic free-for-all; the required UM programs can be important tools for forging a strong group culture. However, economic integration of the salary-based approach may result in more commitment to the group's goals and less focus on individual success.

Examples of each system

Salary-oriented model. In Figure 3 and Table 5, physicians' base compensation is set at 70 percent of the American Medical Association (AMA) median compensation for family practitioners in the Mountain region. Remaining funds (including risk pool proceeds) are allocated based upon

- 50 percent productivity (measured in patient visit RVUs, using resource-based relative value scale)

- 30 percent risk pool performance (in this case, inpatient utilization)

- 20 percent patient satisfaction (measured by regular surveys)

FIGURE 3
Example 3: High capitation, salary orientation

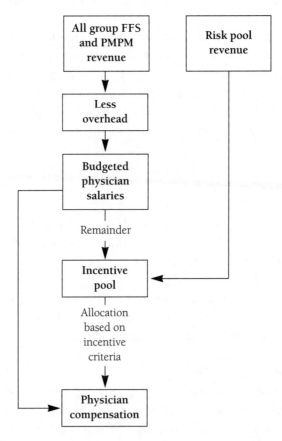

TABLE 5
Example 3: High capitation, salary orientation—calculations

1. Revenue and overhead allocation

	Patient visit FFS revenue (A)	Capitation revenue (B)	Ancillary revenues (C)	Total revenue[1] (D) = (A + B + C)	Overhead (E) = 57.5% × (D)
Physician A	$175,000				
Physician B	$200,000				
Physician C	$225,000				
Physician D	$275,000				
	$875,000	*$464,400*	*$100,000*	*$1,439,400*	*$827,655*

	Physician salary (F) = 70% × $120,000[2]	Remaining funds (G) = (D − E − F)	Incentive pool compensation (H)	Total compensation (F) + (H)
Physician A (cont.)	$84,000		$88,802	$172,802
Physician B (cont.)	$84,000		$98,706	$182,706
Physician C (cont.)	$84,000		$108,903	$192,903
Physician D (cont.)	$84,000		$129,334	$213,334
	$336,000	*$275,745*	*$425,745*	*$761,745*

2. Calculation of capitation revenue

	Assigned lives (A)	Capitation revenue (A) × $12 PMPM
Physician A	725	$104,400
Physician B	775	$111,600
Physician C	825	$118,800
Physician D	900	$129,600
	3,225	*$464,400*

3. Calculation of incentive distribution

Total risk pool revenue (assumption):	$150,000
Total remaining funds:	$275,745
Total incentive pool:	$425,745 (A)

TABLE 5 (CONTINUED)

	Patient visits	Percentage of total visits (B)	Inpatient utilization, days (assumption)	Inpatient days per 1,000 patients	Patient satisfaction score (assumption)
Physician A	3,500	20.0%	150	207	9.25
Physician B	4,000	22.9%	177	228	9.00
Physician C	4,500	25.7%	195	236	9.50
Physician D	5,500	31.4%	260	289	8.50
	17,500	100.0%	782	960	36.25

	Visits-based distribution (C)= (B×A)/2	Utilization-based distribution (D)	Patient satisfaction-based distribution (E)	Compensation, incentive pool (C+D+E)
Physician A (cont.)	$42,575	$24,499	$21,728	$88,802
Physician B (cont.)	$48,657	$28,909	$21,140	$98,706
Physician C (cont.)	$54,739	$31,849	$22,315	$108,903
Physician D (cont.)	$66,903	$42,466	$19,966	$129,334
	$212,874	$127,723	$85,149	$425,745

1. Excludes risk pool revenue, which is allocated through the incentive pool.
2. Median compensation for family and general practitioners in the Mountain region.
Source: American Medical Association, *Socioeconomic Characteristics of Medical Practice 1995* (Chicago: AMA, 1995), 145.

Productivity-oriented model. In Figure 4, a physician compensation budget is created based upon projections of revenue (including all capitation and FFS revenue) and overhead for the year. Compensation is calculated based on total RVUs generated by each physician, with each RVU worth one point. Medical group income is allocated based upon the relative number of points generated by each physician. Physicians are paid a relatively small draw amount, with quarterly bonuses to reconcile against money already paid. As indicated in Table 6, the physicians are involved in rigorous UM to guard against overutilization and other undesirable effects.

In this example, all available group revenue flows into a compensation pool distributed based on productivity measures such as RVUs. Physicians may be paid a relatively small monthly draw, with quarterly reconciliations and bonuses. A strong UM program is required to ensure appropriate utilization.

FIGURE 4
Example 4: High capitation, productivity orientation

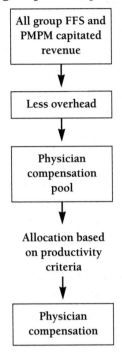

TABLE 6
Example 4: High capitation, productivity orientation—calculations

1. Summary: revenue and overhead allocation

	Fee-for-service production (A)	Capitation revenue (B)	Ancillary revenues (C)	Risk pool revenues (D)
Physician A	$175,000	$104,400		
Physician B	$200,000	$111,600		
Physician C	$225,000	$118,800		
Physician D	$275,000	$129,600		
	$875,000	$464,400	$100,000	$150,000

	Total revenue (E) = (A + B + C + D)	Overhead (F) = (E − D) × 57.5%	Physician compensation pool (G) = (E − F)
Physician A (cont.)			
Physician B (cont.)			
Physician C (cont.)			
Physician D (cont.)			
	$1,589,400	$827,655	$761,745

TABLE 6 (CONTINUED)

2. Calculation of physician revenue allocation

	Physician RVU production	Percent of total RVUs	Physician compensation
Physician A	3,500	23.7%	$180,753
Physician B	3,000	20.3%	$154,931
Physician C	4,250	28.8%	$219,486
Physician D	4,000	27.1%	$206,575
	14,750	99.9%	$761,745

Other considerations

Two other factors will help to ensure the group's mixed environment compensation plan is a success: paying PCPs at an appropriate level and monitoring the compensation plan on an ongoing basis.

Today multispecialty groups must recognize that no matter what the formula says, PCPs must be paid at least the market rate. Managed care will tend to increase the incomes of PCPs and reduce those of specialists. In addition, specialists need PCPs to ensure access to the contracts to provide patients. Therefore, groups that have higher managed care penetration are more willing to subsidize PCP incomes. Several highly successful systems have consciously paid PCPs more than the going rate to ensure the systems' abilities to attract and retain PCPs.

Two methods of providing these subsidies are revenue sharing and expense sharing. Revenue sharing provides that a portion of the revenues specialists generate be allocated to PCPs. For example, 10 percent of all group revenues could be placed in a pool to be allocated equally among all physicians. In this case, the higher-producing specialists would be providing an explicit subsidy to lower-producing PCPs.

Expense sharing, on the other hand, takes advantage of the differing levels of overhead between PCPs and specialists to provide an implicit subsidy. PCPs often have higher overhead rates because of a greater office visit volume and the smaller dollar amount generated by each visit. If the physicians in a group are charged a flat overhead rate, the lower-overhead physicians (generally specialists) will subsidize the higher-overhead PCPs.

Physician groups should monitor compensation plans to ensure original objectives remain fulfilled. If the compensation plan is showing signs of stress, this does not mean the system has failed; due to continual changes in group composition and the business environment, a group will seldom achieve the perfect system. The following signals may indicate the plan needs to be changed:

- Physician complaints regarding inequity, lack of potential to improve incomes, or improper exploitation of incentives

- An inexplicable increase in utilization of ancillary services, as may be shown through payer reports

- Poor financial performance of undercapitated contracts (by measuring FFS equivalent, for example, 90 percent of charges) could indicate improper utilization incentives

- A sudden, significant increase in capitation revenue, as could occur when a group begins to accept managed Medicare or when a large FFS contract converts to capitation

Conclusion

In a market evolving from FFS to capitated reimbursement, it is important for a physician group to ensure its compensation plan is appropriate for its payment environment. The plan should reflect the group's strategic objectives as well as realistically assess its future. As the group becomes more dependent on capitation, physicians need to ensure that compensation becomes less oriented toward traditional methods of measuring physician activity and more aligned with the incentives of prepaid medicine, especially with attention to appropriate utilization. An evolving compensation system tied to the capitation level can help the group accomplish this goal.

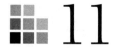 11

Staging the transition to capitated medical groups

Dale Bradford
Vice President and General Manager

James A. Hester, Jr., PhD
Vice President of Network Development
ChoiceCare
Cincinnati, Ohio

CHOICECARE, AN INDEPENDENT IPA-model HMO, has developed a unique network strategy to support its four commercial product lines for 290,000 members in and surrounding Cincinnati. This network strategy, implemented in 1993, is built around a network of independent, physician-controlled group practices with preferred but nonexclusive relationships with ChoiceCare. The financial incentives of these groups are realigned from the current fee-for-service system by a staged implementation of capitation programs that gradually decentralizes the responsibility for medical management to the physician groups and builds their capability to manage care more effectively.

This chapter outlines the major elements of ChoiceCare's strategy, summarizing its results. It will elaborate on ChoiceCare's vision of a high-performing delivery system, summarize the current status of both the Cincinnati marketplace and ChoiceCare, discuss ChoiceCare's core beliefs and its plan for the transition, and discuss some of the issues in applying ChoiceCare's strategy to other markets.

The Cincinnati metropolitan area is located in a tri-state area encompassing southwestern Ohio, northern Kentucky, and southeastern Indiana. It has a population of about 1.7 million, a fairly diverse and slow-growing economy, and a tradition of changing slowly. Consistent with that tradition, although managed care has been present in the city for close to 20 years, the care has not been tightly managed, and utilization rates have thus remained high until recently. HMO penetration is about 25 percent and total managed care penetration, including preferred provider organizations (PPO) and point of service (POS), is about 55 percent.

The city has only one multispecialty group practice, with 50 primary care physicians (PCPs) and 30 specialists. Virtually all of the 950 PCPs are in small (less than 10 physicians) single-specialty practices. The 1,800 specialist physicians have consolidated somewhat into a number of medium-sized (10 to 20 physicians) single-specialty groups, but more than half are still fragmented into small practices of less than 10 physicians. Capitation, especially among the PCPs, is virtually nonexistent except for the one multispecialty group.

Cincinnati hospitals are under increasing pressure to consolidate due to waning revenues from decreasing inpatient days and are pursuing different avenues to maintain revenues, such as expanding into specialty areas or services (e.g., focusing on the senior population). Others are attempting to increase their outpatient market share, with one popular strategy being to purchase physician practices to assure a continued revenue.

Hospitals are also coming together into joint ventures that look more like mergers. Two of the major hospitals have announced a consolidation to a single board and a single management structure with a sharing of bottom line income statements. They have begun joint planning to quickly eliminate duplicate services, both in medical and administrative areas. A second alliance has combined three hospitals, including the University of Cincinnati Medical Center, into a single system under one CEO. These consolidations should result in lower costs and eventual hospital closings.

Cincinnati's main managed care players are ChoiceCare, Community Mutual Insurance Company (CMIC—a Blue Cross affiliate), United Healthcare, Prudential Health Plan, Aetna Health Plan, FHP, and Cigna. CMIC has the largest overall book of business with large indemnity penetration and some managed care. ChoiceCare is the largest managed care company with 290,000 members. There is also a large PPO in the city, Health Services Affiliates.

Building a high-performing delivery system

In order for ChoiceCare to succeed over the long term it must build its products and services around high-performing delivery systems—integrated networks of care to meet its customers' demands for high levels of patient satisfaction, excellent clinical outcomes, and low costs. This elusive "integrated delivery system" represents the current Holy Grail thinking in healthcare policy to reorganize the current "dis-integrated" healthcare networks characterized by fragmented relationships between PCPs, specialty physicians, hospitals, and health plans. Today there is broad agreement on the need for a more effective network structure, yet there are many questions, including what exactly is the vision of the new delivery system and what are the best steps to get there? Nationally, there are a variety of models and approaches to develop an IDS where usually one of three players—medical groups, health plans, or consolidated hospital systems—assumes overall ownership and control.

ChoiceCare's vision of a high-performing delivery system relies on a balanced partnership between the three players who remain independent in order to focus on their separate, complementary roles and responsibilities. The delivery system is primary care medical group driven—built around a network of independent primary care group practices—but depends on strong, effective linkages between PCPs, specialists, and hospitals. The glue that bonds the physicians and hospitals together comes from a global capitation program, aligning financial incentives instead of just transferring risk to the providers to make them a mini-insurance company. If properly designed and implemented this global risk/reward program provides the driving force for a provider-driven cycle of continuous process improvement—the engine that powers the improvements in competitive medical management.

A key concept in this implementation is to provide a reliable reward system to providers for managing behavioral change—both theirs and their patients'—and to minimize providers' actuarial risks. Effective, independent medical groups and a properly designed global incentive program are the twin pillars that support the high-performing delivery system of the future. The rest of this chapter expands these concepts by outlining major elements of the transition plan being implemented at ChoiceCare.

STANDARD MANAGED CARE APPROACH

In general, a standard approach in managing healthcare quality and cost is to capitate PCPs, pay specialists fee for service (FFS), be able to put PCPs at-risk for specialist and hospital costs as needed, pay hospitals per diem, and manage utilization tightly. What are the problems with this standard approach?

When PCPs are capitated, they are financially motivated to provide as little care as possible because their revenues are capped—additional care adds to their costs. If they are put at-risk for specialist costs, they are pulled in both directions, financially motivated to minimize the care they provide and to limit referrals. When PCPs are at-risk for hospital costs, it can be frustrating because specialists are more often the ones who hospitalize, and it becomes very difficult for the PCPs to manage hospital utilization when they are no longer the primary managers of the care. HMOs may argue that PCPs should be more involved in care management, but when patients are hospitalized, their condition is usually severe enough to warrant specialist care. It is hard for PCPs to get back into managing the care, and it may not even be appropriate for them to do so.

Meanwhile, the specialists and hospitals are financially motivated to maximize utilization because they are compensated on a FFS and per diem basis, respectively. Since the incentives are misaligned, the HMO must manage the utilization very tightly, often creating tension in the system and widespread dissatisfaction with HMOs among the providers.

CORE BELIEFS AND APPROACH

The need for a high-performance delivery system stands in stark contrast to the present reality of Cincinnati's current environment. How can the gap between the two be closed? More importantly, how to close the gap in a way that minimizes the unexpected surprises to patients and employers, increases the likelihood that better performing providers will survive, and results in steady improvements in the performance of the healthcare system for the community? ChoiceCare's approach operates using following core beliefs:

1. *Align financial incentives.* Gradually align the financial incentives of physicians, hospitals, and health plans by providing an incremental transition from fee for service to global risk sharing

2. *Develop independent primary care driven medical groups.* Physician-controlled groups will perform better over the long term. Help physicians restructure into independent, physician-controlled groups that are primary care driven but create focused, effective relationships with specialists and hospitals

3. *Establish long-term preferred relationships.* Establish long-term preferred but nonexclusive relationships between the health plan and its providers. Create a capability to identify and respond to the needs of those providers while meeting the demands of customers—employers and members. ChoiceCare recently created a formal Preferred Group Agreement for its key primary care groups because of the importance of its primary care base and the vulnerability of having the base of independent physicians eroded through acquisition by other parties. In exchange for financial and developmental assistance from ChoiceCare, these groups give ChoiceCare the right of first refusal for the purchase of the group and have a long-term (seven-year) agreement to participate in ChoiceCare's products

4. *Decentralize medical management.* Supports evolution of providers' capabilities for medical management of a defined population versus a Darwinian struggle for survival. Many plans have used capitation to simply transfer risk to providers and have done little to teach them how to manage successfully under this new responsibility. ChoiceCare has already developed strong tools for medical management that can be transferred to the medical groups, with the role of ChoiceCare's staff evolving from micromanager to facilitator and consultant. It is also developing new tools to manage defined populations (e.g., using risk assessment tools to manage acute health problems before they become chronic)

5. *Develop a continuous improvement process.* ChoiceCare has achieved modest initial savings in the implementation of these programs. The initial target performance levels for providers are a compromise between current performance and benchmark data on the best performance observed anywhere in the country. ChoiceCare created a group structure, an incentive system, and management information and supporting services that drive performance toward "best practices" over time through a continuous improvement process

MANAGING THE TRANSITION

While these core principles are easy to describe, they are difficult to implement. The following describes the specific tools ChoiceCare used to implement its network strategy.

Align financial incentive

Most managed care organizations have misaligned incentives that result in frustration for the HMO and the providers. The HMOs believe providers are acting inappropriately, yet the providers are being responsive to the incentives in place. In the optimal system of care, however, financial and behavioral incentives motivate all parties in the delivery system to adopt the same behavior and goals. In this system, provider groups receive a global capitation for all or most medical care, and risk for financial performance of the global capitation is shared by the provider group, hospitals, and HMO. But this is not pure capitation. In pure capitation, the provider is paid a capitated amount and is fully at-risk for financial performance, with no one else participating in that risk. If financial risk is to be shared, a pool must be capitated, the providers must be paid out of the pool, and the parties must share in the financial performance of the pool. If all sharing parties do not share in the risk, financial incentives will not be aligned.

Today most physicians in Cincinnati are still in solo or small group practices, not in groups prepared for global capitation. They are rapidly forming groups, but it will take years, and many groups will have to be formed two or three times in different configurations before they find one that will endure.

How can an HMO compensate physician groups in a manner that encourages preparation for global incentives and provides the appropriate incentives for providers still in solo or small group practices? Choice-Care is taking the following three-stage approach:

- *Prelude:* the initial development of limited scope capitation programs

- *Active development:* the implementation of global incentive programs for lead medical groups

- *Maturation:* expanding the global incentive programs to more providers and new product lines

Each of these phases are discussed below by highlighting the key activities for physicians, hospitals, and the health plan.

Prelude (January 1993 to July 1997)

ChoiceCare developed its network strategy and began implementation. It completed the realignment of the physician fee schedule to the resource-based relative value scale (RBRVS) and introduced its initial limited scope capitation programs. Its key actions to date

- Develop a network strategy and obtain senior management and board buy-in through an annual strategic planning process and series of special board meetings and retreats

- Develop ChoiceCare's infrastructure. Supporting a network of medical groups paid on a capitated basis requires major changes to the infrastructure developed to pay individual physicians on a FFS basis. Obtain commitment for additional staffing and begin cross-functional development for project teams to implement required changes in all major operating departments, including management information systems (MIS) capabilities

- Pay all physicians FFS on RBRVS. Four years ago ChoiceCare paid all physicians on a FFS basis with an average of a 20 percent withhold, which was returned in whole or in part at year-end based on health plan performance for the year. But physician costs were increasing much faster than medical CPI and all industry standards. To manage the increase in physician fees and to rationalize the flow of compensation among PCPs versus specialists, an RBRVS payment mechanism was implemented over a three-year period. It was staged over three years because it had a substantial reduction in specialist compensation that was inappropriate to make in one year

- Pay physicians individual incentive payments around quality and customer satisfaction indicators for specific performance improvements in the areas of patient satisfaction, access, and initial quality indicators such as medical records

- Capitate specialists and ancillaries one by one, but keep PCPs FFS

- Encourage formation of group practices

- Pay hospitals on a per diem basis combined with an annual collective target for inpatient care using limits for hospital and medical CPI

Active development (August 1995 to January 1997)

- Phase in a global incentive program for PCP groups and have physician groups, hospitals, and HMO share in hospital pool risk

- Capitate PCP groups only when they are formed and prepared for capitation

- Encourage strong interaction among PCPs and specialists

- Renegotiate long-term hospital contracts to align their incentives with the physician groups and HMOs. The method of compensating hospitals to assure aligned incentives is a particular challenge. ChoiceCare has renegotiated its contracts using a method of payment that combines per case and per diem payments. This fulfills two goals: it encourages hospitals to minimize length of stay, and it allows for hospitals, physicans, and ChoiceCare to share in hospital cost savings, thus aligning incentives. It is a challenge, because in an ideal system, hospitals see themselves as cost centers not as revenue centers. This change in acumen will be a difficult transition for most hospitals

Maturation (post-1997)

Expand the global incentive program to a larger cross-section of PCPs as medical groups continue to develop. Incorporate its new product lines such as Medicare risk and managed disability from the outset.

There are several advantages to this three-stage approach

- PCPs and specialists are appropriately compensated under RBRVS

- PCPs paid under FFS are financially motivated to maximize the care they provide

- Capitated specialists are financially motivated to minimize unnecessary care and motivated to train PCPs to provide as much of the care as possible

- Specialists and PCP groups are put into the role of utilization manager causing providers also to be managers. This reduces the need for external utilization managers

- Physicians focus on quality and customer satisfaction, not only cost

- Hospitals are financially motivated to decrease their costs and length of stay

ChoiceCare believes this approach provides the incentives to physicians and hospitals to move to an ideal system of care, providing high-quality care at the lowest cost while maintaining high customer satisfaction.

Create independent primary care driven medical groups

Until recently, all group development was single specialty. Now multi-specialty primary care groups are beginning to emerge and combine family practice, internal medicine, and pediatrics.

The next stage of physician network development is to create larger primary care groups of 15 to 30 physicians. Each of these groups will probably have multiple offices with a cluster size of five to eight physicians. A group of this size is large enough to support a high-level business manager and supporting administrative systems and enable a physician to focus on delivering care while maintaining an attractive lifestyle. A large practice has a population base large enough to support a global capitation program and the management tools required to succeed under such a program.

However, even with a global capitation and a large managed care population, it is not clear that primary care groups will evolve into large multispecialty groups that employ their own panels of subspecialists. The restructuring of PCPs is being paralleled by a similar consolidation of specialists into larger groups as they prepare to compete for referrals on the basis of performance, instead of personal relationships or hospital privileges commonly used in the past. The more progressive single specialty groups, selective in the physicians they attract, package complementary medical expertise into a single group and add supporting information and patient management systems that will be difficult for a multispecialty group to match.

For example, under managed care staffing guidelines, a primary care group of 30 physicians could support two full-time orthopedic surgeons. An alternative would be to contract on a subcapitated basis with an eight- to ten-physician orthopedic group that could provide a much more complete range of surgical specializations, be involved in creating and improving both inpatient clinical pathways and outpatient practice guidelines, and provide a higher level of expertise to the primary care group. Given the two options, primary care groups will not likely form long-term, contractual relationships with a network of separate single-specialty groups because of better performance.

The key, however is twofold: ensure that multiple options exist in each specialty so there is effective competition for the primary care relationships and that primary care groups obtain performance data on these. The excess supply of specialists could be resolved by consolidating the best-performing specialists into larger groups and by primary care groups selecting the best of those groups.

Establish a physician network strategy
and group development programs

ChoiceCare recognizes its participating physician network is an important asset, has formulated a physician network strategy, and is using programs to implement that strategy. Its main elements are to

1. Develop support for the formation and management of independent physician groups. ChoiceCare has provided a broad array of group practice support services including

   - Educational programs at Xavier University in group practice development. Two hundred physicians have attended a special eight-session program for physicians on the formation of physician group practices

   - Short-term technical assistance groups to develop consolidation plans

   - Development of a practice support organization to provide both group practice development and ongoing management services for physician-controlled primary care and specialty groups

- Affiliation with Health Partners Inc., of Norwalk, Connecticut, (a for-profit medical group development and management company) for groups that prefer an equity model option

- Evaluation and selection of a preferred group practice MIS that includes billing, scheduling, and computerized medical record modules

- Assistance in recruiting new primary care capacity

- Lines of credit at preferred rates and an array of specialized financial services at a major local bank

2. Create long-term preferred but nonexclusive relationships with primary care groups. Groups that sign a preferred group agreement give ChoiceCare a right of first refusal to purchase the group and agreement to participate in ChoiceCare products for seven years. In return, they receive financial assistance to recruit PCPs, pay for transitional management expenses, and convert and install MIS

3. Develop support for small primary care offices. For the foreseeable future, ChoiceCare will continue to have a substantial portion (one-third to one-half) of its primary care base in small offices of fewer than five physicians. Practice management consulting services and other support programs are being designed to keep these offices healthy and strengthen their ties to ChoiceCare

4. Oppose active recruitment from hospital-controlled primary care groups. In December 1994, ChoiceCare circulated to all of its PCPs a formal statement about the accelerating acquisition of PCPs by a number of local hospitals. The policy included specific limitations on the way in which hospital-controlled primary care groups would be allowed to participate in ChoiceCare. The main changes included freezing membership in existing small-panel products, excluding them from the new Medicare and managed disability products, excluding them from any capitation programs, and requiring longer term contracts with the physicians (who were not coterminus with the hospital contracts)

5. Develop support for specialty care groups. The formation of high-performance specialty groups is a key element in the evolution of an

IDS. ChoiceCare has provided significant assistance to both existing and exploratory specialty groups through its group practice development program and the proposed practice support organization. The specialty capitation programs discussed previously are also intended to stimulate the consolidation of specialists into larger groups, facilitate the development of closer links to PCPs, and create the medical management skills required to function effectively under capitation

This network strategy is consistent with ChoiceCare's core beliefs. It also meets the needs of the Cincinnati area, which were explicitly assessed in two comprehensive physician attitude surveys during the last two years. While it offers the potential of better long-term performance, it also risks key portions of its primary care base being acquired by hospitals or well-financed competitors. Over the next two years, the success of this strategy will be determined by the decisions made by a relatively small group of about 200 PCPs in the greater Cincinnati area as they choose the ownership model under which they will practice.

TRANSFERABLE MODEL

This transition to the ideal system of healthcare is more a philosophy than a model. While the philosophy can be transferred, the HMO's commitment must be long term, well capitalized, and woven into the fabric of care delivery. This is not a short-term tactic, nor can it be used by an HMO that does not have a significant market share since the incentives must be sufficient to drive behavior changes. If sufficient membership or dollars are not at stake, the incentives will be too small to overcome the natural aversion to change.

For the committed HMO that has significant market share, this philosophy can be transferred. However, the motivation is not a financial one; rather, it is part of an overall philosophy of care driven by capitation and global risk sharing and the needs of participating physicians to be full partners while remaining independent from an HMO.

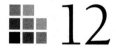

12

Developing a global capitation model for an integrated delivery network

Lori L. Anderson
Assistant Vice President and Senior Consultant
Premier, Inc.
Westchester, Illinois

B ECOME LARGER, CONSOLIDATE, and integrate is a commonly sung theme used by healthcare strategists of the 1990s. However, many hospitals and physician-hospital organizations (PHOs) are looking for ways to meet this market demand without full-asset hospital and PHO mergers.

In 1995, five East Coast PHOs developed a "Super PHO network" called Sea Shore Network (SSN). The Super PHO created common contracting terms and a global capitation model. In this model, SSN was able to accept global capitation for comprehensive healthcare services without consolidating hospital or PHO operations. SSN—consisting of three PHOs representing not-for-profit hospitals, and two PHOs with a for-profit hospital component—was organized to

- Create a common managed care contracting organization without integrating hospital assets or governance

- Gain community health network infrastructure and service capabilities

- Provide HMOs with a "one-stop-shopping" contracting opportunity by covering the market with comprehensive geographic and clinical services

- Ensure market share growth as a result of SSN contracts using a selective panel of PHO providers

- Expand negotiating leverage with payers within the antitrust guide-lines established by SSN's legal counsel

Based on these objectives, SSN developed a global capitation product. This chapter presents a case study at SSN and discusses how its strategy was developed, critical success factors, the global capitation model, and individual PHO capitation results.

The strategy assessment

In 1995, providers in SSN's market were faced with a push by HMOs to move toward capitated provider contracts. This market had moderate managed care penetration, 35.4 percent in 1994, and limited capitation penetration, 16.9 percent in 1994. However, the market also had histor-ically low commercial HMO hospital utilization, 259 days per 1,000 in 1994, prior to any significant penetration of capitation as a form of reim-bursement. SSN's market was also experiencing aggressive market entry by HMOs, which were quickly achieving significant market leverage through consolidation.

SSN's member PHOs evaluated opportunities for partnering and inte-gration options and determined they would gain enhanced appeal as providers by creating a PHO network. In 1995, SSN expanded its nego-tiating leverage by developing a "Super PHO," a linkage of independent PHOs organized to attract patients by providing services as a single net-work, also called an integrated delivery network (IDN). While most experts contend that in the long term, loose voluntary networks will not be able to compete with more tightly controlled systems that can direct care and control service delivery, integrated managed care contracting was seen as a logical first step to approach the SSN marketplace. SSN providers knew that this was only a first step, and managing patient care to produce favorable outcomes and sustaining profit for PHO members would require further integration of healthcare services and PHO oper-ations. During its strategy development phase, the provider group orig-inally considered starting its own HMO to contract directly with employers. However, it ultimately rejected that strategy because it felt the HMO's market control was significant enough that adverse HMO reaction would present a threat of market share loss greater than poten-tial market share gain. Although managed care penetration in this market was moderate, several large, well-capitalized HMOs entered SSN's market in 1994 and were perceived by providers to be quoting premiums under medical cost. Thus, the "entry fee" to the HMO business carried a higher price than the Super PHO could afford.

Determining critical success factors

In addition to an accurate market evaluation and appropriate strategy to respond to market needs, SSN considered the following factors critical to its success.

EXPENSE REDUCTION

Both hospitals and physician groups in the PHOs implemented expense reduction strategies by projecting expected capitated payments and defining global budgets. Targets were based on existing HMO medical expense rates that set a benchmark for budgeting internal provider payments. Expense reduction strategies to adjust to this fixed medical expense methodology were necessary to project any potential surplus in risk pools.

In an attempt to achieve risk pool surpluses, SSN physicians pursued one or more of the following strategies for cost reduction:

- Evaluate economies available in overhead reduction, such as affiliating with multispecialty groups or a hospital-owned medical services organization (MSO)

- Develop appropriate financial incentives for cost reduction (described in risk model section)

- Develop appropriate data-sharing strategies to provide physicians with accurate, timely, risk-adjusted information that may serve as a benchmark for performance improvement

The hospital executives determined an evaluation of appropriate financial incentives as the first step to reduce costs. For example, all hospitals undertook one or more of the following activities:

- Focus on accountability for cost on a per patient basis, not a departmental basis

- Transition cost comparison and benchmarking to a per episode basis, not an admission-procedure basis

- Transition key hospital employees and hospital-based physicians' incentives to a net-revenue basis, not gross-revenue or gross-charge basis (e.g., in one hospital the bonus for the department chair of radiology was based on gross billings. If an increasing portion of the hospital's reimbursement was expected to be capitated, this incentive system would become obsolete. A new revenue-based bonus system took into account the combination of capitated and fee-for-service reimbursement mix and provided bonuses based on net revenue.)

- Develop "capitation readiness" in critical departments' planning including

  admitting and patient registration

  audit and reimbursement

  general accounting

  health information management and medical records

  information systems

  planning and marketing

  patient accounts and business office

  managed care contracting

In addition to creating a capitation implementation work plan involving key hospital departments, each hospital implemented a separate cost-reduction strategy to ensure market competitiveness, including clinical care delivery, clinical and operational support, management, and purchasing contracts. For example, one hospital renegotiated its food, linen, laundry, and office supply contracts with its individual suppliers.

DATA-SHARING STRATEGIES

To manage effectively global capitation, SSN determined the following data elements to be critical:

- Preenrollment data (from each payer) including group specific demographics (e.g., age, sex, zip code, dependent distribution), industry categories for all groups, loss-ratio history, postenrollment reporting from each payer, including claims and utilization management summary reports by provider, employer group, patient age/sex, service type, and diagnostic-related group (DRG)

- Employer-specific data, including billed and allowed charges, actual reimbursement, noncovered charges, inpatient days (i.e., approved, denied, and actual), number of outpatient visits, outpatient surgeries by procedure code, outpatient services by procedure code, admissions and days per 1,000 members by bed type, referrals by provider, and utilization management compliance statistics

By setting this benchmark for its new system, SSN should be capable of capturing all data elements required for physician profiling.

CLINICAL SERVICE EFFECTIVENESS

Many hospitals and physicians, including those represented by SSN, initially fell prey to a "group think" mentality when trying to demonstrate quality of care with an outmoded response of "we know we're high quality because everybody thinks so." While reputation, a subjective value, can never be discounted, SSN providers knew they would be asked to quantify network value. SSN found the following three areas critical to demonstrating value relative to competing networks:

1. *Geographic accessibility.* SSN's geographic accessibility was defined using payer definitions. The market network's coverage required at least two primary care physicians (PCPs) within 8 miles of every HMO member and a hospital within 15 miles of each HMO member. SSN designed its network to fill gaps in any area in advance of marketing the network to payers

2. *Clinical service depth.* SSN included one tertiary hospital and appropriate subspecialists to provide comprehensive tertiary services, requiring almost no out-of-network transfers. SSN contracted for services it did not provide in some pediatric subspecialty areas and selected transplant services

3. *Network efficiency and quality.* Once SSN established its network, its medical leadership established care benchmarking measurements. Those measurements initially included in-network versus out-of-

TABLE 1
Primary care physician profile

	Total $	PMPM	Peer group PMPM	Target PMPM
Number of member months: 1,200				
Capitation payments	$18,000	$15.00	$14.65	$15.00
Fee-for-service equivalents for services covered under cap	$17,124	$14.27	$15.22	$13.50
Net difference	*$876*	*$0.73*	*($0.57)*	*$1.50*
Inpatient by bed type	$38,412	$32.01	$37.00	$33.00
Hospital outpatient services by type	$25,200	$21.00	$23.50	$20.00
Referrals by specialty	$40,800	$34.00	$29.80	$32.00
Other service by type:				
Home health	$600	$0.50	$0.58	$0.55
SNF/ECF	$204	$0.17	$0.20	$0.22
Physical therapy	$300	$0.25	$0.40	$0.27
Vision services	$948	$0.79	$0.76	$0.91
Ambulance/transportation	$204	$0.17	$0.30	$0.28
Appliances/DME	$348	$0.29	$0.30	$0.31
OP mental health	$1,140	$0.95	$0.75	$0.76
OP substance abuse	$480	$0.40	$0.19	$0.19
Prescription drugs	$13,740	$11.45	$11.72	$11.50
Subtotal	*$17,964*	*$14.97*	*$15.20*	*$15.00*
Total in-network	$140,376	$116.98	$120.15	$115.00
Total out-of-network	$13,440	$11.20	$13.60	$11.50
Total medical expenses	*$153,816*	*$128.18*	*$133.75*	*$126.50*
Admissions per 1,000 members		94.6	98.9	95.9
Days per 1,000 members		246.1	272.0	259.0
Referrals by specialty per 1,000 members		4,469.2	4,956.0	4,425.0
Outpatient services by type per 1,000 members		618.1	624.7	657.5
Encounters per member per year (includes well-baby visits)		2.8	3.0	2.6
Patient satisfaction survey results		4.5	4.2	4.0

Note: With the exception of patient satisfaction scores, all data are from PHO information system.

network hospital costs and physician performance criteria. Physician performance criterion measurements included

- Financial results (i.e., per patient per episode or per procedure)

- Inpatient utilization, including admissions per 1,000, bed days per 1,000, and average length of stay

- Patient satisfaction survey results

- Compliance with precertification

- Open practice

Evaluating the market

After evaluating the steps necessary to quantify market value, SSN evaluated the market itself prior to developing managed care models or products. To evaluate their current market, SSN had to answer the following questions:

- Who is offering capitation in this market?

- What is their track record for accurate and timely provider payments and incentive payouts?

- What portion of the premium can SSN expect?

- When does each PHO need to be ready to manage capitation?

- What is each SSN facility's competitive cost position?

The information needed to answer these questions came from state HMO rate filings; hospital profiles (e.g., AHA guides, CON applications, bond issues); area physicians (e.g., AMA master files, hospital staff rosters, state licensing boards, yellow pages); competitor networks (e.g., physician directories); employer and payer market profiles; industry publications (e.g., *Interstudy, SMG Marketing Group, Advisory Board Company, Medical Benefits*); consultants including actuaries, attorneys, and managed care consultants; and other providers contracting with SSN-targeted HMOs in other markets.

Upon the conclusion of the market assessment, SSN determined there was market demand for a well-managed, clinically comprehensive network willing to accept global capitation. SSN's next challenge was to develop the internal controls necessary to establish a loose but well-managed voluntary affiliation.

This effort required redefining healthcare service delivery methods, financial incentives, and accurate expense forecasting for probable or even potential success.

TABLE 2
Capitated contracting shared risk

Shared loss	$12.41 PMPM
Pharmaceutical contractor loss	$11.28 PMPM ↑ 10%
Pharmaceutical contractor gain	$11.28 PMPM ↓ 10%
Shared gain	$10.51 PMPM

Contact can
  Be diagnosis specific
  Exclude outliers or certain drugs

To predict potential losses and gains before the first capitated contract was executed, SSN, in 1995, began to evaluate the project under capitation by comparing historical performance under managed fee-for-service contracts to projected capitated contract performance. SSN also worked with payers to identify potential "ease in" strategies to capitation (e.g., in one PHO's contract, which started in the first year with a risk-sharing arrangement, risk was shared within a corridor). Savings under the corridor were retained by SSN, and expenses over the corridor were assumed by the payer as depicted in Table 2.

This type of risk-sharing strategy allowed SSN to gain experience managing a capitated budget with limited exposure for loss. This contract will expand the risk corridor in year two and evolve into full capitation in year three. Once all of SSN's risk management strategies were in place, SSN developed its global capitated model, which covered all services within the medical expense portion of premiums.

Developing the risk model

SSN was confronted with numerous issues about developing a common capitation distribution model for all participating entities. It had several key issues to address, including

- *A common capitated rate for hospital services.* Participating hospitals had divergent cost structures, and the higher-intensity, higher-cost hospitals did not believe that application of a DRG methodology alone would address cost differences created by the varying case mix between smaller community hospitals and larger urban hospitals

- *A common physician reimbursement methodology.* Some PHOs had more than five years of experience with capitated contracts, some had experience with capitating PCPs only, and some had no capitation experience at all

- *Negotiating thresholds and authority.* The PHOs' ability to bind physicians to a contract at the SSN rate was inconsistent. Some allowed individual physicians to reject any capitated contract regardless of rates, while others completely delegated contracting authority to the PHO Board

- *Consistent reimbursement.* SSN providers comprised physicians and hospitals dispersed across five distinct communities. A range of historical capitated payment rates offered by the same HMOs had been established. SSN had to blend these rates to achieve a regionally competitive rate. This resulted in SSN requiring some capitated providers to reduce their capitation rates with a payer in order to be part of the SSN Super PHO contract

To develop a targeted global capitation rate SSN made the following assumptions:

- Targeted global capitation would be set at 10 percent under the current HMO market for total medical cost expenditures. The target rate was determined by aggregating the HMO medical expenditures using 1994 state rate filings with the state insurance department in SSN's service area

- HMOs would require a premium percentage for administration of 15 to 20 percent, thus reducing base premium price by this amount to estimate global provider payment rates

- SSN would serve as the insurer for the tertiary risk pool and the reinsurer of all medical claims over $50,000

- All other risk for medical expenditures would be managed by the individual PHOs

This last assumption was inherently problematic because one of the five PHOs had no infrastructure in place to manage risk. This issue was resolved by this PHO engaging one of the more mature PHOs to provide "service bureau support" for capitation administration and reporting services. Aggregate risk sharing would be based on the following model:

Total annual medical expenses

equal   Total actual fees paid on capitation, set at 75 percent of physician fees and a global per diem of $1,500 for hospitals

minus   • Copay income
         • Stop-loss recoveries
         • COB recoveries
         • Surplus remaining in medical services fund, if any

plus   • Stop-loss premiums paid
         • IBNR
         • Deficit remaining in medical services fund, if any

Total medical services revenue to PHO *equals* fees on capitation paid out to PHO *plus* any bonus paid during the year.

Establishing the risk model development process

SSN decided to develop a capitated risk model in advance of HMO contracting so that targeted reimbursement could be agreed upon and funds distribution among providers could be determined prior to actual payer negotiation. The goals SSN set for the model were to establish

• Market competitive medical expense

• PCP capitation equal to the highest HMO capitation currently offered

• Specialist reimbursement equal to the average HMO reimbursement currently offered

• Hospital reimbursement that blended reimbursement needs based on divergent hospital cost structures, yet was perceived as fair by the participating institutions

• Other reimbursement (the category of capitation for all other medical expense) capitated in some way that appropriately incented the prudent use of these services

- Risk that was difficult to predict, such as tertiary care, pooled at the SSN level so that it could be shared across the network

- Risk that was more predictable, such as hospital inpatient and outpatient specialist and primary care expense, capitated at the individual PHO level for two reasons: it places risk at a decentralized level with the individuals in the best position to manage it, and as a new and nonasset-integrated partnership, SSN's members were not willing to share risk on a fully integrated level

Next, SSN evaluated infrastructure needs at both the SSN level and the PHO level to determine the capabilities required for risk management. Based on this model, SSN infrastructure requirements were

- Management of the tertiary risk pool, which included sophisticated case management capabilities

- Accepting a single check from payers and distributing funds to the PHOs

- Reinsurance administration or purchase

- Data collection from PHOs, data aggregation and evaluation, and reporting to payers on cost and quality indication

The first step to develop the ability to manage the tertiary pool was to define the included providers and procedures. Two of SSN's PHOs provided tertiary care, one in cardiology only, the other in all areas of tertiary service. Tertiary services were defined as any services within the DRGs as depicted in Table 3.

Next, SSN conducted a "make or buy" evaluation of medical management systems for capitation check distribution and data collection and reporting. It decided to outsource this service, paying a per member per month (PMPM) administrative fee to a service bureau until SSN's volume warranted development of internal capabilities.

SSN also decided to purchase reinsurance rather than serve as the reinsuring agent of the PHOs. This decision was based on SSN's ability to aggregate the Super PHO's volume, enabling it to obtain a more competitive rate than the PHOs would be able to on their own.

TABLE 3
High risk cardiology pool DRGs

Category	DRGs
Cardiac surgery	104–108
Angioplasty	112
Diagnostic cardiology	124–125

TABLE 4
Capitation categories

Type of service	Net PMPM	Percentage
PCP	$15.00	13.0%
Specialist	$32.00	28.0%
Hospital inpatient	$33.00	29.0%
Hospital outpatient	$20.00	17.0%
Other services	$15.00	13.0%
Total	*$115.00*	*100.00%*

Tables 3 and 4 courtesy of Reden & Anders Consultants & Actuaries.

Target capitation development

Based on state HMO rate filings, SSN determined its reimbursement floor of market rate less 10 percent would yield a total medical reimbursement of $115 PMPM. Projected capitation distribution is depicted in Table 4.

Once a target cap was developed for each service category, the individual PHOs, in theory, could distribute the cap using any methodology they wished. However, SSN was required to develop a common capitation methodology and rates because of crossover of PCPs in two of the five PHOs. Under most payer contracts in this market, payers would be administering FFS payments and would want to administer claims payment of any providers under FFS methodology (e.g., noncapitated specialists) uniformly.

Payers were initially skeptical of loosely integrated networks such as SSN, because they viewed a large group of providers with the ability to accept risk as a threat. They were also suspicious that SSN was organizing to gain negotiating leverage. Therefore, consistent and appropriate provider incentives in the risk development model were important to

FIGURE 1
Surplus distribution model

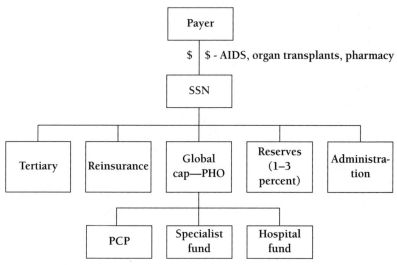

the payers, even though SSN was accepting global medical risk. As a result of these market realities, SSN developed the global risk distribution model shown in Figure 1.

Primary care physician

PCPs were capitated with adjustments based on patient demographics for enrollment with each PCP, group, or site. SSN realized that demographic adjustments would become increasingly important as the PHOs began to serve different communities under the same risk pool structure. These enrollment-based adjustments were especially important because the physicians could adversely select high-risk patients based on the level of services provided by hospitals. Primary care capitation rates, adjusted by age and sex, were calculated as depicted in Table 5.

Specialist capitation

Initially, SSN was not able to capitate all specialists, because the five PHOs had different levels of negotiating leverage with their specialists. For example, PHO A, in existence for many years, was moving PCPs back to FFS and specialists toward capitation, thus adopting a "reverse

TABLE 5
Demographically adjusted capitation rates

Age/sex distribution	Percentage	Standard age/sex factor	$5 Copay	$15 Copay
<2	3.00%	2.500	$35.00	$28.75
2–5	7.00%	1.350	$18.90	$15.53
6–19	21.00%	0.800	$11.20	$9.20
20–44 M	23.00%	0.700	$9.80	$8.05
20–44 F	25.00%	1.000	$14.00	$11.50
45+ M	10.00%	1.150	$16.10	$13.23
45+ F	11.00%	1.250	$17.50	$14.38
Total or average	*100.00%*	*1.000*	*$14.00*	*$11.50*

Services covered:
Office and home visits
Hospital visits
24-hour and emergency care
Other hospital care provided by PCP
Usual service provided in office, immunizations, injections, preventive care
Excludes cost for injectible materials
Lab tests if U&C less than $35.00
Excludes obstetrical neonatal care

Courtesy of Reden & Anders Consultants & Actuaries

capitation" methodology. This change in direction was based on a belief that PCPs needed to be incented to provide more care and refer less readily. This PHO also believed that specialists needed stronger incentives to monitor expenditures and resource use. Operating in a political environment where, as a low-intensity community hospital dominated by primary care providers, the PHO could afford for some specialists to drop out of the PHO if they would not accept capitation. It was also expecting high-enrollment volumes due to the large number of PCPs and, therefore, could capitate most specialists with a reasonable level of predictability of resource utilization.

PHO B was in an opposite market situation. The hospital component is a tertiary facility with an 80 percent specialist and 20 percent PCP distribution. The specialists dominate medical leadership and use their contribution to hospital revenue as potential leverage. This was done in light of the political issues of some of the PHOs and to balance market demands with an operational goal of a common reimbursement methodology. SSN decided to capitate specialty care at the PHO level but pay specialists FFS based on a budget calculated annually.

Fee schedule development

SSN developed a relative value unit (RVU)-based fee ceiling in which specialists were paid at charges or the ceiling amount, whichever was lower. Capitated specialty risk was taken at the PHO level. The fee ceiling was also used to reprice PCP claims to charge them back against the PCP's capitation rates to determine profit or loss. The fee ceiling was developed using a relative value methodology adjusted to the region's Blue Cross/Blue Shield (BCBS) managed care fee schedule. This methodology was agreed upon because

- The RVU methodology created some reimbursement equity among physicians and smoothed historical disparity between primary care and specialist reimbursement

- The BCBS fee schedule was used as a benchmark and adjusted the RVU methodology so that the reimbursement ceiling had relevance to a market standard. In addition, ceiling fees could be adjusted to more closely align with market rates for the few subspecialties with high demand and low supply

This methodology balanced pure equity standards (RVUs) with historical reimbursement (BCBS schedule) to move reimbursement toward relative value without ignoring historical reimbursement.

Hospital capitation development

First, a budget for each hospital's inpatient services was established by looking at projected and historical hospital service expenditures from the state rate filings. Next, PHOs were asked to propose desired hospital reimbursement rates to determine if the hospital's reimbursement requests could be met within the limits of the projected hospital budget. SSN hospitals proposed reimbursement on both a per diem and DRG basis for comparison purposes. Although some hospitals preferred DRGs, SSN members realized HMOs would push for per diem rates for comparability and ease of administration. SSN's actuaries established a global per diem target of $1,500 and established per diem categories for reimbursement by type of service as shown in Table 6.

TABLE 6
Hospital rate development

Service type	Per diem
Medical	$1,100
Surgical	$1,650
High-risk cardiology	
Cardiac surgery**	$25,000–$37,000
Angioplasty**	$10,000–$15,000
Diagnostic cardiology*	$5,000
Deliveries	
Vaginal*	$2,700
Cesarean*	$5,700
Neonate	$1,500
Behavioral	$775
Rehabilitation	$800

*Represents case rate.
**Represents case rate range.
Courtesy of Reden & Anders Consultants & Actuaries.

In the analysis, SSN realized that one of its hospitals provided high-intensity cardiology services with an average length of stay (ALOS) lower than the market. Therefore, the cardiology per diem reimbursement was inadequate for some services. Because SSN did not want to provide one of its PHOs with higher hospital capitation than its partners, it established case rates for outlier services that did not fit within the cardiology per diems. These outliers included cardiac surgery, angioplasty, and diagnostic cardiology. Because of their low length of stay and high intensity, one hospital had market competitive case rates but not market competitive per diems. To keep reimbursement fair, the risk for these cardiology cases was moved up from the PHO level so that all SSN hospitals with admissions for these DRGs would be paid the same. Also, under this methodology, the hospital with significant exposure for these types of cases could accept the same hospital capitation as its partners.

A market rate for outpatient hospital capitation was also created, with a corresponding internal distribution methodology of discount off charges. This methodology will evolve into ambulatory payment groups (APGs) as the market more uniformly adopts this payment methodology.

SSN's hospitals also agreed to assume risk for the "other medical services" category (e.g., durable medical equipment, home health). The hospitals feared that if they asked physicians to take risk for these services, physicians would most likely shop rates within the partner hospitals, a negative since most of these services were hospital owned.

Surplus and deficit distribution

Once SSN established its risk pool structure, the next step was to develop risk pool distribution scenarios for surpluses and deficits. Pool reserves were generated through capitation withholds of 10 percent for primary care, 15 percent for specialists, and 20 percent for hospitals. Distribution of withholds is based on the model depicted in Figure 2. Sample surplus and deficit results are shown in Tables 7 and 8.

In a market where utilization was sure to decline, creating hospital pool surpluses, SSN's hospitals viewed global capitation as an advantage. Under SSN's global risk pool, 40 percent of hospital pool surpluses are returned to the hospitals. In a typical HMO capitation arrangement, the HMO shares pool surpluses with physicians, and hospitals receive no portion. A typical HMO surplus payout would be arranged as indicated in Figure 3.

FIGURE 2
Surplus distribution model

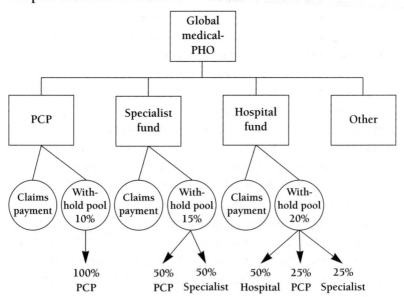

TABLE 7
Risk sharing examples

Hospital risk sharing

	PMPM	Total amount
Member months	120,000	
Hospital fund	$53.00	$6,360,000
Less reinsurance	($3.50)	($420,000)
Net hospital fund	*$49.50*	*$5,940,000*
Actual claims paid	$39.60	$4,752,000
Less pooled claims	($2.45)	($294,000)
IBNR	$9.90	$1,188,000
Net hospital claims	*$47.05*	*$5,646,000*
Fund gain/(loss)[1]	$2.45	$294,000
Fund gain/(loss)—sharing[2]		
PCPs (25%)	$0.61	$73,500
Specialists (25%)	$0.61	$73,500
Hospital (50%)	$1.23	$147,000
Total	*$2.45*	*$294,000*

Specialist risk sharing*

	PMPM	Total amount
Member months	120,000	
Specialist fund	$32.00	$3,840,000
Actual claims paid	$29.44	$3,532,800
IBNR	$1.47	$176,640
Net referral claims	*$30.91*	*$3,709,440*
Fund gain/(loss)[1]	$1.09	$130,560
Fund gain/(loss)—sharing[2]		
PCPs (50%)	$0.54	$65,280
Specialists (50%)	$0.54	$65,280
Total	*$1.09*	*$130,560*

Total PCP reimbursement

	PMPM
Capitation	$15.00
Risk-sharing gains	
Hospital	$0.61
Pharmacy	$0.20
Specialist	$0.54
Total	*$16.35*

Total specialist reimbursement

	PMPM
Capitation	$32.00
Risk-sharing gains	
Hospital	$0.61
Pharmacy	$0.20
Specialist	$0.54
Total	*$33.35*

TABLE 7 (CONTINUED)
Total hospital reimbursement

	PMPM
Capitation	$53.00
Risk-sharing gains	
Hospital	$1.23
Total	$54.23

1. Reflects share of funds available to distribute to each group. Actual distributions to a particular provider may vary depending on provider profile, adherence to preventive care, and utilization management guidelines.

2. Typically, calculation is performed two or three times a year, with a final settlement well after year-end. During periodic calculations, 50% of year-end funds could be distributed, with remainder held until the final settlement.

TABLE 8
Risk-sharing examples

Hospital risk sharing

Member months	120,000	PMPM	Total amount
Hospital Fund		$53.00	$6,360,000
Less reinsurance		($3.50)	($420,000)
Net hospital fund		$49.50	$5,940,000
Actual claims paid		$42.08	$5,049,000
Less pooled claims		($2.45)	($294,000)
IBNR		$10.52	$1,262,250
Net hospital claims		$50.15	$6,017,250
Fund gain/(loss)[1]		($0.64)	($77,250)
Fund gain/(loss)—sharing[2]			
PCPs (25%)		$0.16	($19,313)
Specialists (25%)		$0.16	($19,313)
Hospital (50%)		$0.32	($38,625)
Total		$0.64	($77,250)

Specialist risk sharing

Member months	120,000	PMPM	Total amount
Specialist fund		$32.00	$3,840,000
Actual claims paid		$31.36	$3,763,200
IBNR		$1.57	$188,160
Net referral claims		$32.93	$3,951,360
Fund gain/(loss)[1]		($0.93)	($111,360)
Fund gain/(loss)—sharing[2]			
PCPs (50%)		$0.46	($55,680)
Specialists (50%)		$0.46	($55,680)
Total		$0.93	($111,360)

TABLE 8 (CONTINUED)

Total PCP reimbursement

	PMPM
Capitation	$15.00
Risk-sharing gains	
Hospital	($0.16)
Pharmacy	($0.17)
Specialist	($0.46)
Total	*$14.21*

Total specialist reimbursement

	PMPM
Capitation	$32.00
Risk-sharing gains	
Hospital	($0.16)
Pharmacy	($0.17)
Specialist	($0.46)
Total	*$31.21*

Total hospital reimbursement

	PMPM
Capitation	$53.05
Risk-sharing gains	
Hospital	($0.32)
Total	*$52.73*

1. Reflects share of funds available to distribute to each group. Actual distributions to a particular provider may vary depending on provider profile, adherence to preventive care, and utilization management guidelines.

2. Typically, calculation is performed two or three times a year, with a final settlement well after year-end. During periodic calculations, 50% of year-end funds could be distributed, with remainder held until the final settlement.

FIGURE 3
HMO surplus payout

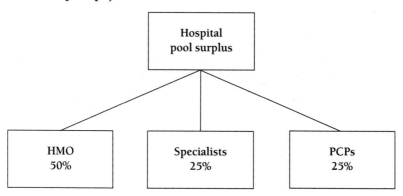

Therefore, by aggressively entering the marketplace with a global capitated product, SSN's hospitals could participate in potential financial
surpluses generated by declining hospital utilization. SSN's hospitals felt
that their alternative was to stand by, as HMOs and physicians gained
financially from dropping hospital utilization with the hospital accepting the loss with no opportunity for any gain.

Conclusion

Effective gains, losses, or risk model adjustments as a result of SSN's
experience are not reportable at this time. There is lack of statistically
significant experience of their members and limited payments flowing
through this model over an adequate period of time. However, lessons
learned by the physician leaders, hospital executives, and PHO executives who participated in the merger of SSN's managed care contracting
about the initial process of early integration are as follows:

1. *Pick partners wisely.* Provider cost is not the only issue. Effective management decision-making processes, physician-hospital relations,
   and partner trust and managed care sophistication all play a role in
   successful integration

2. *Pick consultants wisely.* Actuaries, attorneys, and managed care consultants can jumpstart an integration effort and facilitate the provider's
   movement into more competitive market positions. These same pun-
   dits can consume significant partner goodwill and integration energy,
   to say nothing of the expended opportunity cost, if they are not effective in consulting or providing the appropriate expertise to accomplish the effort

3. *Resolve strategic issues in the planning phase.* The SSN hospitals made a
   commitment to their physicians that the physicians could more easily agree on than the physicians could collectively approve of their
   reimbursement. In fact, hospital capitation development took six
   months because, as the hospital CFOs moved through the capitation
   model options, unresolved strategic issues kept presenting road-
   blocks for the process of developing and implementing capitation

For example, throughout the 14-month Super PHO development phase, SSN never addressed the fact that one hospital was significantly higher cost than the rest. Whether this hospital should or would accept the same capitation as its hospital partners was never resolved in the entire development period. As a result, the hospitals struggled through this issue repeatedly as the capitation budget was prepared, which significantly delayed implementation. The hospitals finally negotiated a compromise whereby one hospital was paid a higher hospital capitation that still equated higher discounts than those required by the rest of the hospitals in SSN. This capitation will be equitably adjusted based on actual experience once the hospital's claims history becomes credible

4. *Conduct an appropriate market assessment.* SSN developed its strategy based on what its members saw happening in other parts of the country not using its own market as a strategic planning benchmark. However, a high-quality market assessment may have led SSN to different conclusions regarding who, how, and what to capitate than the conclusions it drew initially

5. *View networking and capitation development as a process, not an end point.* At first, SSN's providers looked at the capability to provide services under one global, capitated methodology as an end, not to an enhanced market share or greater cost effectiveness. As they worked through the process, SSN providers realized the goal was still better patient care. Global capitation motivates more competitive cost through appropriate financial incentives and creates flexibility in managed care contracting. A bigger network simply facilitates the spreading of risk and creates negotiating leverage. Even though SSN achieved these goals in the process, SSN leaders recognized that creating or enhancing SSN's ability to contain cost, provide quality care, work together to create benchmarks, and serve the community will determine its ultimate success

EXHIBIT 1
Sea Shore Network
DRG analysis by attending physician for Hospital A

DRG 127	Physician 1	Physician 2	Physician 3
Number of discharges	76	48	37
Number of days	271	155	114
ALOS	3.6	3.3	3.1
Average per patient costs			
Operating room	$8	$13	$14
Lab	$565	$525	$628
Radiology	$340	$274	$335
Prescription drugs	$300	$304	$241
Supplies	$15	$17	$27
Other ancillary	$740	$718	$735
Total ancillary	*$1,968*	*$1,851*	*$1,980*
Routine nursing	$2,645	$2,933	$2,970
Special nursing care	$768	$852	$863
Total nursing	*$3,413*	*$3,785*	*$3,833*
DRG total	*$5,381*	*$5,636*	*$5,813*
Average per diem	$1,495	$1,708	$1,875
PMPM expense	$0.14	$0.09	$0.07
Severity adjustment	1.00	0.94	1.01
Adjusted average per diem	$1,500	$1,836	$1,855
Adjusted PMPM expense	$0.14	$0.10	$0.07

Note: All data are from PHO information system. If the PHO system cannot severity adjust data, data may require severity adjustments through a third party such as Dun & Bradstreet Health Information, LP.

Physician 4	Physician 5	Physician 6	DRG total
24	20	13	215
100	67	46	753
4.2	3.4	3.5	3.5
$7	$5	$14	$10
$725	$400	$454	$563
$399	$458	$294	$339
$217	$375	$476	$299
$29	$18	$27	$20
$689	$710	$773	$728
$2,066	*$1,966*	*$2,038*	*$1,959*
$2,550	$3,117	$2,805	$2,805
$741	$906	$815	$815
$3,291	*$4,023*	*$3,620*	*$3,620*
$5,357	*$5,989*	*$5,658*	*$5,579*
$1,275	$1,761	$1,617	$1,594
$0.04	$0.04	$0.03	$0.42
1.05	1.00	1.04	1.04
$1,209	$1,745	$1,554	$1,527
$0.04	$0.04	$0.02	$0.40

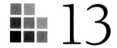 13

Budgeted capitation as a transition model

Margaret L. Houy
Manager, Network Development

Christine Profita
Joint Venture Program Specialist
Harvard Pilgrim Health Care, Inc.[1]
Quincy, Massachusetts

THIS CHAPTER IS DIVIDED INTO TWO major sections. The first explains a budgeted capitation model used successfully by Pilgrim Health Care (PHC), an IPA model HMO located in Quincy, Massachusetts. This model was used to introduce physicians and hospitals to managed care and to educate them on needed changes in practice patterns. PHC has effectively employed this model as a transitional step for bringing physicians under a direct capitation model and for creating locally managed physician-hospital risk-sharing groups. The second section explores the dynamics necessary for a group to operate successfully under budgeted capitation and highlights the ways in which PHC is moving to strengthen its budgeted capitation model to incorporate direct capitation components.

Historically, local physicians have been reluctant to participate in a direct capitation program (under which they would receive monthly predetermined payments) for fear of not knowing how to bring their practice patterns into line with the capitation amount. In 1988, PHC developed a budgeted capitation model that allows providers to be paid on a fee-for-service (FFS) basis and be at-risk for inefficient care or share surplus for efficient performance. Today results have been tighter management of care, higher provider satisfaction, and increased administrative efficiencies.

Transitional model

DEFINITION

Budgeted capitation, also called "phantom" capitation, has the following key characteristics:

- A specified dollar capitation amount is credited through a book entry to a local risk-sharing group of providers that PHC calls a joint venture (JV). The amount credited to the JV is based on the number of members choosing primary care physicians (PCPs) associated with a particular JV

- Healthcare expenses are debited against the JV account as they are paid by PHC on a claims submission basis. Payment rates are determined by fee schedules and contracted rates. Payments are made at fee schedule allowables, minus a percentage withhold amount. The withhold is retained by PHC until the year-end settlement

- One hundred and twenty days after the end of PHC's fiscal year, each JV's total healthcare expenses are calculated and compared against the total credited capitation amount. Settlement is delayed 120 days to allow all but a minute number of claims to be processed. Based on the settlement outcome, the JV has an opportunity for full or partial return of withhold and for risk or surplus sharing with Pilgrim

JOINT VENTURE COMPOSITION

To be responsive to its healthcare community, PHC has emphasized flexibility in the composition of its JVs. All JVs must have PCPs, since PHC operates on a gatekeeper or care manager model. However, since local physician communities vary in their interest in and ability to participate in a risk-sharing venture with the local hospital and specialty physicians, PHC has JVs composed of PCPs only; with PCPs and specialists; and with PCPs, specialists, and hospitals. Each JV participant is linked together by contract to a budgeted capitation rate and to surplus- and risk-sharing terms.

Budget capitation rate

The budgeted capitation rate is derived from PHC's premium yield in the following manner. First, PHC determines its average annual capitation amount by converting its premium yield into a capitation amount by eliminating the family premium subsidy.

Second, PHC retains a small percentage for its overhead expenses with the remaining large percentage of premium allocated for all healthcare costs, including medical, surgical, outpatient, and prescription drug costs. PHC currently retains approximately 11 percent for overhead and contribution to reserves with 89 percent of the capitation amount allocated for healthcare costs.

Third, PHC determines the per member per month (PMPM) capitation rate for each JV based on the average annual capitation adjusted for geographic location, benefit mix, age/sex, and group size. Pilgrim then credits each JV with a monthly capitation rate for each member selecting a PCP participating in a JV.

JV membership is determined by the number of members choosing JV PCPs. For example, if the PCPs in JV A are responsible for providing the care to 5,000 members and the capitation level for their JV is $100 PMPM, JV A would receive monthly credit revenues in the amount of $50,000, or $600,000 annually.

PHC also makes an additional 1 percent of its premium revenue available to each JV if the JV meets established performance criteria. To date, the performance criteria are expressed in terms of percentage improvements in costs and utilization experience from the previous year for established JVs and over planwide costs and utilization experience for new JVs.

Budgeted capitation services

PHC's JV model is based on a global capitation to emphasize the need for coordination among all participants in the healthcare system.

This model provides strong incentives for the various provider groups to work as a system. Therefore, all services provided as a benefit to members are covered by the JV capitation rate with one exception: mental health services (including both psychiatric and substance abuse inpatient and outpatient services) are carved out of the capitation rate and are entirely administered by PHC. The health plan has found that few local providers have the programs and experience to efficiently manage mental health services, and few JVs are willing to accept this risk. Under the global capitation model, the JV is responsible for the cost of all medical services of their members regardless of location of services.

PHC mandates a stop-loss reinsurance program to protect the JV against high-cost cases, including outpatient prescription drug expenses. JVs are charged a premium for the stop-loss coverage. The stop-loss coverage has established inpatient and outpatient deductibles and coinsurance obligations.

For example, JVs with more than 2,000 members have an outpatient deductible of $16,500 per member per year, a 10 percent coinsurance obligation for costs above the deductible, and an inpatient deductible of $35,000 with the same 10 percent coinsurance obligation. The combined premium for that coverage is approximately $9.00 PMPM. JVs with fewer than 2,000 members have a combined inpatient and outpatient deductible of $16,500 with a 10 percent coinsurance obligation for costs above the deductible. The premium for that coverage is approximately $17.00 PMPM. Pilgrim prices the stop-loss or reinsurance coverage at its cost.

Provider compensation and withhold amounts

Under Pilgrim's budgeted capitation model, providers continue to submit claims and be paid on a FFS basis. In-plan physicians are reimbursed for services on an established fee schedule, less applicable withholds and member copayments, coinsurance, and deductibles. In-plan hospitals are paid in accordance with negotiated rates and established outpatient fee schedules, less applicable withholds and member copayments, coinsurance, and deductibles.

All providers participating in a JV are subject to a withhold on claims payments. Physician withhold for services performed in-office (including all obstetrical physician services) is 10 percent of the allowed fee for the procedure and 20 percent for all physician services provided in a hospital setting. Physician withhold amounts are deducted at the time of payment and retained by PHC.

The JV hospital withhold for all hospital services provided to JV members averages 15 percent. The hospital withhold is a booked liability and is not actually withheld on a claims-paid basis as is the case with physician withhold. If, at the time of settlement, the JV owes risk monies to PHC, it bills the JV hospital for the amount owed.

Risk and surplus sharing

At the fiscal year's end, the budgeted yearly capitation revenue is compared against actual claims payments made to all providers for services rendered to JV members, excluding mental health services for which the JV is not at-risk. Healthcare expenses include services provided by any provider rendering services to a JV member, including out-of-plan providers, community and tertiary level services provided outside of the JV, ancillary providers, and skilled nursing facility providers.

If expenses are less than the yearly capitated revenue amount, then the JV experiences a surplus. Each JV provider will have all of his or her withhold returned, and the JV will share in the surplus amount with PHC.

Historically, PHC has shared surplus equally with JV participants, although JV determines how it wishes to distribute to its provider members its share of the surplus. Some JVs distribute the surplus proportionately, according to billed amounts, while others distribute surplus based on PCP panel size and performance criteria specific to the goals and objectives of the JV.

If the expenses are greater than the capitated amount, then the JV experiences a loss. The JV providers assist in funding the loss up to the amount of the JV providers' withhold balance. For example, if the withhold pool contains $10 PMPM and the deficit amounts to $5 PMPM, PHC would retain $5 PMPM of the withhold amount and distribute the remaining $5 PMPM to JV providers in proportion to their contribution to the withhold pool. If the JV's loss exceeds the withhold, PHC is responsible for covering that "excess" loss. Therefore, if the JV loss were $15 PMPM and the withhold pool was $10 PMPM, PHC would retain the entire withhold pool of $10 PMPM and pick up the additional $5 PMPM of loss.

In PHC's JV model, providers' ultimate level of financial exposure is limited to their contribution to the withhold pool. Figure 1 summarizes the funds flow in a budgeted capitation model.

FIGURE 1
Joint venture funds flow

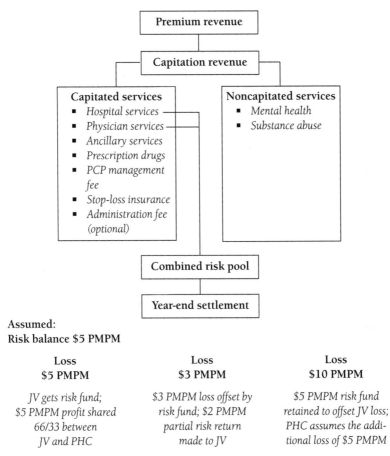

Premium revenue

Capitation revenue

Capitated services
- *Hospital services*
- *Physician services*
- *Ancillary services*
- *Prescription drugs*
- *PCP management fee*
- *Stop-loss insurance*
- *Administration fee (optional)*

Noncapitated services
- *Mental health*
- *Substance abuse*

Combined risk pool

Year-end settlement

Assumed:
Risk balance $5 PMPM

Loss $5 PMPM	Loss $3 PMPM	Loss $10 PMPM
JV gets risk fund; $5 PMPM profit shared 66/33 between JV and PHC	*$3 PMPM loss offset by risk fund; $2 PMPM partial risk return made to JV*	*$5 PMPM risk fund retained to offset JV loss; PHC assumes the additional loss of $5 PMPM*

Dynamics of a successful joint venture

A successful JV also needs appropriate support programs, performance data, providers committed to managed care, and supportive market dynamics.

SUPPORT PROGRAMS AND PERFORMANCE DATA

Joint venture medical director

Each JV is expected to identify and appoint a local medical director, most often a PCP. A strong JV medical director is essential to work with PCPs to help make difficult managed care decisions such as identifying the most appropriate facilities for member care, addressing aberrant practice patterns, and working with the managed care company to communicate management issues.

Standard reports

PHC provides three performance management reports on a monthly basis: a profit and loss statement (see Table 1), an inpatient utilization report (see Table 2), and a PCP referral management report. These monthly reports provide the JV with an overview of its performance.

On a quarterly basis, PHC produces a budget-to-actual capitation analysis (see Table 3) that includes information on 74 different categories of inpatient, outpatient, physician, and ancillary services. The report delineates three types of information about each category of service: average unit cost, utilization per 1,000, and PMPM costs. This quarterly report enables the JV to quickly identify areas associated with significant capitation expenses in which either cost or utilization experience is out of line with budgeted expectations.

TABLE 1
Statement of revenue and expenses
JV NAME
7/01/94 through 4/30/95

	Current month	PMPM	Year to date	PMPM
Revenue:				
Capitation—basic	$664,114	$143.65	$6,831,813	$146.60
Reinsurance cost	($40,775)	($8.82)	($411,038)	($8.82)
Net Capitation—basic	*$623,339*	*$134.83*	*$6,420,775*	*$137.78*
Capitation—drug	$65,739	$14.22	$627,610	$13.47
Reinsurance recoveries	$26,419	$5.71	$353,170	$7.58
Total revenue	*$715,497*	*$154.76*	*$7,401,555*	*$158.83*
Expenses:				
Inpatient services	$74,123	$16.03	$1,725,204	$37.02
Medical and surgical	$391,310	$84.64	$4,054,402	$87.00
Prescription drug	$72,516	$15.69	$761,055	$16.33
Management fee	$5,807	$1.26	$58,307	$1.25
Total expenses	*$543,756*	*$117.62*	*$6,598,968*	*$141.60*
Net income (loss)	*$171,741*	*$37.14*	*$802,587*	*$17.23*
Physician withhold	*$9,538*	*$2.06*	*$97,658*	*$2.10*
Total membership	4,623		46,603	

TABLE 2
HMO joint venture inpatient utilization February 1995

Days per 1,000	JV A	Total JV	PIPA[1]	Total plan
Adult medical	93	97	107	104
Adult surgical	51	58	75	67
Obstetrics	27	32	34	33
Pediatric medical	23	31	38	35
Pediatric surgical	10	6	5	5
Rehab	6	7	13	10
Skilled care	33	17	10	14
Total medical	*243*	*248*	*282*	*268*
YTD	*302*	*274*	*283*	*279*

Admissions per 1,000				
Adult medical	19.9	23.1	23.3	23.5
Adult surgical	7.7	15.6	17	16.4
Obstetrics	11.1	13.3	13.2	13.4
Pediatric medical	10	5	7.6	6.3
Pediatric surgical	3.3	1.8	1.3	1.6
Rehab	1.1	0.5	0.6	0.5
Skilled care	1.1	1.1	0.6	0.8
Total medical	*54.2*	*60.4*	*63.6*	*62.5*
YTD	*69.8*	*65.2*	*68.6*	*67.1*

Average length of stay				
Adult medical	4.67	4.21	4.58	4.42
Adult surgical	6.57	3.68	4.43	4.09
Obstetrics	2.4	2.42	2.53	2.47
Pediatric medical	2.33	6.32	4.94	5.49
Pediatric surgical	3	3.46	3.47	3.4
Rehab	5	14.33	21	18.14
Skilled care	30	16	17	16.36
Total medical	*4.47*	*4.12*	*4.41*	*4.28*
YTD	*4.33*	*4.2*	*4.12*	*4.16*

Surgical day care				
Monthly days per 1,000	37			
YTD days per 1,000	46			

Member months	JV A	Total JV	PIPA	Total plan
Monthly member months	10,844	157,211	155,816	313,027
Fiscal YTD member months	85,297	1,141,537	1,237,584	2,379,205

1. Pilgrim Independent Practice Association is composed of physicians not in JV arrangement.

TABLE 3
FY95 YTD budget to actual
Capitation analysis for fully insured HMO product

Type of service codes	Type of service	Frequency per 1,000	Average unit cost	Capitation
			Budget FY95	
	Hospital inpatient*			
1,4	Obstetrics	32.00	1,468.00	3.91
2	Inpatient medical	145.13	1,220.43	14.76
70	Rehabilitation administration	13.69	801.37	0.91
3	Inpatient surgery	114.00	1,718.29	16.32
7	Surgical day care	48.39	1,623.79	6.55
9	Skilled nursing facility	9.94	389.01	0.32
	Total hospital inpatient*	*373.91*	*1,418.85*	*44.21*
	Hospital outpatient*			
17	Emergency room in area	197	95.77	1.57
	Total hospital outpatient*	*390.06*	*127.20*	*4.13*
	Medical and surgical*			
19	Physician visits	3,091.65	51.28	13.21
44	Inpatient medical care	317.78	74.69	1.98
	Total medical and surgical*	*4,962.88*	*95.70*	*39.58*
	Other medical services*			
12	Laboratory	6,806.33	17.19	9.75
13	Radiology—professional and technical	417.5	116.23	4.04
14	Radiology—technical	565.73	201.16	9.48
15	Radiology—professional	683.43	49.71	2.83
	Total other medical services*	*11,821.32*	*41.43*	*40.82*
	Medical PMPM	84.53		
	Management fee	1.15		
	Rx drug	22.12		
	Total medical PMPM*	*107.80*		
	Grand total*	*152.01*		

*Type of service line items and category of services have been abbreviated for the purposes of this sample and will not calculate to totals.

Actual 7/94-4/95			Variance from budget increase/(decrease)			Percentage variance from budget increase/(decrease)		
Frequency per 1,000	Average unit cost	Capi-tation	Frequency per 1,000	Average unit cost	Capi-tation	Frequency per 1,000	Average unit cost	Capi-tation
19.50	1,311.67	2.13	(12.50)	(156.33)	(1.78)	(39%)	(11%)	(46%)
122.83	1,459.57	14.94	(22.30)	239.14	0.18	(15%)	20%	1%
70.19	755.58	4.42	56.49	(45.79)	3.50	413%	(6%)	383%
132.58	1,294.03	14.30	18.58	(424.26)	(2.03)	16%	(25%)	(12%)
76.04	883.57	5.60	27.65	(740.22)	(0.95)	57%	(46%)	(14%)
0.00	0.00	0.00	(9.94)	(389.01)	(0.32)	N/A	N/A	N/A
421.13	*1,180.29*	*41.42*	*47.22*	*238.57*	*(2.79)*	*13%*	*(17%)*	*(6%)*
177.87	118.75	1.76	(19.13)	22.98	0.19	(10%)	24%	12%
915.35	*92.11*	*7.03*	*525.29*	*(35.09)*	*2.89*	*135%*	*(28%)*	*70%*
3,131.78	55.75	14.55	40.13	4.46	1.34	1%	9%	10%
325.77	67.41	1.83	7.99	(7.28)	(0.15)	3%	(10%)	(7%)
4,526.79	*90.83*	*34.26*	*(436.09)*	*(4.87)*	*(5.32)*	*9%*	*(5%)*	*(13%)*
8,683.85	17.06	12.35	1,877.52	(0.13)	2.60	28%	(1%)	27%
501.64	91.38	3.82	84.15	(24.84)	(0.22)	20%	(21%)	(6%)
323.77	223.54	6.03	(241.95)	22.39	(3.45)	(0.43)	11%	(36%)
485.66	37.08	1.5	(197.78)	(12.63)	(1.33)	(0.29)	(25%)	(47%)
12,531.12	*37.18*	*38.82*	*709.80*	*(4.25)*	*(1.99)*	*6%*	*(10%)*	*(5%)*
80.11			(4.42)			(0.05)		
1.17			0.02			0.02		
16.95			(5.17)			(0.23)		
98.23			*(9.57)*			*(0.09)*		
139.65			*(12.36)*			*(0.08)*		

Using a capitation amount of $1.50 PMPM and a percentage budget variation of plus-25 percent has proven effective to identify areas requiring examination and improvement. Ad hoc reports are run to further identify the source of budget-to-actual variation and to develop effective corrective actions. These standard reports are reviewed in a meeting with each JV medical director on a regular basis. Depending on the needs of the JV, the meetings may occur on either a monthly or quarterly basis.

JV program team

A managed care company establishing a budgeted capitation model also needs to provide and support new programs on an ongoing basis. To meet this objective, PHC has created a cross-functional team that has top-level representation from PHC's financial reporting, medical services utilization analysis, JV development, and JV management departments. This JV program team is responsible for the following activities:

- Companywide JV policy development, such as determining the appropriate manner for protecting patient confidentiality while providing JV providers with needed data on their own members

- Management support, including coordinating year-end settlement and risk-return processes

- Creating and implementing an analytic support initiative that makes available specialized ad hoc reporting, monthly claim downloads, and analytic support

- Holding regional data needs assessment meetings to improve the data and reports provided to JVs

- Holding quarterly JV medical director meetings to convey program information and receive feedback from providers

- Support monthly performance review meetings held with each JV medical director to review monthly financial and utilization reports.

Medical services support

PHC provides each local JV medical director with a monthly stipend. The amount of the stipend varies with the number of members assigned to each JV to ensure that JV medical directors are adequately compensated for their services.

PHC also administers a voluntary case management program for complex or high-cost cases. Cases that meet predetermined criteria are assigned specially trained case managers to maximize efficient provision of care.

A major area of medical services support is PHC's pharmacy administration program, which is an aggressive cost-saving effort built around the promotion of prescribing "preferred" drugs. The program is supported through outpatient prescription reports that show, on a monthly basis, the prescription pattern by PCP of preferred and nonpreferred drugs and the potential savings if the use of preferred drugs were increased. Each JV medical director also receives a summary of his or her PCPs' prescription patterns.

The pharmacy unit identifies lesser-cost equivalents to guide prescription practices. It also publishes a quarterly pharmacy bulletin that identifies additional areas of potential cost savings, new drug information, and PHC policy changes.

PHC is implementing a formulary program in fiscal year 1996 that will have differential member copayment amounts to encourage use of drugs included in its formulary.

Finally, PHC has partnered with a major drug manufacturer to introduce through the JVs a new, lower-cost ACE Inhibitor, a high blood pressure medication. The introduction of this partnership through the JVs has required extensive physician education and resulted in significant cost savings for JVs that have successfully converted members to the new ACE Inhibitor.

Utilization management program

Hospital support for the JV centers on effective utilization management (UM) and quality assurance (QA) programs. The managed care company's and hospital's QA and UM programs must be coordinated to maximize the efficient provision of care, to identify alternative site locations, and to develop effective discharge planning.

MARKET DYNAMICS

To maximize the coordination of care, there is a need for consistent referral patterns within the JV. This means that patients need to utilize the JV hospital and associated specialists, specialty groups and PCPs need to support the hospital, and PCPs need to support the JV specialists. JVs

FIGURE 2
Dynamics of a successful joint venture

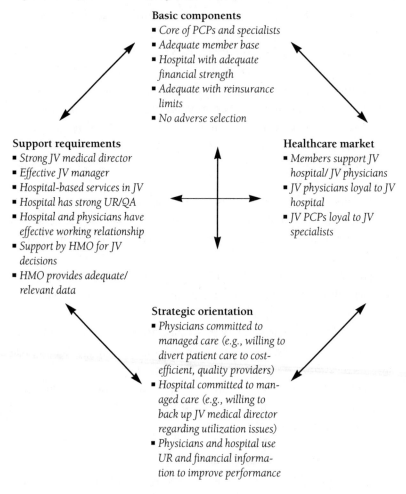

Basic components
- Core of PCPs and specialists
- Adequate member base
- Hospital with adequate financial strength
- Adequate with reinsurance limits
- No adverse selection

Support requirements
- Strong JV medical director
- Effective JV manager
- Hospital-based services in JV
- Hospital has strong UR/QA
- Hospital and physicians have effective working relationship
- Support by HMO for JV decisions
- HMO provides adequate/relevant data

Healthcare market
- Members support JV hospital/ JV physicians
- JV physicians loyal to JV hospital
- JV PCPs loyal to JV specialists

Strategic orientation
- Physicians committed to managed care (e.g., willing to divert patient care to cost-efficient, quality providers)
- Hospital committed to managed care (e.g., willing to back up JV medical director regarding utilization issues)
- Physicians and hospital use UR and financial information to improve performance

with many referrals out of the JV are not as successful in developing and integrating a healthcare team to provide efficient care. The dynamics of a successful JV are summarized in Figure 2.

Budgeted capitation strengths

A budgeted capitation model has enabled PHC to develop a partnership with local providers focusing on shared risk and surplus. This model strengthens a mutual commitment to successful utilization management.

PHC has been working with JVs since 1988. Over this time, Pilgrim has seen JVs move through several stages of development as they mature in their understanding of how to effectively manage care. Mature, successful JVs are increasingly interested in managing under direct capitation to maximize local control of the delivery of healthcare. As such, the budgeted capitation model has been successful as a transitional step toward direct capitation.

The budgeted capitation model also has promoted local autonomy for providers, encouraged local medical leadership, and identified opportunities for service improvement. These benefits have been realized under a system of manageable risk, limited to the amount of the provider's withhold.

PHC's budgeted capitation model emphasizes flexibility to maximize its attractiveness to local provider groups. Through its global capitation approach, PHC has integrated provider incentives by emphasizing the interrelationships of all caregivers.

Budgeted capitation is an evolutionary step, designed and implemented to develop an understanding of current practice patterns and the impact of changes in those traditional patterns. The success of PHC's JV is in the utilization numbers. Overall, JVs have consistently experienced lower utilization than providers not in such arrangements.

Budgeted capitation weaknesses

Budgeted capitation has weaknesses that should be acknowledged. First, it retains the traditional FFS incentives to bill more to earn more. This weakness underscores the importance of strong local leadership and the need to have relevant data to educate providers on needed changes in practice patterns.

Budgeted capitation also leaves the insurer potentially at greater risk, since the insurer is responsible for all risk beyond the withhold. It becomes critical to set the budgeted capitation level appropriately, to provide effective administrative support, and to work closely with providers to bring about necessary changes in practice patterns.

The need for committed providers is critical, but not always present. Similarly, the presence of strong, determined, local physician leadership is critical but not always available. Finally, a budgeted capitation model is not appealing to those providers who are uncomfortable in a team environment. This approach involves regular review of providers' practice patterns, suggestions of changes to be made, and give and take on arriving at decisions that are beneficial for the patient as well as for the JV. A brief case study will give context to the concepts discussed above.

Case study

PROBLEM

The JV in question became part of the PHC network through an acquisition. (As such, its original financial structure varied from the standard model discussed above. The manner in which that model was changed will both emphasize the points detailed previously and demonstrate the flexibility of the budgeted capitation model.) The JV has 10,000 members and includes PCPs, specialists, and a hospital. The PCPs are on a direct individual capitation with no withhold, the specialists are paid on a fee schedule with a withhold, and the hospital is at-risk for all losses beyond the provider withhold. The hospital has noncompetitive rates.

The JV has experienced a high number of specialty referrals and inpatient admissions. The JV has a high rate of adult and pediatric medical admissions. It also has weak physician leadership, so it is unable to effectively address any of these issues.

Given the financial structure of this JV, the capitated PCPs had an incentive to refer patients to the emergency room and to specialists and had no vested interest in the overall experience of the JV.

The hospital's incentive was to maximize revenues through admissions. The specialists were incented to maximize FFS billings. Not surprisingly, the JV had experienced losses for five years.

CHANGES

At the time the JV agreement between PHC, the hospital, and the physicians was up for renewal, PHC decided to take the initiative to restructure the relationship. Fundamental to creating a successful JV were aligning incentives and establishing local leadership to build commitment to managed care.

PHC and the hospital began the process by renegotiating competitive hospital rates and reducing the hospital withhold liability, with PHC picking up losses beyond the withhold. PHC also assisted the hospital with cash flow needs by advancing its portion of the expected surplus six months into the fiscal year. The hospital-based physicians also joined the JV and agreed to established fee schedules. Finally, the financial structure was changed by bringing the capitated PCPs under a withhold.

Aggressive support programs were put into place by first identifying a strong JV medical director and by increasing the financial support of the JV medical director to do local data collection and analysis. The hospital agreed to provide an administrative assistant to the JV medical director. With the help of PHC, the hospital strengthened its internal UR and QA programs. PHC also supported local initiatives to reduce medical care costs by implementing observation bed reimbursement arrangements to divert care to a less costly placement. Information provided to the JV was enhanced by supplying analytic resources to assist in the interpretation of monthly reports and the development of specialized report formats.

The local physician-controlled IPA increased its commitment to managed care by establishing a managed care steering committee to review all data, developing IPA policies regarding the JV's management, and reviewing information on physician practice patterns. Through the actions of the JV medical director, the IPA management committee identified high-admitting pediatricians and worked with them and the hospital to process admissions through the ER and eliminate direct admissions from the pediatricians' offices.

The hospital took specific steps to improve its market image by recruiting new physicians in key specialty areas where patients previously had gone to other facilities. The hospital also affiliated with a major teaching hospital and brought in tertiary specialists to provide specialty services within the community on a regular basis.

In 18 months, the JV participants (i.e., IPA physicians and hospital) developed a strong sense of local ownership. The IPA did innovative data analysis to identify opportunities for improvement, and the hospital developed a strong commitment to the JV's success.

In all, the changes paid off, and the JV has consistently earned substantial surpluses as a result of these efforts.

Areas of model improvement

The key area of its budgeted capitation model that PHC identified as needing improvement is performance incentives. PHC is considering substantially increasing the amount of the capitation tied to more focused performance standards.

For example, Pilgrim is considering tying 1 to 2 percent of capitation to an acceptable level of patient satisfaction measured through an annual, professionally administered survey. An additional percentage point might be tied to achieving a defined level of performance relating to preventive health initiatives (e.g., achieving an 80 percent rate of mammographies for female members more than 50 years of age).

Finally, a portion might be tied to achieving a specified level of inpatient days per 1,000 or by having less than a specified percent of denied days based on specified utilization review criteria.

PHC is looking at these options to link the JV's financial achievements more directly to physicians' changes in practice patterns. PHC believes that such an approach will demonstrate the benefits of local provider units working together.

Conclusion

The budgeted capitation model has the flexibility to be attractive to local providers inexperienced with managed care and to evolve over time to support a very tightly managed care system. The FFS incentives inherent in the budgeted capitation model need to be offset by strong local medical leadership, effective reporting by the managed care company, and financial incentives for the local providers to work effectively as a group.

NOTES

1. On January 19, 1995, Pilgrim merged with Harvard Community Health Plan (HCHP), a combined staff and group model HMO. The new company, Harvard Pilgrim Health Care, is now the largest HMO in Massachusetts.

14

Medicaid capitation and information management

Susan J. Fox, PhD
President
Fox Systems Inc.
Scottsdale, Arizona

L IKE MANY PRIVATE PURCHASERS and healthcare insurers, the Medicaid program is moving to capitation as a preferred model for delivering services to its eligible population. In doing so, federal and state agencies that administer the Medicaid program recognize the challenge of delivering quality services, providing broad access to care, and managing costs.

Medicaid agencies have a federally mandated benefit program to provide primary healthcare services to indigent mothers and children and blind and disabled Americans who meet eligibility requirements. States quickly developed the operational capacity to reimburse providers on a fee-for-service basis. The Medicaid Management Information System (MMIS) emerged as a federal standard for processing, maintaining, and reporting provider, beneficiary, and claims history data. Today, a variety of Medicaid delivery models spans a continuum from traditional fee-for-service (FFS) providers to fully capitated, prepaid, at-risk health plans, with many hybrid blends in between.

This chapter describes states' experiences with managed care, the gradual shift from FFS to capitated (fixed fee per member per month— PMPM) reimbursement, and the changing roles and responsibilities of state agencies and health plans. It also describes how data play a key role in shaping, assessing, managing, and monitoring delivery systems. A historical perspective on the meaning of "management" in Medicaid capitation and the case for state agency access to detailed data is also presented. What, who, and how Medicaid is being managed, are explored. Answers to these questions provide the platform to examine the importance of state agency access to and use of detailed data, leading to the conclusion that Medicaid capitation has fundamentally changed the way Medicaid agencies do business, including management of information.

Managed care models

Managed care is a global category used in state Medicaid programs to define a wide range of healthcare delivery options in which the common denominators are

- Enrollment of a beneficiary with a provider (ranging from single primary care physician to prepaid health plan)

- Payment of the provider for part or all of the services covered on a predetermined, prepaid, fixed rate PMPM basis (ranging from a simple case management fee to full benefit coverage under a prepaid health plan—PHP)

While there are a number of managed care models used by Medicaid state agencies, the dominant model is shifting toward capitation and full risk.

State Medicaid agencies have created models along all points of the Medicaid managed care continuum, as illustrated in Figure 1. This figure represents the continuum of managed care options from the FFS payment of a primary care physician (PCP) to the fully capitated reimbursement of the PHP.

The bottom of the continuum represents PCPs who bill FFS and receive an additional administrative PMPM fee to coordinate primary care services, write prescriptions, and arrange referrals to other providers. Primary care services not authorized by the PCP are not reimbursed by the state Medicaid agency.

The mixture of FFS payment and capitated PMPM payment changes along the continuum with progressively more risk and responsibility passing to the provider. As a rule of thumb, if the provider shares equally, at a minimum, in the risk of healthcare costs, there is enough incentive for the provider to actively manage patient care and costs.

FIGURE 1
Managed care continuum

Total risk
No reinsurance
No risk sharing

Full risk prepaid health plan/HMO	Comprehensive services. Contractor at-risk for PMPM fee.
Health insuring organization	Administrative services for an annual budget of services and administrative fees; completely at-risk. Providers have some risk sharing. Range: IPA, coalitions, health plans.
Partial risk prepaid health plan	PHP at-risk for medical services, but some benefits may be excluded (e.g., pharmacy, long-term care, mental health, dental).
Capitated benefit	Carve out of a single benefit (e.g., dental, pharmacy, or mental health). At-risk contractor receives PMPM capitation fee.
PCP network	A group of PCPs or PCCMs administered by an organization.
Primary care case management	Individual physician at-risk for primary care services. Receives PMPM capitation.
Primary care physician	Fixed fee for referral management (typically $2.00 to $3.00). No risk. State may provide incentives for reduction in total patient cost.
Fee for service	No provider risk. Traditional care management.

At the top of the continuum, the PHP or HMO assumes the majority of the risk for a designated PMPM fee. The state may share in the cost of catastrophic cases through a reinsurance policy for member expenses exceeding a threshold, and PHPs and HMOs adversely affected by a higher percentage of high-cost patients may receive risk pool compensation.

These models have been developed over 25 years in response to increasing pressures to manage program quality, service, and costs. Along the continuum of approaches there is an ever-increasing shift in financial risk and management responsibility from the state agency to the provider. When the state agency ceases to pay directly for rendered services, issues about ownership of and access to data come to a head. The following discusses questions of data access and management.

Data management

WHY MANAGED CARE?

Managed care models are attractive to state agencies for several reasons.

Federal and state revenue savings

Capitation offers states savings by shifting provider payment away from fees for services rendered to a predetermined rate per enrollee per month (capitation), thus placing the health plan at-risk for the delivery of care. Total capitation payments are fixed at levels lower than the FFS equivalent or, at a minimum, are budget neutral.

Predictability of expenditures

A monthly capitation payment is paid to the health plan based on the number of enrollees and associated premium rates. States can project expenditures based on trends in eligibility.

Delegation of administrative functions

States require health plans to plan, build provider networks, ensure access, promote education, reimburse providers, and perform utilization and quality management. It is the PHP's responsibility to deliver appropriate quality services and to reimburse its providers.

Reduction in state administrative burden

The increase in capitated contracts reduces the relationships the state agency has to maintain. Rather than contracting with and processing claims for 10,000 providers, the state agency maintains a relationship with perhaps 12 health plans, which either employ or contract with individual providers.

Best alternative under block grants

Sharing the financial risk with providers makes managed care a prime candidate for maintenance of health benefit programs under Medicaid block grants. In fact, states with successful prepaid health plan experiences may be disadvantaged under block grants. Their success in managing costs results in lower overall healthcare expenditures—the determinant for block grant allocations or capped federal contributions.

WHAT IS BEING MANAGED?

All healthcare services are authorized through a benefit design package and with administrative oversight. Under FFS reimbursement, the state agency is directly responsible for all administration and payment of service. As the contract model moves closer to full capitation, the burden of management shifts from the state agency to the capitated organization. The following are examples of the transfer of management responsibility.

Patient care management

In the FFS model, the provider is responsible for the services rendered and receives payment for these services. The state agency oversees the appropriateness and quality of care through a combination of claims edits and postpayment review functions. In capitated contracts, however, a health plan agrees to provide all services for a predetermined monthly fee per enrollee and accepts the responsibility for daily monitoring of appropriateness and quality. The state continues to perform overall monitoring.

Utilization management

The state uses all available tools to manage the utilization of services, including sophisticated claims-processing operations, program analysis, audits and investigations, and other strategies to restrict the number and cost of services. The at-risk health plan assumes the responsibility for utilization management. Unnecessary or inappropriate service, or over-utilization, results in higher costs and reduced profits for the health plan. To manage the services, the health plan must perform utilization management. However, it is in the state's interest to ensure its contracted health plans are managing utilization without reducing the level of care required for their enrollees.

Cost management

For nearly three decades, state agencies have been developing and using sophisticated approaches to managing FFS costs, including fee schedules, fixed dispensing fees, formularies, diagnostic-related groups (DRGs), and other reimbursement policies. Through managed care, the state can simplify its cost-management activities by focusing on an actuarially determined or negotiated PMPM rate and can substitute a set of capitation rates for thousands of individual service fees. Then, the health plan can manage its own costs. The state may intervene to manage distribution of high-risk cases or equalize payment for providers disadvantaged by higher numbers of enrollees requiring high-cost care.

Consumer satisfaction

The state agency and the health plan recognize the importance of retaining the enrolled member. Turnover and loss of members can jeopardize health plan financial stability. Therefore, states with capitated contracts periodically conduct consumer surveys to learn and report enrollee satisfaction. Managing consumer satisfaction becomes a primary concern for the at-risk managed care contractor who will seek to maintain enrollment levels during the year and retain membership during the period of open reenrollment—when individual members can choose to switch to another plan.

WHO IS THE MANAGER?

There is an inherent dualism in the Medicaid managed care model. For health plans, financial risk and management responsibility are intertwined. Public trust makes the Medicaid model of managed care different from commercial healthcare plans. No matter how much risk the provider assumes, the Medicaid agency remains the final guardian of the beneficiary's rights to access to medical care and the keeper of the tax-payer's purse.

There are also differences in roles shared by the provider and the state agency. For instance, both the provider and the agency have quality-of-care functions, financial management responsibilities, consumer satisfaction interests, and provider credentialing activities. However, the at-

TABLE 1

Responsibilities shared by providers and the Medicaid agency

Responsibility	Provider organization		State agency
	Low risk (PCP)	*Full risk (HMO)*	
Patient care management	Responsible for delivery of primary care	Responsible for providing all prescribed benefits	Defines benefit package
	Responsible for appropriate referrals	Usually assigns a PCP for care management	Defines rights of beneficiaries to receive care
		May define care management protocols	Audits managed care providers
			Hears beneficiary grievances regarding care
Utilization management	PCP may be at-risk for some part of the cost of referred services	For a fixed fee PMPM, must deliver necessary services	Monitors utilization through statistical analysis, comparison of health plan experience and health plan versus FFS, and on-site audits
	PCP authorization required for payment of referred services	Monitors all services for appropriateness	Responsible to the beneficiary for access to and quality of service
		PCPs and hospitals may share risk for appropriate utilization and cost containment	Responsible to taxpayer for maintaining savings in the capitation rates
			Monitors utilization to ensure health plan capability in cost management
Network management	Individual PCPs may form referral pools	PHP/HMO employ and maintain contracts with providers; own or contract with facilities	Establishes network rules, obligations
		Responsible for maintaining network	Contracts with, manages, and maintains PCP networks
		Network obligations established via contracts	Contracts with PHPs, HMOs
			Network requirements are part of PHP/HMO contract
			Approves network contracts

TABLE 1 (CONTINUED)

Responsibility	Provider organization		State agency
	Low risk (PCP)	Full risk (HMO)	
Network management (cont.)		Motivated to limit network to acceptable provider partners Maintains provider services	Monitors PHP/HMO for network compliance (e.g., number of providers by type, ratio of members to providers, access, licenses, sanctions) Must ensure adequacy of the network Hears appeals regarding provider complaints
Financial management	May have some risk for referred service costs related to fee withholds	At-risk for cost of care within revenue fixed by capitation payments Controls administrative overhead May contract with key provider partners to meet financial capitation targets	Establishes reimbursement policy, fees, rates for FFS, PCP administrative fee, and capitation rates May share in risk by paying for catastrophic care or managing risk pools to compensate for providers adversely affected by higher numbers of high-cost patients Ultimately responsible for overall program expenditures May be subject to state or federal mandates for cost savings, budget-neutral expenditures, or cost management within a budget fixed by a block grant ceiling
Quality-of-care management	Subject to audit and consumer satisfaction surveys	Must perform quality assessment internally May monitor outcomes Responsible for quality of care throughout the participating provider network Maintains member services Has grievance procedures	Audits providers Conducts consumer satisfaction surveys Wants to perform outcome measurement Hears beneficiary appeals regarding complaints and grievances Oversees enrollment and disenrollment process

risk provider must have daily operational control over the delivery of healthcare services, whereas the state oversees and monitors these activities from a distance. Table 1 illustrates the dual roles of providers and the state Medicaid agency.

HOW IS DATA MANAGED?

As the traditional management functions performed by the state agency shift to the health plan, the state's role changes from that of detailed manager to macromanager. This new role requires new skills, different business processes, and a strong dependency on data.

Program management begins with access to data and use of tools to transform data into information and information into knowledge. Data management is the tool to manage effectively the multitude of healthcare options. Technological advances, a refocusing of healthcare data analysis, and reporting have broadened states' data access options.

Twenty-five years ago, capitated health plans contracting with state Medicaid agencies negotiated to report utilization data in a high-level summary format, quarterly. In general, states agreed to this arrangement because

- Health plans said there would be significant costs to collect, convert, and submit detailed data

- Health plans used a wide range of data collection approaches (e.g., paper medical records and paper or automated claims from contracted providers)

- Plans collected different data elements and used different data structures

- Some plans had no automated information system; those that did used diverse vendors and products

- State agencies lacked system capacity to manage intake of health plan data including extraction, conversion, editing, storing, and reporting. There were no rigorous standards for FFS claims or health plan service data

Some states believe that health plan application evaluation, contractual requirements, periodic audits, and summary reports provide an adequate base for state monitoring of health plan contractors. That is, a health plan is awarded contracts because it has the administrative structure, provider network, management procedures, and proven track record to provide the covered benefits at a cost lower than the capitation revenue.

The barriers listed above prevented states from collecting detailed data at the beginning of managed care implementation. Rather, contracting health plans provided quarterly summary utilization and financial reports and underwent state audits. In the absence of real data, states rely on adjusted FFS data as a surrogate for capitated program utilization.

In the 1980s, Arizona, Missouri, Michigan, and Minnesota began prepaid health plan contracting and required detailed encounter data from the onset. Although the debate continues today, the trend is to collect detailed information from health plans (as is done in Hawaii). As a sign of the changing times, a task force is now working on a joint Medicaid/Medicare standard encounter data set.

Technological changes

Over the last three decades, computer technology has undergone dramatic change, and the healthcare industry has been a beneficiary. Some changes have had a positive effect on the management of health information, including

- Use of mainframe to client/server environments and personal computer workstations

- Hard-coded application programs replaced by flexible, user-friendly software applications

- Reliance on programmers to make any changes superseded by end-user control

- Manual data entry eliminated by electronic data submission, swipe cards, and point-of-service devices

- Separate files replaced by the ability to integrate databases

- Creation of electronic highways linking information systems of multiple organizations, including provider and payer

- Electronic Data Interchange standards applied to automated transaction transmission and processing

With the technical advances comes pressure exerted by employers demanding detailed reporting, which has resulted in comprehensive, efficient, accurate, and cost-effective collection, retrieval, and analysis of data. Whereas in the 1960s and early 1970s submitting detailed data may have been an administrative burden to both health plan and state for most managed care organizations, this is no longer true. Technology now makes it possible for health plans to fully comply with state data requirements and to satisfy employer reporting demands.

Standardization of data

In addition to technological changes, progress toward standardization enables states to integrate health plan data statewide. Receipt of standardized data allows states to compare health plan performance. Uniform data elements and claim and encounter format discussions have been under way over the past decade. While progress to standardize data has been slow, these efforts are beginning to bear fruit. States are participants in defining electronic data transmission standards and minimum data sets.

Pharmacy point-of-sale systems illustrate the advances in technology and standardization of data. Pharmacy benefit management organizations are electronically connected to pharmacies nationwide to perform eligibility verification, drug utilization review, provider profiling, and claims payment all in a single transaction initiated at the pharmacy. This capability is possible through an established, standardized, nationwide pharmacy data structure and use of state-of-the-art telecommunications. Linking the prescriber to the pharmacy electronically will complete the information loop between the state, health plan, physician, and pharmacy.

Refocusing data analysis and reporting

From the state's perspective there is a different focus in the analysis of FFS models versus capitation. For example, in the traditional FFS model, data analysis focuses on overutilization, fraud, and abuse of benefits. In the fully capitated, at-risk model, data analysis shifts to underutilization, quality of care, healthcare outcomes, rate setting, access to service, and comparative performance. Along all points of the managed care continuum, states have been experimenting with methods of managing the program through collection and analysis of data.

WHO GETS THE DATA?

A key to effectively managing the Medicaid program is the question of who owns or has access to the data: federal agencies, state agencies, the health plan, the provider network, consumer organizations, or the public? While states in the 1970s and 1980s may have believed that detailed data were not needed, most states today accept the need for information but still deliberate about what should be required.

State agencies have 25 years of Medicaid experience collecting and analyzing FFS claims data containing specific service and payment information. These agencies have more experience managing utilization and costs than any other healthcare financing organization through maintenance of information on population demographics, services rendered, and providers.

Although PCP model programs continue to generate claims, under full capitation programs claims are not submitted to the state. In lieu of claims data, some states require capitated health plans to submit encounter data. The term "encounter" refers to the patient and describes the physician-patient visit and associated services in a closed panel setting. This word has also been adopted in capitated Medicaid managed care programs to refer to the detailed record, equivalent to a claim, that describes a service rendered, such as a physician office visit or lab test. The encounter record, which contains a subset of claimlike data and may contain equivalent FFS dollar values, is used exclusively for reporting since payment to health plans is achieved through the prepaid capitation fee.

Information management is needed by participants at all administrative levels of the capitated Medicaid managed care program. Managed care challenges each stakeholder—the provider, the health plan, and the state agency—to use information to manage effectively business processes and treatment outcomes for Medicaid recipients. Table 2 describes potential use of data by each stakeholder in the Medicaid program.

Each stakeholder shares the responsibility for managing its share of the program prudently. The level and amount of detailed data required by healthcare management partners should be commensurate with the amount of risk assumed by the participant. The state agency can never

TABLE 2
Use of data by stakeholders

Stakeholder	Use of detail data
Provider—PCP (no risk)	Case load, referral statistics, income analysis (FFS, case management fee), proper payment, internal financial management, patient intensity, types of services rendered
Provider—PCP (partial risk)	Case load, case mix, personal performance ratings (report card), referral patterns, peer comparison, risk pool analysis, income analysis
Provider— subcapitated or performance-based (PCCM)	Case load, case mix, personal performance ratings (report card), referral patterns, peer comparison, PMPM utilization
Capitated health plan	Utilization management: provider profiling, referral management, prescription utilization patterns, disease management, case mix analysis, PMPM utilization statistics, HEDIS reporting and monitoring, quality of care and outcome analysis, case mix adjusted treatment outcome analysis, consumer satisfaction Financial management: comparison of costs to capitated payment, IBNR Other: provider contracting and credentialing, marketing and enrollment analysis, provider network performance, provider satisfaction
State Medicaid agency	Health plan profiling and comparison: utilization, quality of care, treatment outcomes Health plan medical and facility audits Federal reporting requirements: Office of Research and Development (ORD) with focus on access, utilization, and cost analysis; Health Care Financing and Administration (HCFA) with emphasis on total expenditures, audit of federal financial participation, and waiver approval Rate analysis Health plan financial analysis Fraud and abuse (PCP programs) Trend analysis: utilization, financial, and outcomes Patient access to care, quality of care, and satisfaction Evaluation of capitated expenditures versus the FFS equivalent Enrollment, disenrollment, auto-assignment analysis Case mix and adverse selection analysis Reinsurance payments Risk pool maintenance and distribution Adequacy of provider network, credentialing, performance monitoring

delegate all risk and responsibility because of its ongoing role of public fund trustee and public welfare guardian.

Access to health plan data

Variation in risk-sharing arrangements and their context have shaped contractual agreements between states and providers. The fundamental premises of managed care drive the continued need for detailed cost and utilization data.

Under block grant allocations or a capped federal contribution, more states may turn to the higher levels of managed care risk sharing with the provider community to operate within their fixed budget. In this case, the importance of information accessible to the responsible state agency is paramount. At the same time, advances in technology make access to uniform data more efficient.

The following are examples of how states use data analysis. These apply to both healthcare reform and block grant distribution.

FINANCIAL VIABILITY ANALYSIS

There will be an increase in the number of new players as more states initiate risk-sharing contracts. But many contracting health plans are not experienced in the management and delivery of prepaid services. With access to detailed service data, agency staff can examine the utilization of services reported by individual plans and compare plans against each other and FFS experience. Agency staff can assist plans to identify areas of potential overutilization and excessive subcontractor costs so corrective actions can be taken.

ADVICE FOR START-UP AND SAFETY-NET PLANS

Smaller health plans, start-up health plans, and safety-net providers (i.e., federally qualified health centers, public health service sites, and rural health centers) may lack sophisticated management information tools or systems. These plans are at greater risk of becoming insolvent and realize their precarious cash flow position too late to implement corrective actions.

Health plans do not have equivalent program management skills or ability. In the early stages of implementing managed care programs, states may, out of necessity, contract with start-up health plans, and even the best qualified health plans may find themselves in financial trouble. As risk-sharing partners, states should be able to provide technical advice on health plan management, but will be limited if they lack the necessary information. With the right information, states will be in a better position to provide the necessary advice to health plans.

HEALTH PLAN PERFORMANCE COMPARISON

While individual plans cannot compare their own detailed data with other plans' experience because they lack access to other plan data, the state agency may be able to provide this service. The value of the data comparison will be only as good as the detail and quality of the data submitted by the individual plans.

Advances in technology, communication systems, and standardization of data make it feasible to provide a database that both state agencies and participating at-risk providers can access, as long as provider specific and client identification information is protected.

RATE ANALYSIS AND DEVELOPMENT

As the population enrolled in prepaid health plans increases, the FFS pool is reduced. If the FFS pool cannot be used to derive a base FFS equivalent rate by age, sex, or zip code, it is important to have useable statistics on utilization and cost of services for actuarial analysis and PMPM rate determination.

QUALITY ASSESSMENT

Detailed service data allows the state agency to identify, in advance of an audit, those health plans, providers, or recipients whose profiles indicate aberrant or unusual patterns of utilization, especially in underutilization, inappropriate procedures, and inappropriate referrals.

Quality is a key factor in demonstrating the value of capitated managed care to providers and consumers. The managed care industry and Medicaid agencies have been working to define data reporting requirements, including quality of care indicators and using Health Plan Employer Data and Information Set (HEDIS) models, and other report card formats to track utilization and performance. Medicaid agencies are adopting and modifying these requirements for the Medicaid managed care plans.

Other quality indicators such as access to care, patient satisfaction, facility review, medical record review, and documentation practices require specialized auditing methodologies. Health plans are required to conduct regular and continuous quality improvement studies and report results to the states, benefit managers, employer groups, and regulatory and oversight commissions. Encounter and claims data are required to support quality assessment activities.

MODEL PRACTICES

States can take a leadership role to develop "best practices" if they can access detailed data. Best practices include identifying managed care organizations that demonstrate exemplary patient management and disease management practices. Both the medical community and state policy analysts regard best practices as important tools to reduce undesirable variations in medical treatment and promote optimal treatment outcomes.

ACCESS TO HEALTHCARE

With detailed data, reports demonstrating access to healthcare can be produced. These reports may include

- Unduplicated count of recipients receiving care from each PCP

- Ratios of beneficiaries to users for each major category of service

- Number of office visits, lab, and x-ray procedures PMPM

- Number of emergency room and outpatient hospital visits PMPM

- Across-plan comparisons of utilization

- Comparison of providers' utilization patterns within health plans

Without detailed data, the state must rely on independent surveys, at additional expense to the state, to determine customer satisfaction and quality and utilization of service.

VALIDATE REINSURANCE CLAIMS

With detailed data, the state can determine where limits for reinsurance should be set, what changes should be made, and which contractors have cases approaching stop-loss limits. In reviewing a reinsurance claim, states can access other recipient service history to compare treatment and related costs. Reference to other cases with the same demographics and diagnosis can help the state evaluate the merit of the claim.

COMPARATIVE ANALYSIS

With access to a database of service information, the state can produce periodic reports on utilization, health plan comparisons, most frequent diagnoses, trend analysis, and changes in patterns of utilization.

States with access only to periodic summary statistics are severely limited in this activity. Special studies conducted in lieu of access to detailed data require the cooperation of health plans, are labor-intensive, and become an extra expense for the state.

In all, states gain several management benefits from analyzing detailed service information. Detailed claims data from contracting health plans support the state's ability to manage utilization, quality improvement, actuarial and financial risk, and monitor treatment outcomes. Without detailed data the state has no means to perform essential planning activities, such as policy analysis, trend identification, and rate adjustment.

DATA ACCESS BARRIERS

There are several challenges that offset the argument in favor of state access to detailed health plan data. The issues listed below are being addressed by proponents of data access and information management.

Uniformity of data

Requiring detailed data from health plans imposes standards on contractors' record-keeping procedures. In states where detailed data are not required, each contractor has acquired or designed its own system, with different record formats, codes, and data elements. Thus it becomes extremely costly for the state to re-create uniform data by abstracting or extracting data from different medical record systems and healthcare MMIS.

However, as a prerequisite for electronic data transmission, Medicaid systems developers are undertaking efforts to standardize the medical record and healthcare information data sets. These standards will impose data uniformity. Data uniformity lowers the cost of collecting and integrating data from a variety of sources. The state and participating at-risk providers will benefit from these decisions.

Reversing decisions to forgo detailed data

If the state decides not to require detailed service data from contracting health plans, the decision cannot be easily reversed. Health plan contractors may resist and demand additional administrative fees for complying. States can overcome this resistance by lowering the cost of compliance and providing access to the resulting database.

Data accuracy and timeliness

Both health plans and states point out that detailed data supplied by health plans may be untimely and inaccurate. If detailed data are flawed, then summary statistics also may contain the same flaws. The state is then even further removed from a correct picture of utilization of services. The solution is to incentivize the provider to submit edited data according to the terms of its contract.

Some states have instituted incentives, as well as sanctions, for health plans' performance in providing accurate and timely encounter data. Health plans are encouraged to submit data because the state publishes report cards, which include submission of data as an item to be evaluated. Some states have also proposed monetary rewards for the submission of data. As an additional incentive, health plans may have access to summary statistics from competing health plans. If health plans do not provide data in a timely and accurate manner, states may impose sanctions, such as monetary penalties.

Defining the data set

State agencies must refine and standardize reporting elements. Data collecting builds historical experience to understand relevant elements and to understand changes in care and utilization. Several states, including California, Arizona, and Hawaii, have developed definitions of a minimum encounter data set. A major initiative was recently launched to create a Medicaid/Medicare version of a minimum encounter data set, nicknamed "McData." At the core of such data sets are basic FFS claim data elements such as patient and provider information and services performed, disease state, date, and location.

Differences in health plan data sets are found in data not obtainable (or not obtained) through routine claim submission, such as

- First examination for pregnancy in the second trimester rather than the first trimester

- Mammography exam results that indicate cancer

- Outcomes of treatment associated with the cancer and linked to the exam identifying the disease state

Future outlook

Changes taking place in healthcare technology and financing, coupled with the move toward health reform at the state level and the possibility of block grant allocation, are accelerating the conversion from FFS reimbursement to provider risk-sharing arrangements. Twenty-five percent of Medicaid eligibles today are enrolled in some form of managed care arrangements with more states planning or implementing managed care programs.

This move to managed care will catapult Medicaid agencies with model capitated managed care programs into national leadership roles. These state agencies are laying the groundwork for others to build upon. Their success in managing these large and complex programs will serve as models for the rest of the country. If state agencies gain access to health plan data they can then share their knowledge and expertise with others.

CHANGING MANAGEMENT ROLE

The growth of capitated managed care has fundamentally changed the shape of the Medicaid organization and its approach to management. Under capitation, health plans assume the risk and accountability of the Medicaid population. Claims are no longer submitted to the state for payment and day-to-day program decisions shift from the state to health plans and providers. In the end, the state remains the primary stakeholder, guardian of public welfare, and trustee of public funds. Thus the state continues to be responsible for

- Ensuring the quality of health services received by Medicaid beneficiaries

- Ensuring access to the healthcare delivery system

- Achieving its budgetary goals

- Awarding provider contracts to qualified organizations

- Managing expenditures

- Establishing capitation rates and reimbursing health plans

- Providing information (public accountability)

- Sustaining consumer satisfaction (beneficiary and taxpayer)

- Ensuring the ability of the delivery system (ensuring against interruption of service)

- Monitoring enrollment and disenrollment of members

- Managing member grievances and appeals

- Conducting health plan profiling and comparisons

- Conducting provider auditing

To manage the change process, state agencies have recognized the need to undergo some form of business reengineering and information engineering to facilitate the move from FFS to managed care.

Prognosis

State agencies implementing capitated programs in the 1980s reflected on lessons learned from the pioneers in the 1970s. States in the 1980s strengthened the contracting relationship with the health plans, required detailed encounter data, and expanded PCP networks as an alternative to full capitation. In the 1990s, managed healthcare is expanding rapidly and more states are calling for state-of-the-art decision support systems for their entire book of business—fee for service, capitation, and hybrid risk-sharing models. If managed care industry and public sector service delivery integration increases, there may be regional coalitions of employer, individual subscriber, and publicly financed healthcare programs that will purchase services collectively and draw management information from an integrated database.

The potential to build a comprehensive healthcare delivery system is strengthened by technology, which includes improvements such as

- Lower cost

- User workstation system architecture

- Speed and efficiency of point-of-sale transaction processing

- Linked referral information systems (e.g., physician, lab, pharmacy)

- Access to the information highway for additional sources of data

- Data uniformity

- Powerful decision support tools

Technology is bringing stability and predictability to the risk-sharing partners. Capitated delivery systems are maturing, and Medicaid administrators have learned that information is essential to rational risk management.

In the next few years, Medicaid agencies will increase the rate of conversion to capitated managed care; all urban areas are likely to have shared-risk arrangements involving government agencies (at a regional level) and provider organizations. There will be regional data exchanges, based on standardized data sets combining Medicaid, Medicare, CHAMPUS, and private payer data. Outcome data will be collected, providers will be profiled and assessed, and effectiveness of treatment will be measured. Complex security measures will be in force to protect the data from inappropriate use and to ensure provider and patient confidentiality. Paper will virtually disappear as medical records, referrals, and prescriptions are stored and transmitted electronically.

Access to and use of data will be the key to manage the twenty-first century's healthcare delivery program.

▪▪ 15

Case study: capitation, collaboration, and economic Darwinism

Cal James
Principal
APM Incorporated
San Francisco, California

I N L A T E 1 9 9 0 , T H E A L T A B A T E S Health System (ABHS) in Berkeley, California, began to lose its primary care physicians (PCPs) to Kaiser Permanente Medical Group (KPMG) in nearby Oakland. Capitation in the East Bay marketplace was less than 10 percent of most physicians' practice revenue. Kaiser's presence was monolithic, with more than 50 percent of the managed care marketplace, and Hill Physicians Medical Group (HPMG), with headquarters in San Ramon, was rapidly increasing its influence over private practice physicians through its fee-for-service reimbursement model. ABHS knew that to survive as a fee-for-service reimbursement system turned full risk capitation, it would have to dramatically increase the size of its PCP referral base and begin to add new business partners, including other hospitals and insurance companies.

ABHS first turned to the needs of its own physicians. It established a management services organization (MSO), Alta Bates Medical Resources (ABMR), to provide turnkey administrative services for fully integrated PCP practices across the East Bay. The MSO was also the administrative mechanism for Alta Bates Medical Group (ABMG), an IPA. At that time, having a single MSO serving the needs of both the IPA and fully integrated group practices was novel. IPAs and fully integrated groups are competitive in most communities, and it is difficult to create a management company to serve the needs of both. The president/CEO of the MSO was designated as the executive director of each of the client medical groups to maximize administrative coordination and minimize territorial conflict as the various organizations pursued their managed care goals.

ABMG had 275 physicians in 1990 and by 1996 has grown to almost 550 physicians through affiliated IPAs in the nearby cities of Pinole and San Leandro. Physicians affiliated with the ABHS through these IPAs currently manage more than 90,000 HMO enrollees in the East Bay, compared to an enrollment of 150,000 for HPMG and 700,000 for KPMG. Alta Bates Medical Associates (ABMA), a fully integrated primary care medical group affiliated with ABMR, grew from 29 to 35 physicians during this period, with a goal of 50 physicians by the end of 1997. Two more fully integrated primary care groups, Pinole Medical Group (PMG) and Alameda Medical Group (AMG), both with 10 physicians, are also served by ABMR. The PCP leaders of these three medical groups work together closely and may eventually merge to simplify administrative systems and governance.

The MSO model chosen by ABHS differs dramatically from the administrative models of its two main competitors, Hill Physicians and Kaiser. ABHS-affiliated physicians govern themselves, determine their own compensation schemes, own their contracts, and direct the course of managed care development. Physicians affiliated with HPMG are contracted individually by the medical group and have less to say about the management company's (Pri-Med) direction as it contracts with various health plans on their behalf. Kaiser offers a foundation model, where the medical group and hospital are business partners with the health plan. This merger of the providers with the health plan sets the stage for significant administrative economies and simplification of systems, giving Kaiser a potential competitive advantage.

Since the early 1990s, the three East Bay medical group competitors—Alta Bates, Hill, and Kaiser—have tried to enroll as many members as possible in order to achieve bargaining leverage with employers and payers. Since there was so much excess capacity of physicians and hospital beds in the East Bay, the three competitors have been locked in a premium price war, and significant reductions in health plan payments have been made to both physicians and hospitals. As the market continues to consolidate, this price warfare will likely accelerate and then stabilize as the three competitors try to differentiate themselves, ultimately on the basis of access and quality.

When ABHS began to establish the MSO and the affiliated medical groups in 1990, it first convened leaders of its medical staff and mem-

bers of the primary care community to develop a set of guiding principles to bond the professional community with the institution. The goal
was to provide a basis for developing managed care capability and avoid
the fragmentation of specialty, primary care, and hospital interests that
has characterized other managed care markets. The guiding principles
included

- ABMA PCPs and contracting ABMG specialists will deliver high-
  quality, cost-efficient healthcare services

- ABMA will offer an attractive, collegial, and professionally and economically rewarding practice alternative to PCPs

- ABMG's specialists will be offered an opportunity for professionally
  and economically rewarding practices

- ABMA will promote respect and consideration among PCPs and
  ABMG specialists

- The group practice program (GPP), a healthcare partnership of ABMR
  with ABMA, AMG, and PMG, will balance the interests of PCPs,
  specialists, and the hospital

- ABMA managed care contracting will be coordinated and conducted
  through ABMG as long as the IPA meets the established performance
  expectations

- The GPP will consider the interests of the patient first, the group second, and individual physicians third

- The GPP will be operated as an MSO, whereby the MSO represents the
  IPA, the integrated groups, the hospital, and the health system

- The group practices may later consider conversion from an MSO to a
  medical foundation or the creation of multispecialty medical groups

- The GPP will strive to become economically self-sustaining by the
  end of its third year of operation

These guiding principles were aimed to establish a level playing field
for the professional community and the hospital. By concentrating all
professional capitation revenue from the health plans through the IPA
and then on to the component medical groups, the physicians would

address their concerns regarding the historical inequity in income distribution between PCPs and specialists. The IPA would also try to determine how best to

- Incent PCPs to remain in the community

- Compensate primary care and specialty physicians for their services

- Rationalize overcrowded specialty panels

- Address the institutional needs of cutting costs, eliminating excess beds, and reducing utilization

By having one conduit for all capitation, the physicians would have a vehicle to address a multiplicity of concerns, including the division of capitation between PCPs and specialists, the creation of specialty panels, risk pool management, clinical resource management, and liaison with the hospital. By jointly contracting with the hospital under full risk capitation, the institution and the physicians developed a mechanism to divide capitation, rationalize excess capacity, and redirect resources from inpatient to outpatient use, as the pace of managed care change has quickened.

This approach emphasized physicians' local decision-making autonomy, medical management as close to the point of care as possible, and self-discipline across the entire healthcare delivery system. It was also hoped that this approach would help to avoid short-term profit taking and the development of a "spot-market" mentality, where the low bid clinches the deal. Any of the groups or special interests, left to independent decision making, could focus only on their own economic survival and could treat healthcare services only as economic commodities, with little attention to the "public good" role of healthcare in the community.

ABMG and the GPP were interlocked so that board members would understand the issues of both practice venues. In addition, the MSO's board included IPA and integrated medical group representatives and leaders from the hospital and the health system to create an objective arbitrating body if special interests threatened to deter the system from its goals. This interlocking governance and representation by physicians was envisioned as a force to integrate the ABHS and affiliated physicians without ABHS ownership of patient records and contracts—the "continuing value" of the physician's practice.

As the level of managed care competition increased in the East Bay, so did the pressures on the ABHS and its guiding principles. Outside interests from southern California, as well as new proprietary organizations springing up in the Bay Area, put tremendous pressure on the PCPs to consider alternatives that might compensate them better for their services or to offer the possibility of administering the entire capitation stream. In accordance with the guiding principles, ABMG had to regear its governance, ownership, and payment mechanisms to respond to these developments and to offer its PCPs the same level of control and compensation as other alternatives—such as equity model MSOs or staff model HMOs.

ABMG's specialists were willing to support these changes over three years because they realized that the alternative (i.e., concentration of the entire capitation revenue in the hands of PCPs) meant rapid movement to a reduction of subspecialty panels or significant cuts in specialists' capitation payments. The hospital and the health system have continued to support the guiding principles for the same reason—to avoid the kind of spot-market pricing that frequently compensates hospitals at a level below their true cost. As the pace of change has accelerated and more proprietary interests have entered the local market, the governance process requirements for making the ABHS model work have become significant.

Some physicians have complained that they did not have the time or patience to meet as often as necessary to maintain the guiding principles. Other physicians grew impatient with the continual discussions needed to redistribute income and rationalize hospital services. Some physicians considered joining forces and forming cartel-like panels in order to go directly to the health plans for subspecialty carve outs, hoping to garner greater market share at higher prices for their services. These forces tended to fragment the professional community and to create a scenario that enabled health plans to continue offering lower prices for pro-vider services and to achieve their profit maximization goals.

In this environment, ABHS faced organizational stress and some questioning of its guiding principles. Thus far, however, this process has provided a means of solving problems and enabling continued cooperation between physicians and hospitals, and ABHS still believes this is the best approach for developing managed care in the East Bay communities.

Network evolution: East Bay Medical Network/Bay Physicians Medical Group

In 1993, ABHS began discussions with ABMG, East County Medical Group, Pacific Healthcare Medical Group, and a number of East Bay hospitals about establishing a new managed care organization called East Bay Medical Network (EBMN)/Bay Physicians Medical Group (BPMG). This new MSO model would provide a vehicle for joint managed care contracting among the physicians of Alameda and Contra Costa Counties in the East Bay. The physicians formed a new professional corporation, Bay Physicians Medical Group, a super-IPA capable of accepting the professional capitation stream from the payers. The network hospitals became subcapitated entities to Alta Bates Medical Center, the recipient of the hospital capitation stream. EBMN provided contracting services and worked to integrate the IPA administrative functions of the founding medical groups, such as management information systems (MIS), claims processing, member services, and utilization management.

When the network and its affiliated medical groups finalized arrangements in January 1994, they represented 65,000 lives, 800 physicians, and 7 hospitals. EBMN staff immediately began to educate the health plans about the value of the network and its ability to accept full risk for the services it provided to the community. In 1996, EBMN/BPMG physicians provide healthcare services to more than 150,000 health plan members, and membership is expected to grow to 250,000 enrollees by 1997 through internal growth and affiliation with other IPAs and medical groups.

A major component of the EBMN's operating philosophy is that physicians and their local hospitals are best served in managed care by working together as business partners, rather than against each other over issues of price and affiliation.

Throughout the process, the hospitals affiliated with EBMN agreed to form risk pools with their local physicians and in many cases provided support to establish new IPAs within their communities. The physicians and their local institutions also took part in negotiations to determine how to distribute capitation among the hospitals, the physicians, and various subspecialists within the IPA. Local, fully integrated medical groups, including Pinole, Alameda, and ABMA, were linked to the system through subcapitation with their local IPAs with the idea of creating medical communities at full risk for healthcare services.

The capitation streams from the health plans were designed to enter the community through the local IPAs and hospitals. Professional capitation was subdivided among the physicians into predetermined budgets, and hospital capitation was set up to fund a shared risk pool to be divided equally between hospitals and physicians if efficient utilization yielded a surplus. The governance and decision making within these local communities were all linked through EBMN/BPMG to the same basic guiding principles that founded the ABHS system.

In 1996, it is apparent that the future of physician network development and direction of managed care contracting in the East Bay is at the EBMN/BPMG level. The level playing field established among the ABHS organizations has been expanded to embrace all of Alameda and Contra Costa Counties. ABMR's MSO is being reorganized this year so that managed care operations and infrastructure supporting all of the BPMG's IPAs will move to the EBMN (super-MSO) level. GPP development supporting fully integrated primary care groups and related billing, practice management, and consultation for individual physicians will expand to all of Alameda and Contra Costa Counties. GPP operations will also relocate to EBMN as a separate division. Finance and information system activities at the local IPAs will move to the network level over the next year. By broadening the level playing field established by the guiding principles and capitation and by moving the identity of the management services organization and physician organizations to a higher level— EBMN/BPMG—the network can now achieve significant economies of scale and reductions in administrative overhead. At the same time, the network can better serve the payers' needs by functioning as a single, accountable administrative unit and can better serve the enrollees by significantly broadening the network of provider services.

The stage has been set for dramatic payer and provider market consolidation in the East Bay. EBMN/BPMG expects to link with other regional IPAs and medical groups through the California Healthcare System/Sutter and the new California Health Network, a statewide chain of integrated delivery systems, to serve more than 500,000 HMO enrollees in the San Francisco Bay Area by the year 2000.

Capitation funds and the network

Capitation funds from the various health plans flow through EBMN/ BPMG in accordance with the principle that there is a single stream of capitation for all physicians in the network and a single stream of capitation for all hospitals. The capitation funds are subcapitated to local communities, where physicians and hospitals form shared risk pools that are equally divided if appropriate utilization yields an excess.

The flow of money begins with EBMN contracting on behalf of BPMG and ABMC. The California Department of Corporations does not allow EBMN, as an MSO, to accept a single capitation stream for both the medical groups and the hospitals. However, EBMN can instruct the health plans in how to divide the capitation stream into professional and hospital components. Separate checks are then cut to BPMG and ABMC. BPMG subcapitates the professional capitation stream, after a deduction of 1 percent (or less) for network MSO expenses, and the separate medical communities determine the split of professional capitation for primary care and specialty physician budgets. This split is determined by actuarial analysis, historical payment patterns, market prices, and determination of subspecialty specific, annual equivalent payment levels.

On the hospital side, ABMC either subcapitates hospitals that wish to be at full risk with their community physicians or pays the contracting hospital a negotiated per diem rate. Where the local hospital is capitated, it forms a shared risk budget with its local IPA. This pool of money is available for all institutional services ordered by the physicians. The IPA also negotiates a schedule of per diem rates to charge against the shared risk budget in accordance with utilization. Separate rates are negotiated for medical-surgical days, ICU/CCU, neonatal intensive care, psychiatry, and outpatient services. Any money remaining in the budget at the end of the period is divided equally between the hospital and the local IPA.

Within each IPA, the professional capitation is taxed 10 percent or less for administrative services, and the remainder is subdivided into budgets. Between 35 and 50 percent of the professional capitation is paid to PCPs, using an age-, sex-, and severity-adjusted capitation schedule. Between 20 and 25 percent of professional fees are paid out to non-capitated, specialty, and ancillary service providers and to institutions for items such as outpatient facility fees. The remainder of the budget is divided among the various subspecialty panels on the basis of preagreed budgets. The panels, in turn, determine how money is divided among the physicians. Typically, the scheme for subspecialty division involves developing points to be awarded for the number of referrals received from PCPs (such as one point per referral per year), the number of managed care enrollees, the complexity of procedures performed, or any other payment mechanism the physicians feel is equitable and does not closely resemble fee-for-service payment. The subcapitation scheme is determined by a fee and compensation committee of physicians and is approved by the local community IPA's board of directors. By creating capitation budgets by subspecialty, individual physicians within the IPA share some of the risk of the overall enterprise. This keeps the physicians focused on managed care principles and lays the groundwork for ultimately receiving a single payment from health plans, employers, or the government for the managed care of an entire community.

"Economic Darwinism" takes place in this professional subcapitation scheme when details of subspecialty utilization and performance are summarized and reported to the PCPs. Reports will soon go to the various PCP panels that show how the subspecialists order tests, the cost of their hospital and outpatient services, their patient satisfaction levels, and the outcomes of their care. These data will help PCPs guide their referrals to appropriate physicians on the panels. Those physicians on the panel receiving referrals will receive points for work performed, which are used to divide the subcapitation budget. Those receiving few or no points receive little or no money, which will ultimately cause the panel size to decrease as physicians voluntarily opt out. The EBMN and BPMG believe that this economic Darwinism is the most appropriate way to trim specialty panels. When subspecialty panels are trimmed arbitrarily or perfunctorily, referral patterns and quality as well as continuity of care may suffer. At a minimum, relations between PCPs and specialists worsen to the point that mutually beneficial cooperation may become impossible.

Finally, there is the issue of the flow of capitation between the founding IPAs when patients demand to see a PCP in one IPA community and a specialist in another, or when a patient from one community is hospitalized in another community due to its special services or because of an emergency. In these cases, services are compensated in accordance with a discounted RBRVS (resource-based relative value scale) fee schedule where each community agrees to reciprocity. While it is too early to determine the effect of this reciprocity and transfer payment mechanism upon the network, it will be closely tracked to evaluate the best method for managing risk across the network.

Ultimately, the individual IPAs may merge their separate professional corporations to form a single large medical group. If that happens, a single set of professional compensation rules will be developed that can be easily administered by the MSO serving the entire network. The local medical communities will then become operating units of BPMG, responsible for local medical management, utilization review, and quality assurance. This step in administrative and governance simplification will make EBMN/BPMG more competitive in the East Bay.

Keeping the plates spinning

Just as the circus sideshow star keeps dinner plates spinning on the ends of sticks, those developing the EBMN/BPMG often feel they are spread thin running from community to community to maintain managed care's momentum.

Physician education, governance meetings regarding subcapitation, patient education activities, and constant reinforcement of managed care principles all require tremendous time and energy. If any one community is neglected for the benefit of another, its managed care "plate" begins to spin down and threatens to destabilize the professional community. The leaders running from stick to stick, injecting new energy and understanding into the professional communities, hope to maintain a balance across the entire network.

Each of the professional communities made up of physicians and hospitals are akin to a plate on the end of a stick. In this metaphor, there are forces that tend to integrate and balance the community and forces that tend to fragment and destabilize it. As the community plate spins faster with the pace of change in managed care and competition, these forces become more challenging and difficult to manage. The forces that tend to integrate and balance the community are

- The guiding principles

- Interlocking governance

- A single stream of capitation revenue entering the physician community, divided equitably and in response to market forces

- The belief that the physicians have a partnership with their local hospital for mutual benefit

The forces that tend to fragment and destabilize a community include

- Individual self-interest that becomes distructive to the overall professional community

- External forces, including proprietary interests, that tend to concentrate all of the power into the hands of one special interest group (e.g., PCP-dominated IPAs)

- The rapid pace of change in managed care

- The "schizophrenic phase" during the time before the "managed care flip" (the point at which at least 50 percent of all revenues are capitated) in which the physicians and the hospital would prefer to stay with their previous fee-for-service payments and behavior but know they must move toward capitation as rapidly as possible

These opposing forces stay in balance as long as people are willing to communicate, exercise self-discipline, follow the guiding principles, and recognize the value that long-term partnerships can bring to their community.

The forces that tend to integrate and fragment motivate a constant search for alignment of incentives among PCPs, subspecialists, and hospitals. More and more organizations recognize they must find a way either to simulate or embrace a single bottom line, so that all network providers share both risks and rewards of appropriate utilization behavior.

There are many ways to accomplish this goal. Foundations can be developed to own and manage both the professional community and the hospitals. In these cases, the foundation's bottom line becomes a measure of success shared through salary and bonus increases to physicians and shared risk returns to the hospitals. Various public equity models are springing up nationally, where physicians own a healthcare system and hospitals become cost centers, rewarded for their efficiency. ABHS is attempting a "virtual bottom line" by interlocking the governance of the component parts and creating a managed care contracting council to make decisions regarding the split of capitation revenue between physicians and hospital, the removal of excess capacity from the subspecialty network and the hospital, and the balance of interests among all of the network's contracted providers.

Today, it is too early to tell which of these approaches will yield the greatest benefit or which of the models is best suited to a particular community's needs. As the managed care marketplace continues to consolidate, the most robust models for dealing with the transformation from fee-for-service medicine to capitation will emerge. If these efforts to keep the managed care plates spinning are successful, the energy and attention required to keep them spinning must come from the community's physician leadership. The healthcare system will benefit from local medical management and regional administrative coordination, and those forces that tend to integrate will balance against those that tend to fragment.

Payer relationships: maximizing premium to providers while minimizing administrative cost

When EBMN contracts with the various health plans, the discussions focus on how much premium revenue the health plan should keep for its contributions as a broker, a marketer, and a holder of risk reserves and for the use of its HMO license as a risk-bearing mechanism. In the future, the full risk contracts negotiated by the EBMN will likely become percent-of-premium agreements, where the network receives a fixed percentage of health plan premium revenue (with certain stipulations regarding minimum capitation revenue levels, and a scheme for age, sex, and severity adjustment to match the characteristics of the community's population). Depending upon how the California corporate practice of medicine laws develop, EBMN may eventually obtain a wholesale HMO license to allow it to accept a single capitation stream from the health plans to cover both physician and hospital services. This new license capability would work around the current state law that prohibits the corporate practice of medicine. Payers would benefit because one check could be cut for all services rendered, establishing single-point accountability for both professional and institutional behaviors.

Along with a focus on the amount of retention that should be provided to the health plan for its services, there should be no duplication in administrative infrastructure. If the health plan is required, for instance, to report patient care outcomes to the employers under HEDIS 3.0 (performance measurements established by the National Committee for Quality Assurance), then a single system of HEDIS reporting should be established and funded to avoid duplication by providers. This principle of nonduplication also applies to credentialing, member services, eligibility, claims processing, and other administrative functions. The overall administrative fees charged by this form of payer relationship should not exceed 7 to 8 percent of total capitation revenue based upon best practices observed at several large-scale HMO administrative operations across the country.

To negotiate with the health plans, EBMN is establishing long-term contractual relationships with those health plans it believes will most likely survive consolidation of the managed care marketplace. Ideally, administrative fees will be minimized, and there will be an attempt to streamline the accountability infrastructure. Policies and procedures may become standardized in the direction of single-payer simplicity. An early indication of interest in this kind of efficiency is evidenced by some health plans wanting to possess an equity interest in EBMN and sit on its board of directors. Again, the forces at work are natural economic drives that tend to move the interests of the payer and the providers toward a single bottom line, single governance, and single company focus.

Will the competition cooperate?

While the EBMN works to fulfill the needs of its PCPs, specialists, and hospitals according to the guiding principles, its competition is hard at work attempting to capture the dominant share of the East Bay PCP community.

An equity model of physician participation is becoming increasingly popular statewide and throughout the country, as the pendulum swings back toward PCPs as patient care coordinators. In fact, PCPs have a long history of primacy in Western medicine to determine care and treatment paths for patients. As subspecialty medicine began to develop after World War II, there was less emphasis on the role of the PCP as overall care coordinator and more emphasis on the individual choices of the patient to determine the type of provider used. Today, the pendulum is swinging back to the primacy of the PCP.

While this redefinition of the PCP as the arbiter of care is important to the success of managed care in general, it can be dangerous to profession-al communities of physicians and their referral relationships, as well as to their relationships to community hospitals. In an extreme case, all of the capitation revenue is placed in the hands of the PCPs, who are then in a position to deal with only those specialists they choose and potentially to pay a spot-market price for both subspecialty and hospital services, depending upon the level of competition in the marketplace. In this model, healthcare is handled more like a classic economic commodity than the "public good" that it really is. While this model may be extreme-ly efficient in rationalizing the system and eliminating unnecessary specialists and hospital beds, it may also be detrimental to the long-term health and quality of the provider community. In extreme cases, it creates an unhealthy level of antagonism that can be counterproductive to maintaining the professional integrity of the community. In addition, health plans and employers want access to the broadest possible network of specialists to maximize enrollee choice of provider. PCP-driven equity models may inadvertently sacrifice this choice and damage the marketability of the network.

Many of the equity models offered to PCPs provide a compensation scheme that immediately trims five or more percentage points of capitation revenue off the top to compensate shareholders, often in distant communities, and to create public equity value for the contracting MSO. In fact, the only real economic benefit of establishing these equity model MSOs is the percentage points of administrative fees and the shared risk revenues that can be realized early in the process of establishing UM controls. These earnings streams can be leveraged on the open market by "going public." The physicians might be better off avoiding these points of management company profit and keeping the managed care arbitrage resulting from savings in reduced utilization to invest in a diversified portfolio of public HMO and physician management company stock. These earnings could, in turn, be used to recapitalize the managed care infrastructure in the local community.

MSO operations are high-volume, low-margin businesses that are extremely difficult to manage profitably. For this reason, EBMN and ABHS are using the private equity model for physician network development. The five or so percentage points of profit and the managed care arbitrage that would have left the community under an external public equity model can be kept in the community to help recapitalize the local healthcare system and to stabilize payments for services rendered by its physicians and hospital. Given the already high level of premium retention by the health plans, local medical communities cannot afford to pay points of profit to investors in distant markets for the use of their capital. In the long term, EBMN and ABHS believe that this money will be vital to the health and welfare of the provider network.

The fragmentation of the payers, physicians, and hospitals brought about by the pursuit of any single-minded equity interest encourages the various parties to "leverage" other system components. What is needed is less fragmentation through a partnership of physicians, hospitals, and selected payers marketing their distinguishable services to employers and consumers as a more cost-effective healthcare delivery system, sustaining self-discipline, and adhering to guiding principles. Short-term profit taking should yield to self-discipline and long-term stability without ignoring the competitive realities of the marketplace. Proprietary interests will invariably enter the market, and various coalitions of physicians will form self-interest groups to oppose the network's interests. They will do this as they respond to the natural competitive forces of the marketplace. They will also pursue self-interest if the network is unable to deliver an equitable competitive model capable of making decisions fast enough to remove the excess capacity from the system. The question is—is there time to give peace a chance?

Capitation through the ages: the most ethical form of payment for medical services?

Capitation is actually an old concept aimed at fairness and equity. Over several thousand years of Chinese medicine, the patient has paid the physician only when the patient is well. When the patient gets sick, the payment stops and is not started again until the patient is again well. This capitated system of payment for healthcare services has served millions well through the ages. Some argue that the Chinese system of payment for healthcare services should be extended to Western medicine.

Recently, physicians in EBMN have been debating whether or not capitation is the most ethical form of payment for medical services. Recent survey data in the professional journals reveal that consumers are often happier under managed care. This research also contends that physicians are better motivated under capitation to practice preventive care and to minimize unnecessary services and can do better under capitation if they practice appropriate, efficient care and manage appropriately sized panels of enrollees.

It has also been shown that managed care, and capitation per se, saves money. Again, recent survey data from the Rand Corporation indicates that HMO costs are significantly lower than fee-for-service costs in major managed care markets. If the outcomes are the same or better, if patient satisfaction is high, if physicians can do well, and if administrative simplicity and removal of excess capacity on the institutional side are a result of managed care and capitation, then the Chinese have been right all these thousands of years.

Healthcare reform is taking place in California, in the Bay Area, and at the EBMN and ABHS, with the physicians calling the shots. They are meeting to discuss how reform will be carried out, how to pay for it, how they will assure that their patients receive appropriate care, and how to remove excess capacity from the system in response to natural economic forces. EBMN/BPMG and ABHS hope to manage this process in a way that preserves the integrity of the professional community, the relationship of individual patients to their physicians, the referral relationships between primary care and specialty physicians, and the overall quality of healthcare in the East Bay. This will be a difficult challenge at a time when consolidation seems to say that price is paramount. Like in Minneapolis, where price competition seems to have reached an end point, quality will ultimately prevail and will ultimately be used to choose managed care contracting partners. This quality will be determined by the best physicians making their own decisions, in concert with their hospital counterparts, about how to define, deliver, and pay for quality healthcare.

NOTES

1. Alta Bates Health System (ABHS) is a fully integrated healthcare system located in the East Bay of the San Francisco Bay Area of California. The not-for-profit system serves a community of 350,000 patients through the 550-physician Alta Bates Medical Group (ABMG) (an IPA), 509-bed Alta Bates Medical Center (ABMC), Visiting Nurses Association (home healthcare) and Hospice of Northern California, skilled nursing facilities, and other related healthcare entities. Alta Bates Medical Group is affiliated with and subcapitates San Leandro IPA and West Contra Costa IPA. ABHS owns 50 percent of East Bay Medical Network (EBMN) (MSO), a contracted healthcare delivery system in Alameda and Contra Costa Counties that manages the total capitated care of more than 150,000 HMO enrollees through five IPAs and seven hospitals. Three East Bay IPAs—Alta Bates Medical Group, East County Medical Group, and Pacific HealthCare Medical Group—have formed Bay Physicians Medical Group (BPMG), which owns the other half of East Bay Medical Network. ABHS is also affiliated with California Healthcare System/Sutter, consisting of Mills Peninsula, Marin General, California Pacific Medical Center, and ABHS, and the Sutter Health System affiliates. These various affiliations have created a contracting mechanism responsible for over 500,000 lives in the San Francisco Bay Area.

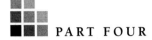

PART FOUR

NETWORK FINANCIAL MANAGEMENT

16

Financial controls and reporting for capitation

Geoffrey B. Baker
Managing Director
Physician Management Alliance
Los Angeles, California

Heather Shupe
Financial Manager, Health Plan Services
Stanford Health Services and
Lucile Salter Packard Children's Hospital
Stanford, California

Contributing comments by
Larry Bonham, MD
Chief Medical Officer
Physician Venture Management

M ANAGED CARE PROVIDERS FACE many challenges in their strategies to reduce prepaid risks. The "managed care experience curve" heightens these challenges further. Without the experience that comes from performing medical management, determining provider reimbursement and risk-sharing methodologies, and processing claims/encounters for data reporting, many providers can stumble. Several capitated independent practice associations (IPAs) and medical groups floundered in the mid- to late 1980s by paying fee-for-service claims without sufficient tracking or knowledge of true specialty referral liabilities.

This chapter introduces these prepaid risks and the financial controls for managing and reducing these risks. This chapter also identifies critical preimplementation considerations before establishing a financial control and reporting system. These preimplementation considerations include (1) developing the financial expertise of management service organization (MSO) staff; (2) delineating business/accounting and organizational relationships; (3) addressing critical business decisions before building the managed care information system tables and dictionaries; (4) drafting procedures and systems to support core managed care flows; (5) developing provider education and training; and finally, once operational; (6) creating the applications, reports, and processes that help physicians and management mitigate capitation risk.

To be successful and limit prepaid risk, capitation requires managed care providers (e.g., hospitals, physicians, and ancillaries) to exercise fiscally conservative reimbursement and tight utilization to limit prepaid risk. This means controlling costs, aligning incentives, tracking costs and utilization to providers, caring for patients in the most appropriate settings, aggressive case management, and preventive care programs. Figure 1 summarizes these prepaid risks and the ability of the provider to manage these risks as controllable, moderately controllable, and uncontrollable. Most of the risks identified in Figure 1 represent a mixture of price, intensity, severity, and frequency risks.

Whether a provider organization (hospital, medical group, or IPA)

FIGURE 1
Major prepaid risks

Controllable	Moderately controllable	Uncontrollable
• Risk-sharing incentives are not aligned among all providers and may lead to overutilization and higher costs	• High overall hospital utilization (bed day per 1,000 members)	• Catastrophic hospital and ambulatory claims
• High specialist referral costs and/or high out-of-network referrals to nonaffiliated providers	• High cost mix of inpatient and ancillary services	• Payer unwillingness to negotiate capitation rates high enough to cover medical and administrative expenses
• High management service organization costs and high administrative retention leaving insufficient capitation to cover medical expenses	• Low enrollment, hence insufficient scale economies and high administrative overhead	• Skewed enrollment, inaccurate actuarial estimates of family size and contract distribution (i.e., age/sex/family size adjusted capitation payment) resulting in insufficient capitation
	• Low copayments or insufficient patient financial incentive and inadequate patient demand management	• Higher percentage of high-risk, high-cost employees in employer groups, resulting in adverse selection and insufficient capitation

can accept the risks associated with capitation contracts and be financially and clinically successful depends on several factors. These factors are illustrated in Figure 2. Developing a detailed strategy and operations framework for managing these factors favorably can reduce prepaid risks and improve clinical and financial performance.

For example, full-risk contracts compel medical groups and hospitals to create a positive contribution margin by delivering care in the most economical setting. The "network scope factor" in Figure 2 illustrates that provider networks with sufficient geographic coverage and the availability of ancillary services (e.g., rehabilitation, skilled nursing, outpatient surgery, laboratory, home health, physical therapy, and radiation therapy) can reduce costs by keeping patients within a network of contracted providers and directing patients to cost-effective providers. Providers who own or have negotiated favorable subcapitation contracts with home health agencies, ambulatory surgery centers, skilled nursing facilities, and reference laboratories are better positioned to control costs at the point of patient entry than providers who rely on hospital settings or out-of-network providers with high per diems or discounted fee-for-service schedules.

Controlling utilization depends on how the provider organization structures its reimbursement and risk-sharing incentives and how it tracks practice patterns (see "payment structure" and "network structure" in Figure 2). As a reimbursement methodology, capitation has proven the most cost-effective approach for managing medical care and directing resources toward wellness and prevention. Capitation increases physicians' awareness of the costs associated with their treatment decisions. Capitation also incentivizes physicians to reduce costs per professional hour, professional hours per visit (use of nurse practitioners), visits per enrollee, cost per ancillary procedure, number of ancillary procedures, and medical office and clinic overhead costs. The decision to capitate providers, however, depends on several considerations.[1] Most of these considerations deal with who can manage risk, accept risk, and take the potential upside gain. Considerations include

1. Sufficient division of service responsibilities and financial responsibilities between specialists and primary care physicians

2. Sufficient practice penetration by HMOs, panel size, and enrollment volume (e.g., more than 8,000 senior risk and 20,000 commercial)

   - Business or referrals can be directed easily

FIGURE 2
Managing costs

Has your organization invested in cost management programs and processes to provide capitated care in a cost-effective manner?

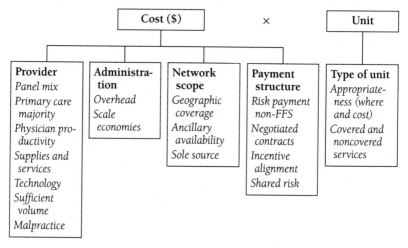

3. Capitation and fee-for-service equivalency

4. Tolerance for risk in terms of individual and aggregate stop-loss levels

5. Impact on production incentives

6. Concern for quality, patient shunting, and adverse selection

   - Parties agree on referral guidelines and criteria in advance (e.g., specialist and ancillary provider demonstrates willingness to work constructively with the primary care physician to assume appropriate referrals)

7. Predictability or variability in services

8. Provider readiness

9. Sizable dollars at stake to justify the specialty capitation process

   - Specialist or ancillary costs are rising monthly

   - Conviction that true reductions in cost are available. Specialist or ancillary provider has unique insights unattainable through utilization review

   - Specialty or ancillary service generates significant volume

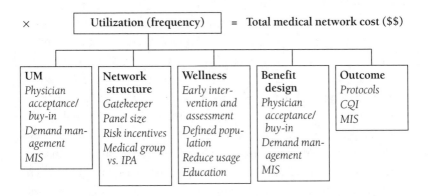

10. Reliable utilization statistics to develop subcapitated rates

The ability to closely monitor patients, measure physician productivity, and provide timely practice pattern feedback to physicians is essential for controlling cost. Providers who invest in decision support information systems that track costs, utilization, and frequency of services accurately are better able to quantify the effectiveness or ineffectiveness of their medical management policies.

Relevant financial controls for managing prepaid risks: preimplementation steps

Before assuming a delegated capitation contract and instituting financial controls, the provider organization needs to complete the following:[2]

1. Secure provider participation agreements on an exclusive basis. This allows the parent organization (e.g., MSO, PHO, or IDS) to negotiate contracts on behalf of participating providers (e.g., IPA-medical group, ancillary providers, and hospitals). Centralizing negotiation simplifies communication, allows combined strategic objectives to be addressed, and strengthens negotiating positions. This assumes that the physician primary care and specialty panel has formed along with the institutional and ancillary network

2. Develop strategies for negotiating full as well as partial risk capitation contracts, encouraging HMO delegation of selected functions,[3] reducing HMO and MSO administrative retention, and optimizing capitated enrollment. For example, in order to encourage HMO delegation to the MSO, the provider network will need to work with the HMO to define their respective operational responsibilities. To optimize enrollment, the provider network will need to determine the potential enrollment associated with the HMO contract(s) to assure a sufficient MSO staffing level and an adequate physician panel size (practice penetration and primary care to specialty representation). Throughout the negotiation process, the provider network must demonstrate its ability to manage capitation (e.g., MSO information system, claims and referral turnaround time, utilization management-quality assessment committee attendance and minutes, and National Committee on Quality Assurance—NCQA—audits)

3. Develop a division-of-responsibilities matrix that allocates service responsibilities among HMOs, hospitals, and medical group participants. (Within the medical group, service responsibilities are divided between primary care and specialist physicians.) This step is vital to identifying responsibility and associated risk among all parties. Member services, liability for out-of-area claims (i.e., claims related to services performed outside of the local service area), health assessment, stop-loss premiums and proceeds, and catastrophic pools (e.g., AIDS and transplantation) are areas for consideration. Others include primary care, specialty care, chronic and subacute care, home health, vision, mental health, and pharmacy benefits

4. Organize the provider network for risk. This includes the following:

- Resolving governance and ownership structure issues. Some of these issues include appropriate primary care representation, lay-physician board composition, membership parameters and scope of authority granted to a cooperative MSO, PHO, or IDS board, financial responsibility and accountability of participants, legal structure of contracting body, and reporting relationships to and from providers

- Restructuring network reimbursement costs as appropriate, by various methods including

a) Identifying internal reimbursement rates and transfer pricing for institutional, ancillary, and medical group services (e.g., diagnosis-related groups [DRG] case rates, resource-based relative value study [RBRVS], and subcapitation)

b) Developing an internal capitation budget process

c) Completing agreements with fee schedules and appropriate participation terms for providers

5. Develop the management service organization (MSO), which includes

- Recruiting MSO personnel with sufficient expertise by functional area (e.g., claims, finance, contracting, provider relations, medical management, eligibility, member services, group practice operations, and information system services)

- Defining the business structure and organizational relationships among MSO participants

- Developing procedures and systems to support core managed care transactions such as enrollment and disenrollment, community-based case management, authorization and referral tracking, claims processing, payment, reporting, capitation payment auditing, and risk pool distribution

- Reengineering to streamline core activities and functions if needed

- Generating critical financial applications and reports for tracking and minimizing prepaid risks

- Installing and configuring the information system (e.g., building module tables and dictionaries)

6. Negotiate and be able to implement appropriate age/sex capitation rates for partial or full-risk contracts with the HMO or payer

7. Identify and communicate HMO contract operational requirements to appropriate constituents (e.g., providers or members). This requires the following:

- A multidisciplinary team approach for addressing hospital-based physicians. This team can educate the referring physicians on appropriateness of various tests or most cost-effective alternatives

- Ongoing performance feedback to physicians (e.g., utilization, cost, intensity, and outcomes) and generating reports that can help to educate and spot problem areas

- Submission of billing versus encounter forms (if the hospital or the physician group is receiving capitation, then it does not file claims for payment to the MSO, yet a claim should be generated to track encounter data)

- Coordination of hospital and IPA-medical group efforts for education and communication purposes (e.g., eligibility verification, case management, and in-network referral)

- Extensive education for frontline administration and nonphysician clinical staff on care delivery under capitation. This includes financial, clinical, and quality indicator factors (e.g., patient satisfaction); specific operational guidelines related to eligibility, authorization, and internal utilization management; referrals to associated (contracted) providers; vendor claims; and benefit management (e.g., mental health cap)

Preimplementation considerations for MSO staff

Figures 3 and 4 show the functions for a typical fully delegated MSO. Because step 5 noted above is pivotal to implementing a financial control and reporting system that reduces prepaid risks, these two figures expand upon each.

Figure 5 shows an example of the type of tasks, frequency of tasks, skill sets, and time needed by title for MSO functions.

ARE THE MSO STAFF TRAINED FOR CAPITATION MANAGEMENT?

MSO fiscal services department staff and physician finance committee members will need training in the financial, accounting, and reimbursement principles of capitation. All MSO personnel will need training on how to use flowcharts, procedure manuals, job descriptions, and on-line system practices. MSOs that educate personnel on transaction flows will have more productive employees and fewer cross-functional coordination problems. For example, if a claims clerk knows how the enrollment

FIGURE 3
MSO organizational functions

Most system operations and infrastructures are housed within the MSO, which provides management services to participating providers (e.g., IPA-medical group, hospitals).

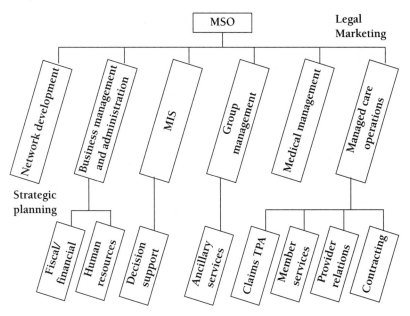

Fiscal/finance
- Capitation reconciliation
- Actuarial analysis by contract
- Stop-loss
- Provider reimbursement
- Budgets
- Billing/collections
- Patient flow

Human resources
- Personnel development
- Network hardware/ software maintenance
- Telecommunications
- Electronic data links
- Development of affiliated physician group relationships
- Facilities
- Compliance
- Quality assurance
- Utilization management

- Patient reporting
- Cost and outcomes
- Continuous quality improvement
- Clinical protocols
- Referral authorization

Claims TPA
- Process claims/encounters
- Clearinghouse
- Claims edit and payment adjudication

Member services
- Enrollment eligibility
- Member satisfaction
- Dispute resolution
- Patient interface/education

Provider relations
- Provider contract database (fee schedule, credentialing information)
- Provider directory
- PCP-member assignment

FIGURE 4
MSO fiscal services department

The MSO fiscal services department will be responsible for business services, financial controls, and reporting functions.

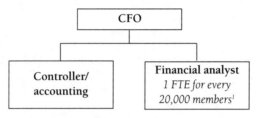

Typical staffing (total department)
.15–.25 FTE per 1,000 enrollees[1]

Responsibilities

- Flexible budget development
- Payroll and physician compensation
- Capitation eligibility reconciliation
- Financial statements
- Actuarial analysis
- Profitability analysis by contract
- Risk pool settlement and analysis
- Stop-loss reporting and recovery
- Provider subcapitation

- IBNR estimation
- Group practice acquisition and valuation
- Special studies
- Business office billing and collections (FFS)
- Accounts receivable management accounts (FFS), accounts payable
- General ledger transactions
- Bookkeeping, bank statements

1. GHAA IPA Staffing Standard, 1993 GHAA Annual HMO Industry Survey.

files are built and understands the process for authorizations, the clerk will be better prepared to answer provider questions more accurately with fewer telephone transfers. Ideally, the financial training program could be designed for participants with the following objectives in mind:

1. Learning how to develop and implement financial controls for capitated provider networks

2. Understanding the organizational structure, roles, and activities that occur in the MSO fiscal services department

3. Understanding and developing an accounting structure for the business relationships among MSO provider participants

4. Reviewing the process and steps necessary to implement financial controls for capitation risk-contracting with the information and general ledger (G/L) systems

5. Understanding the managed care information system and G/L program capitation transaction cycles

6. Understanding the distinction between claims and capitation payments to providers

7. Understanding the importance of coding and establishing appropriate medical classifications for tracking medical and administrative expenses

8. Understanding the proposed chart of accounts, managed care accounting procedures, and risk pool fund structures

9. Understanding the risk pool settlement process

10. Understanding the financial controls reporting cycle and how to interpret key managed care financial reports

11. Communicating financial, clinical, and utilization report results to administrative and physician constituents. Communication should include options and recommendations for follow-up and corrective courses of action

12. Reviewing which key physician and administrative decisions remain outstanding, how they affect the managed care information system implementation effort, and when and how they will be resolved

Ideally, this education effort should begin before installing or configuring the managed care information system. Typically, the information systems vendor cannot install the software and hardware unless the MSO staff have sufficient expertise. At the end of the orientation period, the MSO fiscal service department should know how to handle the following managed care activities (this list is illustrative and not complete):

1. Referral procedures and tracking

2. HMO/MSO eligibility downloading and encounter submission

3. Capitation income tracking and verification

4. Provider reimbursement terms, with terms distinguished by specialty type

5. Stop-loss, reinsurance, coordination of benefits, and third-party liability recovery and development of stop-loss and reinsurance thresholds

6. Risk pool structures, reconciliation, and payout parameters

7. Enrollee assignment to primary care physicians

8. Chart of accounts and fund accounting procedures

9. Integration with other information systems (e.g., clinical, cost accounting, case-mix, billing, and general ledger)

FIGURE 5
Staffing requirements by function

Projected staffing requirements
Capitation operations
1,600 commercial; 4,500 Medicare; 6,100 total enrollees

Staff type	Task	Frequency
Utilization management		
RN	Authorization check	Ongoing
	Concurrent review	Ongoing
	Discharge planning	Ongoing
Administrative	Utilization report	Monthly
Director/Manager	Participation in utilization targets	
	and budget development	Annual
Admitting		
Admit clerk	Authorization check	Ongoing
	Eligibility check	Ongoing
	Copayment collection	Ongoing
Patient financial services		
Capitation specialist	Remittance reconciliation	Monthly
	Eligibility reports distribution	Monthly
	Claims processing (30 minutes per claim)	Ongoing
	Reinsurance billing	Twice per year
General accounting		
A/P clerk	Pay external claims (15 minutes per invoice)	Ongoing
	Remittance reconciliation	Monthly
Reimbursement		
Reimbursement	DRG payment monitoring	10 cases per year
Managed care/Contracting office		
Analyst	Claims reports and data management	Monthly
	Claims lag analysis	Monthly
	Risk share provision	Monthly
	Financial performance	Monthly
Contract manager	Develop budget and utilization targets	Annual
	Negotiate external provider contracts	Annual
	Negotiate risk share agreement	Annual
	Grand total	

10. Relationships between local and regionwide physician and hospital organizations

11. Credentialing

12. Capitation terms and allocation methodologies

13. Subcapitation agreements

Annual hours	FTEs	Skills needed
		Concurrent review process
		Concurrent review process
		Concurrent review process
120	0.06	PC spreadsheet application
40	0.02	
48	0.02	Billing and receivable system
48	0.02	Billing and receivable system
2,269	1.09	Billing and receivable system
40	0.02	Billing and receivable system
528	0.25	Accounts payable system
48	0.02	Billing and receivable system
20	0.01	
120	0.06	Financial spreadsheet
144	0.07	Financial spreadsheet
96	0.05	Financial spreadsheet
96	0.05	Financial spreadsheet
40	0.02	Contracting and budgeting
300	0.14	Contract negotiation
50	0.02	Contract negotiation
4,007	*1.92*	

14. Vendor agreements and payment procedures

15. Interpretation, analysis, presentation, and follow-up of capitation performance reporting

BUSINESS STRUCTURE AND RELATIONSHIPS

Before configuring the information system and producing financial and utilization reports, MSO fiscal personnel must define the business relationships among provider organizations. These are the contractual, risk-sharing, reimbursement, and referral relationships that exist among the provider network (corporate umbrella), medical groups, IPAs, hospitals, and ancillary providers. The business structure of the provider network has significant impact on the way the information system processes financial data. The information system cannot produce financial statements and reports such as profit and loss statements, budgets, and per member per month (PMPM) variance reports if the accounting structure does not relate to the business structure. Without such structure, for example, the information system cannot process claims or subcapitation payments, charge the appropriate risk pool, and assign costs to a cost center. Business units, cost centers, region, and product lines (e.g., Medicare risk, commercial) will be needed for all service regions and within each service region for institutions, ancillary providers, physician organization, and panels of primary care groups.

FIGURE 6
MSO responsibility centers and
business relationships

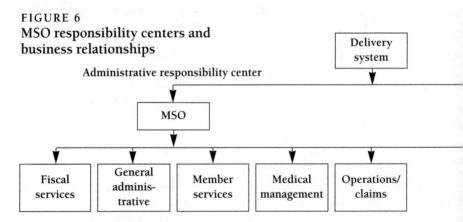

Figure 6 shows how responsibility centers can highlight the business relationships that occur between the MSO and its affiliated provider network. In Figure 6, responsibility centers are used to break out and monitor administrative and medical costs within the delivery system. Each responsibility center may have a department where profits and costs can be reported on financial statements. These departments in turn may charge each other for services rendered based on contracted rates, purchased service agreements, or other internal transfer pricing methodologies.

Key questions that arise from defining the business relationships noted in Figure 6 include, but are not limited to

1. What is the provider network organization and ownership structure? What are the unique business relationships between members, providers, product offerings, and service regions?

2. How will financial reporting for revenues and expenses be recorded— at the aggregate, specific provider organization, or region level? In other words

   ▪ What are the business units and payer organizations (e.g., cost centers, departments, divisions, and companies in an organization)?

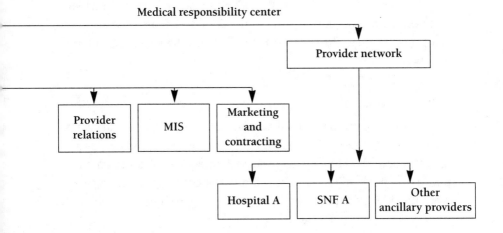

- Which organizations (e.g., local PHO, hospital, clinic, or IPA) are providers affiliated with? How will risk pools be structured around these business organizations? How many pools are necessary? When claims and capitation are paid, will the costs be charged to specific responsibility centers?

- How are the service regions defined? What are the geographic populations whose revenue and utilization may need to be identified and for which provider contracting may vary? How will capitation be allocated by service area?

3. Are the financial activities for the responsibility centers (i.e., provider organizations and risk pools) tied to membership? Can the information and decision support systems provide age/sex and contract adjusted PMPM reporting (i.e., summary PMPM healthcare cost reporting by age/sex cells)?

4. Does the accounting structure relate to the organizational structure? How detailed is the chart of accounts with respect to responsibility centers and the coding structure?

ACCOUNTING CONSIDERATIONS

The MSO fiscal services department will need to develop a managed care chart of accounts to map business structure. The Medical Group Management Association (MGMA) has a chart of accounts that serves as a good starting point. This mapping process includes establishing appropriate accounting procedures, coding, and responsibility centers. Accounting procedures should discuss how the G/L and managed care information systems will record journal entries and G/L transactions to reflect the funds flow through the provider network. The following areas deserve attention.

Risk pool structure

Risk-sharing contracts require that capitation income due to and claims paid from each risk pool be monitored so that surpluses and deficits are allocated according to a predetermined methodology. A fund structure for the risk pools will need to be set up. To align incentives among network providers, the funds structure should include a determination of how risk-sharing surpluses and deficits will be shared among providers. The funds structure may be kept separate from the G/L accounts. Capitation income and claims/subcap payment transactions are recognized in these funds (i.e., PCP and hospital payout) and the G/L. Considerations for various primary care, specialist, ancillary, and institutional pools include

1. *PCP pool.* Should subcapitation pools be established for pediatrics and family practice/internal medicine? Over time, is a primary care pool necessary? If providers are paid on an RBRVS basis, how will this structure facilitate migration to PCP capitation? Can the PCP pool be compartmentalized by PODS (pools of doctors or risk groups)?[4] Will the POD structure allow for PCP profiling? Does the accounting structure and information system permit distribution of pool surplus funds to high-performing PODs without significant spreadsheet and manual manipulation of data?

2. *Specialist pool.* Have subcapitation pools been established for all specialties (OB/GYN particularly)? How will specialist and hospital pool surplus be distributed to these pools? Which specialties should and should not participate in specialist or hospital pool surplus?

3. *Ancillary pool.* Should a separate pool be established for risk-sharing purposes with ancillary providers (e.g., home health and ambulance)?

4. *Institutional pool (inpatient and outpatient services).* For hospital services that are capitated, how will payment and transfer-pricing issues be addressed? Considerations include

   - Creating a transfer-pricing method that results in neutral incentives for patient treatment and referral. Hospital subcapitation remains transparent for the physicians, allowing patients to move anywhere within the provider network

   - Subcapitation may work best for hospitals with distinct, nonoverlapping service areas to reduce duplicate bookkeeping and complex administrative settlement between institutions at year-end

   - Creating a transfer-pricing system that is simple. Administrative simplicity avoids duplicate division of responsibility, elaborate network rates, and bookkeeping to handle buying back of services

Appropriate coding structure

Medical service categories require a coding structure for the medical expense statement. This includes tracking department costs for medical management, claims, provider relations, member services, marketing, information systems, general administration, fee-for-service billing and collections, and facility management. Classification accounts should be developed at a level of detail that is reasonable for the proper administration of individual expense categories.

Financial statements

Statements can include MSO, hospital institution, and physician organization profit and loss statements and balance sheets. Creation of global medical expense and provider summary reports should also be considered.

Bank accounts

The creation of a separate account for claims payments due to high volume is recommended. It also will be important to have electronic reconciliation capability as the volume grows.

Accounting period

Generally, a monthly financial period is appropriate with either a calendar or fiscal year. Usually, the capitation payments are on a one-month lag to actual enrollment. It is customary to pay retroactively for additions and subtract for deletions. It is important that contracts be written to limit any retroactivity to three months.

Figure 7 is a basic chart of accounts structure that allows for financial reporting at the individual provider level as well as at a regional service area. This chart of accounts structure relies on identification as well as use of responsibility centers as key management tools. Responsibility centers are identifiable organizational units through which activities of the various provider organizations are performed (i.e., tracing of all revenues and costs to the center responsible for their occurrence). Developing both the responsibility centers and chart of accounts requires defining the organization's business structure and its external relationships.

FIGURE 7
Basic chart of accounts structure

Region	Division	Site	Department	General	Provider
00	000	00	00	0000	0000
MSA #1	Physician, hospital, MSO, other	Group site, MSO site, hospital site	Individual department	1XXX Asset 2XXX Liability 3XXX Revenue 4XXX Revenue deductions 5XXX Compensation 6XXX Supply expenses 7XXX Purchased services	Provider type

INFORMATION SYSTEM CONFIGURATION:
BUILDING TABLES AND DICTIONARIES

Figure 8 provides an overview of how an HMO contract can relate to business decisions, accounting structure, and the managed care information system. Figure 8 shows how the terms and conditions from HMO capitation contracts and provider reimbursement agreements are translated into a series of financial transactions on the accounting and managed care information system.

Once MSO personnel and physicians agree upon their business structure and accounting procedures, the managed care information system and G/L can be configured. Any limitations on the part of the information system during this process can directly impact an organization's ability to manage information. The limits of the information system's capabilities for recording transactions can and will effectively limit management's ability to improve cost and outcomes performance.

Both the information systems vendor and MSO information systems department will need to build dictionaries and tables for contract terms, credentialing data, reimbursement rates, and negotiated capitation amounts on the managed care information system. As fundamental building blocks, dictionaries and tables organize the information necessary for a managed care information system to process data and produce reports. Dictionaries, for example, help ensure accurate data entry by comparing and verifying incoming claims data against preexisting databases. Dictionaries also allow users to partition the database by

FIGURE 8
Managed care information system implementation

Once physicians and MSO personnel resolve their business structure and funds flow, the managed care information system will need to be configured.

Dictionary and implication

Business structure	*Implication*
▪ Division, region, provider, site	▪ Track performance by medical group/ IPA, POD, risk pool, specialty, in- or out-of-network, medical service category
▪ Provider affiliation	
▪ Provider specialty	
▪ Coding	
▪ Place of services	▪ Adjudication of claim/encounter by division of responsibility
Capitation management	▪ All services at-risk under contract
▪ Provider fee schedule	▪ Cap/member reconciliation
▪ Capitation parameters	▪ Reinsurance recovery
▪ Stop-loss parameter	▪ Verify eligibility and benefits, PMPM reporting information, cap/member reconciliation, and COB recovery
Eligibility	
▪ Member information, PCP assignment	
Referral management	▪ Match claim to authorization
▪ Benefits, protocols, referral reasons	▪ Financial liability (DOR)

organizational structure and service regions. Key configuration steps include the following.

Provider reimbursement

This step includes downloading contract rates, payment methodology, terms, and conditions into the managed care information system. The finance committee and fiscal services department will need to compile the reimbursement rates and complete the provider contracts. These personnel also must decide which procedures and providers are capitated. Capitation presents a series of special configuration issues.

1. How will amounts be allocated among the funds? What is the basis for allocation (e.g., age/sex factors)?

2. How will pools be set up (e.g., by geography, by institution, by members assigned, by PCP selection)? How will the institutional pool be tied to the PCPs and specialists?

3. What are the capitation parameters by risk population, business unit, member class, and age/sex factors?

4. Can the system produce fee-for-service equivalency reporting for the following:

- Physician organization, IPAs, or medical groups (i.e., RBRVS, case rates, and capitation)

- Institutions (i.e., DRGs, per diem, and case rates)

- Ancillary providers (i.e., case rates, ambulatory payment groupings, and capitation)

Stop-loss thresholds and attachment points for reinsurance recovery
Lack of an integrated database can make stop-loss tracking problematic. HMO and individual provider stop-loss methodologies are varied and complex. The managed care information system should be able to track and accumulate allowable expenses on a specific member on an organizationwide basis. The type of services covered and not covered under the reinsurance contract will need to be tracked. For example, out-of-area, PCP, mental health services, and transplants may be excluded for recovery purposes. Expenses for covered services will need to be repriced and calculated according to fee-for-service equivalency parameters. Finally, the system will need to compare reinsurance premium cost with recovery (e.g., 50, 60, or 70 percent recovery rate on reinsurance premium?). Other stop-loss considerations include

1. For the medical group or IPA, the stop-loss limit must be set at an amount low enough to eliminate the effects of random claim fluctuations but not so low as to eliminate variations in experience due to meaningful differences in physicians' practice patterns. The range in cost for commercial population stop-loss insurance is .9 to 4.0 percent of medical group capitation amount depending on the attachment point. Examples of stop-loss terms for a commercial population include

   - $1.50 PMPM cost with an attachment point set at $7,500 of paid RBRVS fee schedule ($0.33 for an attachment point of $25,000)

   - After attachment point is reached, reimbursement will be based at 75 percent of the RBRVS paid fee schedule

   - Total charges against the specialist pool on a specific basis are limited to $10,000 per year

2. For the hospital, the range for the commercial population reinsurance premium is 4 to 6 percent depending on services covered (inpatient

and outpatient) and the attachment point (reinsurance deductible). Based on the California market, the typical hospital reinsurance deductible ranges from $50,000 to $150,000. Examples of reinsurance terms for a commercial population include

- $1.30 PMPM cost with attachment point set at $100,000 of charges

- $1.60 PMPM cost with attachment point set at $75,000 of charges

- $2.75 PMPM cost with attachment point set at $50,000 of charges

- Calculation of charges up to the attachment point can be based on several methodologies such as per diem, DRG case rate, and percent of billed charges up to a maximum dollar amount per day

- After the attachment point is reached, reimbursement will be based at 50 percent of charges

Provider tables

These include relevant credentialing and billing information. Considerations for setting up such tables include

1. Type and classification of provider (e.g., specialist, primary care, and dual role)

2. Handling of multiple billing addresses, provider networks, group practices, and office identification

3. Determining provider financial affiliations, reimbursement methods, and pool class assignment. Will providers be grouped according to PODs for risk pool performance and profiling purposes? How will on-call and cross-coverage be handled? Will reimbursement methods vary by type of HMO and PPO contracts? Will some providers be paid lower rates than others? Are different physician panels used for different programs or product lines (i.e., Medicare risk, commercial, and Medicaid)?

4. Defining providers by business segment unit or geographic region

5. Methodology for assigning members (e.g., geographic, institutional affiliation, member geography, age/sex category, PCP individual, POD, or group)

Allocation of pool funds or deficits and pool structure

The finance committee and IDS fiscal services department staff may need to allocate deficits and surpluses based on a combination of the following variables:

Affiliation status

PCP status

Member status

Member number (i.e., number of assigned enrollees)

Member sex

Group division

PCP affiliation

PCP pool class

Benefit package

Contract type

Risk population

Utilization performance

Productivity

Membership

Tables will need to be developed for the MIS. Membership parameters include, but are not limited to

1. Contract eligibility (family composition, tier type such as subscriber and dependents, and student age cutoffs)

2. Division, medical group, or regional service area changes

3. Member eligibility and PCP changes

4. Benefit eligibility (e.g., covered services, noncovered services, waiting period, service and dollar limits, and COBRA identification)

5. Type of risk population (e.g., Medicare, Medicaid, or commercial)

6. Member on review (e.g., denied or pended claim, problem members)

7. Member claims history

8. Member authorization history

9. Enrollment history (e.g., frequency of changes in plan, PCP, or medical group or panel)

10. Other (secondary) coverage

Coding

The MSO management information systems (MIS) and fiscal services department will need to verify that ICD-9CM diagnoses, CPT-4 procedure codes, specialized codes (e.g., supplies, durable medical equipment [DME], and other), UB 92 revenue codes, and DRGs loaded in the managed care information system are consistent with the codes used to create the medical activity statement (see Report 2). Personnel need to verify that the managed care system can compile and aggregate procedures and outpatient revenue codes into appropriate groupings (e.g., Milliman & Robertson, DRG, MDC).

Benefits management

The vendor and MSO MIS department need to configure the managed care system for benefits offered, copayment, and deductible amounts, limits, and maximums. Based on plan design, counters will need to be defined to accumulate benefit limits and amounts. For example, based on the HMO evidence of coverage (EOC), the mental health visits may be limited to an annual maximum number of 25 visits. This may differ by payer. The MSO will need to "count" the number of visits and determine eligibility for providers before services are rendered.

Downloading and interface with payers

The following issues should be raised and addressed during contract negotiations with payers:

1. Eligibility information downloading directly or via tape. Handling of retroactive terminations and deletions for capitation reconciliation purposes

2. Encounter information uploading back to payers for potential employer HEDIS reporting requirements[5]

3. On-line capability of checking eligibility and claims payment (HMO or MSO service responsibility)

4. Transfer of member service calls to the MSO on provider relations, claims payment issues

General ledger system interface

The MSO MIS staff need to decide how the managed care information system links with the G/L and budgeting system, the hospital, and medical group information systems. Some of the steps include

1. Deciding if the managed care information system has sufficient budget reporting and G/L capabilities, then deciding if the hospital G/L or managed care system is most appropriate for financial reporting and handling of network managed care transactions

2. Developing a flexible budget that incorporates frequency per 1,000 RVU, costs per unit, enrollment, and PMPM assumptions for variance reporting purposes. Downloading the flexible budget on managed care information system or other appropriate accounting systems

3. Interfacing with the MIS database program for ad hoc report writing

4. Interfacing with the hospital clinical information system

5. Interfacing with the medical group information system

Testing

MSO personnel should test managed care transactions and financial reports before adjudicating the first "live" claim. MSO personnel may consider testing in the following areas.

1. Incurred but not reported (IBNR) estimation (i.e., reimbursement rates used and linkage to utilization management authorization system; authorized but not yet billed)

2. Profit and loss statement reporting

3. Actual to expected budget variance reporting

4. Eligibility audit reporting (PMPM months, member retroactive adds
   or deletes)

5. Reinsurance and stop-loss exception reporting for total services rendered to a patient that exceeds specified limits (i.e., indicate need for
   payment above normal capitation or stop-loss threshold)

6. Coordination of benefits (COB); PMPM cost recovery reporting

7. Subcapitation payments

8. Payment of vendor claims (i.e., link to contracted rates for contracted
   providers)

9. Risk pool reconciliation and distribution

Special tracking

For risk pool distribution purposes, the managed care information system may need to link with multiple databases for tracking of risk indicators or HEDIS report card measures (e.g., health risk appraisals—SF 36
form, medical records, and claims data).

SUPPORT FOR CORE MANAGED CARE TRANSACTIONS

Once configured and after conducting trial runs, the managed care information system can now post HMO capitation income, reconcile income
with eligibility, process claims/encounters, pay providers, record transactions, and produce financial reports. Flowcharts should be developed for
core managed care processes. Flowcharts can help identify problems or
opportunities for further streamlining and elimination of manual intervention. Flowcharts of core processes include enrollment, capitation
received, subcapitation payments, member list distribution to providers,
encounter reporting, authorizations, utilization management functions,
scheduling, claims management, COB and third-party liability tracking,
risk pool tracking, IBNR calculation, and management reporting.

The flowcharts of transaction flows should be developed before or
simultaneously with system installation. Such timing can reduce configuration delays and help streamline operations. Flowcharts can contain
descriptive narrative, indicate appropriate control points and procedures, show both input and output from the system, and cross-reference
to both job descriptions and procedure manuals. Examples of input and
output from transaction flows should also include a list of where the

documents or data originate and where they are sent. These listings can later be used as control logs to make sure that all appropriate data is received and also distributed. Figure 9 provides an example of core managed care transaction flowcharts and partitioned database levels for enterprisewide reporting. Enterprise-level reports aggregate individual provider performance (e.g., PMPM, cost per unit, frequency per 1,000, and RVUs) at a macro level. Enterprise reporting establishes a tracking system that identifies patient encounters in multiple settings throughout the provider network by using a single, unique identifier for each member regardless of the point of entry.

INFORMATION SYSTEMS STRATEGY AND DEVELOPMENT[6]

Marketplace solutions for provider-based managed care applications come from two points of origin: claims processing and medical practice billing. The provider network business model will determine which point of origin is used to acquire a managed care information system. For example, the IPA network model can begin on a claims processing

FIGURE 9
Core managed care transactions

Several core managed care transactions generate the data necessary to administer capitation.

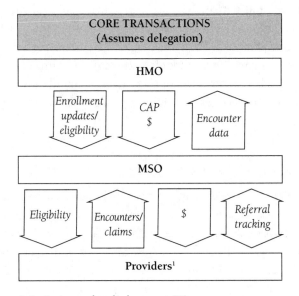

1. Institutions and medical groups or IPAs.

system adapted for enrollment, capitation, and reporting. The system must be equipped to handle large claims and encounter volumes manually. As enrollment builds, the provider network will need to link the managed care information system electronically with physician office practice management systems (e.g., billing and scheduling). For a medical group, the provider network will need an information systems platform that integrates physician billing, utilization management (e.g., referral and service authorizations), claims adjudication, appointment scheduling and patient registration, case management, and care planning under standard protocols.

MSO decision makers need to invest time and resources in the information system's medical management module. In the intermediate to long term, developing a managed care information system that pays claims like a preferred provider organization (PPO) on a fee-for-service basis provides no competitive advantage. The added value of a capitated provider network comes from an ability to substitute less-expensive services and improve prehospital, in-hospital, and posthospital service delivery through superior medical management. For this reason, the implementation of case management systems that complement or integrate with the managed care information system are a key aspect of information systems strategy. The case management module of a managed care information system can assist a provider network in consolidating the inpatient and outpatient utilization management functions. The case management module helps MSO personnel monitor the patient in the hospital and posthospital settings (e.g., skilled nursing, home health). The referral management module permits the authorization of services under a standard of care (criteria). The referral module also supports case management processes by helping managed costs for noncapitated specialists.

DECISION SUPPORT AND THE NEED
TO CAPTURE/CONTROL DATA

Decision support and control of claims/encounter and medical information are critical priorities for an MSO. Decision support provides a meaningful framework for performance and financial problem solving. Without delegation by the HMO of the claims/third-party administrative function to the MSO, the MSO will not have the sufficient CPT-4, ICD-9CM, cost, and membership detail to manage capitation. Even in situations where the payer adjudicates claims or processes encounter forms and provides PMPM reports retrospectively, the provider network may not be able to exercise sufficient control over the IBNR process (e.g., estimating future liability and monitoring authorizations, payment, and costs). Many nonstaff model HMO information systems cannot provide sufficient detail, databases, or reports for providers to improve outcomes and wellness for a defined population. This shortcoming is particularly glaring for integrated outcome databases that require medical records, pharmacy, patient satisfaction (e.g., SF-36 form), and claims/encounter information.[7]

FINANCIAL REPORTING CYCLE AND REPORT DEVELOPMENT CONSIDERATIONS

MSO personnel will need to push financial controls and reporting as a front-end and not a back-end implementation consideration. At the outset, the fiscal services department needs to provide clear direction and set priorities for MIS department and vendor installation efforts. Fiscal services personnel should provide direction on the types of financial applications needed and oversee development of summary and "drill down" reports. Industry experience has shown that most off-the-shelf managed care information systems address up to 75 percent of the desired reporting capabilities for managing capitation. MSO personnel should be prepared to address the remaining needs with internal resources, outside consultants, and programmers. For existing operations, MSO personnel and provider network participants need ongoing performance monitoring. Provider network financial officers, board members, and finance and managed care contracting committee members should review any performance monitoring effort with the following considerations in mind:

1. Who should produce the reports (i.e., key financial and operational responsibilities and assignments)?

2. What should the report track (e.g., financial managed care indicators, reports, education, and interpretation)?

3. Who should receive the reports and when (i.e., report distribution list, production frequency)?

4. How will information be acted upon? What is the continuous quality improvement (CQI) process for MSO administrative and physician

follow-up? What changes in medical management policies and procedures are necessary given current performance?

Figure 10 illustrates the performance monitoring and CQI process going forward. Steps in programming and production include

1. Design reports and applications

2. Identify, build, and test interfaces

3. Make database changes (tables and dictionaries)

4. Create test data

5. Test system reports (prototypes)

6. Create training materials

7. Calculate distribution, frequency, and responsibility

FIGURE 10
Overview of financial reporting cycle
Implementation effort for financial report

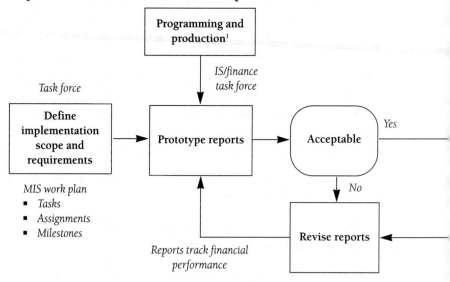

Presentation of financial reporting information

How financial information is captured, reported, and communicated can make or break provider networks' performance under capitation. The MSO fiscal services department should have user-friendly, summary, and drill down financial reports. These reports summarize financial performance at the network level with the ability to derive detailed performance at the POD level. In addition, the information system should stratify, profile, compare, and apply financial data in meaningful formats. These formats include

1. Actual performance (e.g., PMPM, frequency per 1,000 members) versus expected, budgeted, or group mean

2. Longitudinal trends (i.e., monthly, quarterly, yearly) adjusted for seasonality to track increases in costs and utilization

3. Comparisons of costs, intensity, and use between individual and groups of providers

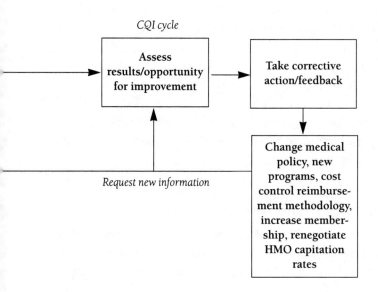

4. Break-out of data (e.g., cost, frequency per 1,000, intensity) by lines of business (e.g., commercial, Medicare risk, Medicaid, HMO payer, employer)

5. Break-out of data by geographic service area

6. Stratification of data (i.e., cost PMPM, frequency) by clinical grouping, DRG, UB 92 revenue codes, MDC, ICD-9CM, and CPT-4 groupings

7. Age/sex risk strata to adjust for case mix and population

Figure 11 provides a helpful explanation of common ratios and formulas used for managed care reporting purposes in steps 1 through 7.

To avoid information overload, financial reporting should be based on a step down approach (i.e., high-level summary information followed by detailed information of interest). The drill down format begins with the fund level and ends at the procedure level. An example of the drill down format is provided in Figure 12.

DATA REPORTING PITFALLS AND TRAPS

Data collection methods must be comprehensive and consistent. To ensure indicator statistics are valid and comparable, all data should be subject to rigorous integrity checks. For example, during the first year of operation, physicians and financial officers should treat financial reports and PMPM results for a start-up IDS with caution. Typically, one year of meaningful experience is needed, with approximately 90 to 180 days for claims run-out or lag to interpret financial performance. The first year may not be comparable to later periods due to new managed care programs and physician introduction to referral protocols. Another concern may be a low enrolled managed care membership (e.g., fewer than 25,000 commercial members) or PCP practice penetration (e.g., fewer than 60 members assigned to the PCP). Low enrollment may skew the statistical validity of utilization and PMPM results. These data considerations are highlighted in Figure 13.

LINKING FINANCIAL AND UTILIZATION REPORTING
TO PREPAID RISK REDUCTION STRATEGIES

This section shows which financial management reports are relevant for controlling and reducing prepaid risks. Secondly, this section provides a listing of these reports and their descriptions, purposes, frequencies,

FIGURE 11
Terminology and formulas
Raw utilization and cost annualized basis

Member months
Number of members × 12
1,000 members × 12 months = 12,000

Frequency units per 1,000

$$\frac{\text{Units x } 1,000 \times 12 \text{ (months)}}{\text{Member months}} \qquad \frac{\text{Cost PMPM} \times 12,000}{\text{Cost per unit}}$$

Cost per unit

$$\frac{\text{Total cost (total units} \times \text{cost per unit)}}{\text{Total units}} \qquad \frac{\text{Cost PMPM} \times 12,000}{\text{Units per } 1,000}$$

Cost PMPM

$$\frac{\text{Total cost}}{\text{Member months}} \qquad \frac{\text{Units per } 1,000 \times \text{cost per unit}}{12,000}$$

$$\frac{\text{Annual utilization rate} \times \text{cost per unit}}{12 \text{ months}}$$

Total variance
(Cost PMPM – budgeted cost PMPM) × member months

Frequency variance

$$\frac{\text{(Actual units per } 1,000 - \text{budgeted units per } 1,000) \times \text{member months}}{12,000} \times \begin{array}{l}\text{Budgeted} \\ \text{cost per} \\ \text{unit}\end{array}$$

Cost variance
Total variance – frequency variance

and possible formats. Figure 14 links major prepaid risks as identified earlier in Figure 1 with reports that track these risks as well as potential risk reduction strategies associated with these prepaid risks.

Top 10 critical managed care reports and applications

The purpose and application of the critical managed care reports for controlling prepaid risks listed in Figure 14 are described in this section.

FIGURE 12
Financial reporting—drill down approach
Framework for solving financial problems

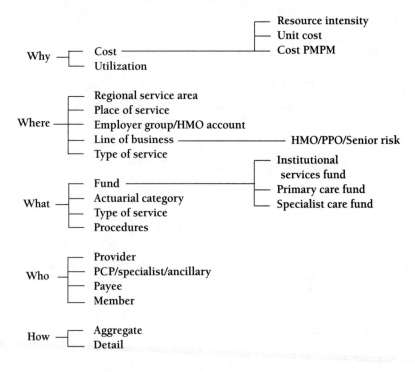

These reports include

1. Managed care network performance report card

2. Medical activity statements

3. Financial performance report by HMO payer

4. Risk pool settlement reports

5. IBNR reports

6. Monthly physician capitation summary report

7. Stop-loss reinsurance recovery report

8. Actuarial age/sex report

9. Capitation payment/member reconciliation reports

10. Enrollment and eligibility reports

FIGURE 13
Avoiding data pitfalls and traps

Data collection methods must be secure. To ensure indicator statistics are valid and comparable, all data should be subject to rigorous integrity checks.

Data comparability
- Time period (data completeness impacted by the claims lag period, 90–180 days required, seasonality)
- Need for one year of meaningful experience. First year of experience may not be comparable
- Differences in patient populations (age/sex, regional pathology, case mix)
- Appropriate population subsets are used for determining utilization rates for specific services
- Changes in benefit design (copayment and benefit structure impacts utilization)
- Appropriateness of grouping methodology used to classify data
- Local billing practices and provider reimbursement

Data accuracy
- Subjectivity and variability in physician/office staff coding (does the encounter/claim adequately portray the patient experience?)
- Properly completed and coded encounter and claim form (keystroke entry errors?)

Data consistency
- Common integrated database for cross-comparison and consistency or were variable sources without a common database used?
- Standard coding convention used across time periods

Data significance and volume needs
- Population with normal distribution more than 40,000 members
- Statistical significance within each specialty (primary care versus neonatology)
- Minimum of 700 member months per PCP (60-plus members) to avoid variation

PHYSICIAN PROFILING REPORTS

Another vital reporting area not covered in detail here is physician profiling. Physician profiling compares physicians within their peer groups, which can be determined by their responsibility centers, PODS, specialty, or the type of patients they treat. After adjusting for case mix (age/sex) and catastrophic outliers (i.e., financially or clini-cally defined), PCP profiles include rankings of PCPs according to individual, referral, ancillary, and institutional cost and utilization. Specialists, for example, can be profiled by their specialty according to patient case cost, patient condition (e.g., MDC, ICD-9CM), and resource utilization. Physician profiling reports or report cards should be understandable, accurate, and discussed with individual providers. Comparative profiling information

FIGURE 14
Linking managed care reporting to reducing prepaid risk

Major prepaid risks	Relevant risk reduction strategy	Relevant managed care reports
Risk-sharing incentives are not aligned among all providers and may lead to overutilization and higher costs	Risk pool structure, design, and participation level Incentives or criteria for surplus distribution and allocation of deficits Reimbursement structure or methodology Funds flow decision points (e.g., reserves, allocation of capitation among medical group, hospital, MSO, ancillaries)	Financial and service responsibilities matrix Funds flow sensitivity "what-if" analysis Risk pool settlement reports • Funds allocated by pool • Paid claims by provider • IBNR lag report • Settlement at pool level • Settlement at the PCP or group level (PODS) • Cap-member reconciliation report
High specialist referral costs and/or high out-of-network referrals to unaffiliated providers	Primary care management and protocols Physician and ancillary panel mix and access Geographic coverage, panel access Medical management Reimbursement structure or methodology	Medical activity and expense statements • Type of service analysis report Specialty activity and expense statements • Flexible budget (actual to expected) IBNR lag study reports Paid claims or capitation by provider report Primary care utilization and cost summary • PCP utilization profile and ranking summary • PCP cost profile and ranking summary • PCP referral and visit activity reports • PCP CPT-4 and diagnosis detail report • Fee-for-service equivalency report • Out-of-area report

FIGURE 14 (CONTINUED)

Major prepaid risks	Relevant risk reduction strategy	Relevant managed care reports
High management service organization costs and high administrative retention leaving insufficient capitation to cover medical expenses	MSO budget, overhead, accountability, performance, and pricing Physician governance and board oversight Reduction of HMO administration retention and duplicative services for fully delegated provider network	Financial statements • Income • Cash flow • Balance sheet Responsibility center accounting and tracking Network performance report card
High overall hospital utilization (i.e., bed days per 1,000 members)	Comprehensive continuum of care Primary care and medical management Wellness, population health status	Medical activity and expense statements Inpatient activity profiling reports Paid claims or capitation by provider report Specialty care utilization and cost reports
High cost mix of inpatient and ancillary services	Provider contracts and reimbursement Reimbursement structure and incentives	Medical activity and expense statements Network performance report card Episode and case activity reports
Inability to meet enrollment objectives, resulting in insufficient scale economies and high administrative overhead	HMO and MSO membership marketing Conversion of indemnity and PPO business to full risk or global capitation contracts Membership satisfaction and retention	HMO plan financial report(s) • Membership and enrollment reports Network performance report card
Low copays or insufficient patient financial incentive and inadequate patient demand management	Benefit design (HMO and employer control) Nurse triage and helpline Wellness programs, patient education	Call and visit activity and tracking reports
Catastrophic hospital and ambulatory claims (e.g., neonatal intensive care)	Case management, early case identification, sufficient reinsurance coverage	Stop-loss reinsurance report • Fee for service equivalency report Provider and PCP patient case detail report Episode and case activity reports

FIGURE 14 (CONTINUED)

Major prepaid risks	Relevant risk reduction strategy	Relevant managed care reports
Payer unwillingness to negotiate capitation rates sufficient to cover medical and administrative expenses	Provider contracting leverage (e.g., PCP exclusivity, network configuration—group versus IPA)	Actuarial (age/sex) risk strata report
Insufficient capitation payment and collection	Eligibility and benefits determination Reconcilement of capitation payment to membership and payment terms Retroactivity determination	Contribution margin report by HMO or payer Cap-member reconciliation report Enrollment report
Skewed enrollment, inaccurate actuarial estimates of family size and contract distribution (i.e., age/ sex/ family size-adjusted capitation payment) resulting in insufficient capitation	Population risk and assessment (claims data, risk assessment surveys)	Actuarial (age/sex) risk strata report PCP expense risk strata profile report
Low penetration or a higher percentage of high-risk, high-cost employees in employer groups, resulting in adverse selection and insufficient capitation	Benefit design, employee health plan selection incentive, large population	Actuarial (age/sex) risk strata report

when combined with financial incentives and helpful medical director guidance has proven very successful in changing physician practice patterns.

MANAGED CARE NETWORK PERFORMANCE REPORT CARD

This report is a high-level summary report card of hospital, medical group, and MSO performance. It compares provider network actual performance with standard/budget and provides intracomparisons between local providers with overall network performance. Individual line items such as membership turnover rate and patient satisfaction rating have considerable impact on network profitability, membership growth, physician satisfaction with network MSO services, patient satisfaction, and quality of care. Criteria for the individual line items noted under the categories of membership, administrative performance, access and primary care network, and quality of care/outcomes management are determined and selected by local provider network participants.

The managed care network performance report card features drill down focus on items with variation of 20 percent or more. The report is accompanied by narrative explaining why deviations of 20 percent or more have occurred for the performance indicator, what type of actions need to be taken, when these actions will be taken to resolve the deviation (if necessary), and who will be responsible for CQI follow-up. Outcomes for all outstanding items from prior reports are noted.

This report is used by provider network board members, senior management, and physician leadership on a monthly basis. Benefits include

1. Shows variance between projected enrollment and actual enrollment levels by membership type (e.g., Medicare, Medicaid, commercial)

2. Shows variance between projected catastrophic cases per 1,000 members and actual for case management and stop-loss reinsurance recovery purposes

3. Shows age/sex case mix variance between a normalized population and actual population served

4. Provides a high-level profit and loss statement for all HMO contracts. Expense categories also include administrative and out-of-area expenses

5. For management of specialty referral costs, provides high-level snapshots of professional referral categories such as radiology, surgery, emergency room, ancillary services, and physician visits

MEDICAL ACTIVITY STATEMENTS

The medical activity statement is a type of service analysis report similar to the GHAA reporting format. This can also include a specialty activity statement that sorts by type of professional service. The flexible budget compares actual with expected (budget) utilization (days per 1,000, frequency per 1,000, average length of stay), intensity (relative value units per 1,000), and cost (cost per unit PMPM). The statement also identifies claims settled by major service categories (CPT-4 professional), UB-92 revenue codes, and DRGs for institutional services. As a claim is adjudicated, the procedure or code for service and place of service is grouped by medical service categories for reporting purposes. Medical activity statements can be generated by service region, physician POD, and primary care physician and are useful for drawing comparisons between

REPORT 1
Managed network performace report card
Quarterly performace report

Indicator	Network YTD actual	Network YTD budget	Actual percent of budget
Membership			
Membership			
Commercial	13,000	18,000	72%
Senior	0	0	0
Total	13,000	18,000	72%
Member turnover/total membership	6.0%	5.0%	120%
Member grievance per 1,000	1.5	2.0	75%
Average days for resolving grievances	2.29	3.5	65%
Age/sex case mix index			
Commercial	$1.07	$1.00	107%
Catast cases per 1,000	$9.40	$7.20	131%
Catast case PMPM	$4.27	$3.58	119%
Network profit and loss			
PMPM performance			
Average HMO capitation	$109.78	$102.88	107%
Inpatient hospital	$(22.22)	$(18.49)	120%
Outpatient hospital	$(8.87)	$(8.56)	104%
Ancillary	$(2.39)	$(1.79)	133%
Primary care	$(14.41)	$(15.26)	94%
Specialist care	$(37.58)	$(28.94)	130%
Out of area	$(4.48)	$(3.08)	145%
Out of administration	$(15.83)	$(15.43)	103%
Total surplus/deficit	$4.00	$11.33	35%
Cost and efficiency			
Inpatient			
Total bed days	292	242	121%
Admits per 1,000	71.07	70.50	101%
LOS	4.40	3.43	128%
PMPM	$21.16	$18.00	118%
Cost per admit	$3,680.00	$3,064.00	120%
Authorized hospital cost/actual cost			95%
Outpatient			
Radiology			
Frequency per 1,000	176.9	130.0	136%
PMPM	$3.07	$2.37	130%
Surgery			
Frequency per 1,000	77.3	70.0	110%
PMPM	$2.18	$2.27	96%

REPORT 1 (CONTINUED)

Indicator	Network YTD actual	Actual YTD budget	Actual percent of budget
Cost and efficiency (cont.)			
Outpatient (cont.)			
Emergency room			
Frequency per 1,000	141.1	140.0	101%
PMPM	$1.16	$0.99	118%
Ancillary services			
Frequency per 1,000	324.8	271.3	120%
PMPM	$2.37	$1.75	136%
Authorized outpatient cost/actual cost	98.0%		
Physician services			
Visits per 1,000	3,099	3,114	100%
Visits per member	3.10	3.11	100%
RVU per visit	1.32	1.20	110%
Visits PMPM	$13.12	$12.45	105%
PCP PMPM	$14.27	$14.96	95%
Referral costs and utilization			
Referrals per 1,000	1,222	1,009	121%
Referrals per visit			
(% of visits referred)	45%	32.4%	139%
Adult	7.8%	8.5%	92%
Pediatric	87%		
Authorized referral—professional			
cost/actual cost	$30.27	$22.03	137%
Specialist PMPM	$7.66	$6.34	121%
Ancillary PMPM	$37.93	$28.37	134%
Total referral PMPM—difference	$9.56		
Out of area			
Out-of-area PMPM/total medical PMPM	5.8%	3%	193%
Out-of-area bed days/total bed days	2.7%	3%	90%
Out-of-area referrals/total referrals	6.3%	3%	210%
Administrative performance			
Days turnaround referral request			
Routine	3.26	2	163%
Urgent	1.02	1	102%
Average days turnaround claims	18.36	30	61%
Provider grievance rate per 1,000	24.07	30.3	79%
Average days for provider			
grievances resolved	2.30	2.5	92%

REPORT 1 (CONTINUED)

Indicator	Network YTD actual	Network YTD budget	Actual percent of budget
Access and primary care network			
PCP to specialist ratio	40%/60%	45%/55%	88%
Average percent of total PHO patients—PCP	6%	25%	24%
PCP per member ratio	1/867	1/1,800	48%
PCP turnover percent per total PCP	0.06	0.03	200%
PCPs within 10 miles of member	1.2	2	60%
PCP closed practice per PCP total practice	7%	15%	47%
Average members per PCP	110	450	
Quality of care/outcomes management			
Patient satisfaction survey	84%	90%	93%
90% agree/strongly agree	1.5%	2%	75%
Readmission rate	24%	15%	160%

network participants by service region. Special considerations need to be made for treating IBNR, out-of-area expense, COB, copayment, and reinsurance recovery items.

Medical activity statements are used by the provider network CEO and CFO, MSO and/or medical group/IPA medical directors, provider network boards, and participating IPA-medical group board members on a monthly basis. The key benefits of the medical activity statements are that they

1. Show variance between actual and expected utilization and PMPM costs. Useful for identifying problems or opportunities for improvement by major medical service category. Major variations can lead to further investigation followed by recommendations for changes in reimbursement or medical management policy before deficits are incurred

2. Show where services are performed by type of provider. Help users see if the network is fully leveraging its continuum of care (e.g., ancillary network) and directing patients to the most appropriate setting

3. Specialty activity statements allow IPAs and medical groups to develop subcapitation rates for specialists

FINANCIAL PERFORMANCE REPORTS AND CONTRIBUTION MARGIN REPORT BY HMO PAYER

HMO payer reports include provider network, physician organization, and MSO financial statements based on a separate chart of accounts. Profit and loss statement parameters will need to be defined and tables on the managed care information and G/L system will need to be established. An example of a simplified profit and loss statement includes the following items:

1. Capitation revenue

2. Fee-for-service revenue

3. Interest from cash assets

4. Risk pool proceeds

   <minus>

1. Billing and accounts receivable charges

2. Capitation expenses

3. Claims expenses (hospital, medical/outpatient)

4. IBNR expenses

5. Pending referral liabilities

6. Administrative expenses

7. Risk pool expenses

8. Other expenses

   = Profit/loss

These reports also show the contribution margin by HMO plan and type of contract (i.e., Medicare, Medicaid, commercial). Analysis shows growth in membership year to date, prior year, PMPM revenue, and expense; enrollment information by plan during a specified time period; and age/sex membership by plan as well.

Financial performace reports are used by provider network CFO, MSO administration, contracting personnel, provider network board members,

REPORT 2
Medical activity statement
Comparision of actual to budgeted performance

	Actual		
Type of service	Annual utilization per 1,000	Average cost per service	PMPM cost
Inpatient hospital			
Nonmaternity			
Medical	77.0	$2,800.00	$17.97
Surgical	87.0	$3,450.00	$25.01
Psychiatric	21.0	$1,365.00	$2.39
Alcohol and drug	12.0	$1,000.00	$1.00
Maternity			
Mother	60.0	$1,900.00	$9.50
SNF/ECF	3.0	$450.00	$0.11
Subtotal	260.0	$2,583.71	$55.98
Outpatient hospital			
Emergency hospital	127.0	$350.00	$3.70
Outpatient surgery	52.0	$2,200.00	$9.53
Radiology	104.0	$550.00	$4.77
Pathology	132.0	$180.00	$1.98
Other		$165.00	
Maternity	7.0	$785.00	$0.46
Subtotal	422.0	$581.29	$20.44
Physician			
Inpatient surgery			
Primary surgeon	45.0	$1,200.00	$4.50
Assistant	7.0	$665.00	$0.39
Anesthesia	29.0	$630.00	$1.52
Outpatient surgery			
OP facility	99.0	$450.00	$3.71
Office	249.0	$125.00	$2.59
Anesthesia	35.0	$400.00	$1.17
Maternity			
Deliveries	22.0	$1,400.00	$2.57
Cesarean deliveries	5.0	$1,600.00	$0.67
Nondeliveries	13.0	$300.00	$0.33
Inpatient visits	270.0	$95.00	$2.14
Extended care visits	2.0	$95.00	$0.02
Emergency room visits	130.0	$110.00	$1.19
Office visits	3200.0	$65.00	$17.33
Home visits	1.0	$112.00	$0.01

Budgeted			Variance	
Annual utilization per 1,000	*Average cost per service*	*PMPM cost*	*PMPM cost*	*Percent PMPM cost*
71.2	$2,800.00	$16.61	($1.36)	−8.2%
54.9	$3,450.00	$15.78	($9.23)	−58.5%
13.8	$1,365.00	$1.57	($0.82)	−52.2%
4.7	$1,000.00	$0.39	($0.61)	−156.0%
32.0	$1,900.00	$5.07	($4.43)	−87.4%
4.8	$450.00	$0.18	$0.07	38.8%
181.4	*$2,620.06*	*$39.60*	*($16.38)*	*−41.4%*
95.0	$350.00	$2.77	($0.93)	−33.6%
54.0	$2,200.00	$9.90	$0.37	3.7%
90.0	$550.00	$4.13	($0.64)	−15.6%
95.0	$180.00	$1.43	($0.55)	−38.5%
100.0	$165.00	$1.38	$1.38	100.0%
4.8	$785.00	$0.31	($0.15)	−48.4%
438.8	*$544.48*	*$19.92*	*($0.52)*	*−2.7%*
24.4	$1,200.00	$2.44	($2.06)	−84.4%
5.7	$665.00	$0.32	($0.07)	−21.8%
22.4	$630.00	$1.18	($0.34)	−28.8%
104.0	$450.00	$3.90	$0.19	4.8%
152.0	$125.00	$1.58	($1.01)	−63.9%
39.0	$400.00	$1.30	$0.13	10.0%
16.0	$1,400.00	$1.87	($0.70)	−37.4%
4.0	$1,600.00	$0.53	($0.14)	−26.4%
10.0	$300.00	$0.25	($0.08)	−32.0%
155.0	$95.00	$1.23	($0.91)	−73.9%
3.4	$95.00	$0.03	$0.01	33.3%
100.0	$110.00	$0.92	($0.27)	−29.3%
2,750.0	$65.00	$14.90	($2.43)	−16.3%
0.7	$112.00	$0.01	($0.00)	−42.9%

REPORT 2 (CONTINUED)

Type of service	Annual utilization per 1,000	Average cost per service	PMPM cost
		Actual	
Critical care	13.0	$183.00	$0.20
Consultation	125.0	$190.00	$1.98
Therapeutic injections	119.0	$30.00	$0.30
Allergy tests	19.0	$200.00	$0.32
Allergy immunotherapy	225.0	$32.00	$0.60
Physical medicine	330.0	$60.00	$1.65
Cardiovascular	108.0	$150.00	$1.35
Diagnostic testing	70.0	$157.00	$0.92
Dialysis	9.0	$232.00	$0.17
Chiropractor	262.0	$58.00	$1.27
Radiology	790.0	$85.00	$5.60
Pathology	2,400.0	$16.00	$3.20
Immunizations	263.0	$33.00	$0.72
Well baby	151.0	$30.00	$0.38
Vision exams	240.0	$70.00	$1.40
Speech exams	10.0	$40.00	$0.03
Hearing exams	94.0	$52.00	$0.41
Physical exams	150.0	$45.00	$0.56
Podiatrist	52.0	$100.00	$0.43
Outpatient psychology	320.0	$105.00	$2.80
Outpatient alcohol/drug	30.0	$124.00	$0.31
Subtotal	*9,887.00*	*$76.12*	*$62.72*
Other			
Prescription drugs	4,983.00	$41.00	$17.03
Home health or PDN	20.0	$200.00	$0.33
Ambulance	25.0	$400.00	$0.83
DME	45.0	$288.00	$1.08
Prosthetics	4.0	$715.00	$0.24
Eyeglasses and contacts	143.0	$195.00	$2.32
Subtotal	*5,220*	*$50.19*	*$21.83*
Total	**15,789.0**	**$3291.31**	**$160.97**

	Budgeted			Variance	
Annual utilization per 1,000	*Average cost per service*	*PMPM cost*		*PMPM cost*	*Percent PMPM cost*
6.0	$183.00	$0.09		($0.11)	−116.7%
80.0	$190.00	$1.27		($0.71)	−56.3%
80.0	$30.00	$0.20		($0.10)	−48.8%
17.0	$200.00	$0.28		($0.03)	−11.8%
155.0	$32.00	$0.41		($0.19)	−45.2%
200.0	$60.00	$1.00		($0.65)	−65.0%
95.0	$150.00	$1.19		($0.16)	−13.7%
51.0	$157.00	$0.67		($0.25)	−37.3%
7.0	$232.00	$0.14		($0.04)	−28.6%
270.0	$58.00	$1.31		$0.04	3.0%
600.0	$85.00	$4.25		($1.35)	−31.7%
1,900.0	$16.00	$2.53		($0.67)	−26.3%
360.0	$33.00	$0.99		$0.27	26.9%
107.0	$30.00	$0.27		($0.11)	−41.1%
227.0	$70.00	$1.32		($0.08)	−5.7%
5.0	$40.00	$0.02		($0.02)	−100.0%
78.0	$52.00	$0.34		($0.07)	−20.5%
190.0	$45.00	$0.71		$0.15	21.1%
40.0	$100.00	$0.33		($0.10)	−30.0%
240.0	$105.00	$2.10		($0.70)	−33.3%
25.0	$124.00	$0.26		($0.05)	−20.0%
4,733.0	*$74.06*	*$50.11*		*($12.61)*	*−25.2%*
3,000.0	$41.00	$10.25		($6.78)	−66.1%
30.0	$200.00	$0.50		$0.17	33.3%
10.0	$400.00	$0.33		($0.50)	−150.0%
30.0	$288.00	$0.72		($0.36)	−50.0%
2.1	$715.00	$0.13		($0.11)	−90.5%
142.0	$195.00	$2.31		($0.02)	−0.7%
3,214.1	*$53.15*	*$14.24*		*($7.60)*	*−53.4%*
8,567.3	**$3,291.75**	**$123.87**		**($37.12)**	**−30.0%**

REPORT 3
Summary HMO contribution margin report
All payers

	Total cost	Percent of revenue	PMPM	Cost per encounter
Revenue:				
Capitation				
Copayment				
COB				
Stop-loss				
Total capitation revenue	*$18,450,180*	*100%*	*$61.50*	*$228.49*
Expenses:				
Primary care physician				
shared risk cost	$4,224,780	22.9%	$14.08	$52.32
Referral cost	$9,191,700	49.8%	$30.64	$113.83
Direct operating expenses	$1,809,360	9.8%	$6.03	$22.41
Other medical expenses	$1,355,760	7.3%	$4.52	$16.79
Total medical expenses	*$16,581,600*	*89.8%*	*$55.27*	*$205.34*
Contribution margin (loss)	$1,868,580	10.1%	$6.23	$23.14
MSO administrative expense	$1,563,660	8.5%	$5.21	$19.36
Net income (loss)	*$304,920*	*1.6%*	*$1.02*	*$3.78*

Member months	300,000
Members	25,000
Encounters per member	3.23
Total encounters	*80,750*

and finance and contracting committee members on a monthly basis. Some key benefits include the following:

1. In order to monitor profitability by health plan, revenue data including capitation and copayment income, risk settlements, and stop-loss income must be tracked against expenses, including claims paid to outside providers, costs of services provided internally (encounter and/or claims information), and stop-loss premiums. This information is critical at contract renewal time to be able to negotiate capitation rate increases and can be easily accessed with financial performance reports

2. Tracking of profit and loss by benefit plan, health plan, and overall can be very useful for individual negotiations with each health plan.

RISK POOL SETTLEMENT PROCESS AND REPORTS

Risk pool reconciliations can present MSO personnel with a host of challenges. Failure to complete risk pool reconciliations in a timely manner can have negative financial implications and generate provider dissatisfaction, particularly when reimbursement is low. MSOs that have shared risk pool arrangements with HMOs may not be processing institutional claims. As a result, MSO fiscal service department personnel may face the challenge of generating a risk pool reconciliation report with missing institutional data or incomplete HMO data.

Typically, under the risk pool reconciliation accounting procedure each provider participant risk pool is debited monthly with an actuarially determined amount for each member and then reduced by those members' actual provider reimbursements. The credits are adjusted based on the age and sex characteristics of the membership to reflect differences in members' expected PMPM costs. Reductions to the respective provider pools are based on negotiated provider rates incurred during the accounting period. Settlement occurs three to four months after the experience period.

Report 4 provides an example of risk pool settlement and reconciliation process. This example includes

1. Backing out catastrophic days

2. Settlements for the medical group will be made quarterly:

   - Based on cost and quality data compiled during the prior quarter

   - It is not believed that the IBNR "tail" existing after 90 days will be significant enough to pose a financial risk to the medical group pool

3. If an aggregate deficit exists after the interim payments are disbursed, it will be applied to the following quarter's surplus or deficit

4. Excessive shortfalls will be covered with short-term borrowing at the medical group or IPA level

5. Estimated surpluses and deficits beyond a specific percent of budget will be applied to the quarterly adjustment of PCP and specialist compensation

REPORT 4
Risk pool settlement
reconciliation of referral experience pool to actual

	Actual	Projected	Variance (Projected– actual)
Capitation revenue professional cap	$1,085,543	$1,042,121	$43,422
Total	$1,085,543	$1,042,121	$43,422
65% allocation to claims expense	$705,603	$677,379	$28,224
Less:			
Referral claims paid	($199,775)	($199,775)	$0
Specialist subcap payments	($152,347)	($152,347)	$0
Positive/(negative) balance	$353,481	$325,257	$28,224
50% risk pool distribution Annual allocation	$176,741	$162,629	($14,112)
Total	$176,741	$162,629	($14,112)
Less:			
25% payout primary care	($44,185)	($40,657)	($3,528)
25% payout specialist	($44,185)	($40,657)	($3,528)
Balance risk pool	$88,370	$81,314	($7,056)

6. Year-end settlements will call for reconciliation of any deviation from budget. Outstanding surpluses or deficits will be contributed to the medical group and institutional pool according to the distribution methodology

Risk pool settlement reports reconcile capitation revenue and other income with claims expense paid (i.e., provider claims and subcap payments for each pool). This requires information from the IBNR lag report and paid claims by provider report. This type of report also shows that certain reserves may be retained for IBNR purposes so that surplus pool funds are not fully paid out. Surplus monies are paid out of pools and distributed according to the risk-sharing distribution formula.

Risk pool settlement reports are used by MSO CFO, MSO fiscal services department, provider network board, and finance and contracting committee members on a quarterly basis.

Another type of risk pool settlement report is that which is performed at the provider organization detail level. This report displays a summary of a local provider entity's distribution and depletion of risk pool funds over the reporting period. The local provider organization can include individual PCPs, primary care PODs, IPAs/medical groups, or regional service areas. This report is used to determine pool account balances, monitor budgeted versus actual risk pool results, track stop-loss, provide fee-for-equivalency reporting, and control claims costs.

It is used by MSO fiscal services department, medical director, finance and contracting committee members, and participating primary care physicians on a quarterly basis.

INCURRED BUT NOT REPORTED REPORTS

Typically, long periods of time transpire between the time a noncapitated provider submits a claim for payment and the time service was rendered. The MSO fiscal services department must rely on a method for adjusting from a cash basis to an accrual basis. In other words, MSO finance personnel must make accurate estimates of all potential liabilities resulting from services rendered. To calculate risk pool balances correctly, estimate financial liability and monitor costs, the MSO fiscal services department must estimate the claims outstanding—incurred but not reported, (IBNR). IBNR represents the liability for services that are the organization's responsibility under capitation but have not been recorded by the claims department yet. This would include all out-of-area claims, out-of-network payments such as emergency rooms, and services that were authorized and performed but have not yet been submitted.

Some early pioneers in managed care failed because they did not properly accrue for IBNR claims. IBNR is a critical area that requires accurate, timely, and conservative calculation. Common methods for calculating IBNR or medical accrual include actual utilization, lag schedules, and historical PMPM. Under actual utilization, pending liability can be determined from outstanding referrals. Estimated pending liability is determined from the original liability minus any approved dollars from claims linked to the referral. This method and these reports allow the finance department to determine the potential liability and to estimate how long it will be take for pending liabilities to be recorded. Lag schedules are discussed in further detail below.

Typically, there is a 60- to 120-day lag in receiving and processing claims. After the end of 120 days, one can anticipate approximately 80 percent of claims being paid. During the first 18 months of taking full risk, the actuarial analysis percentages of non-subcapitated providers should be used along with at least a 10 percent cushion factor. After one year of experience, actual finished (i.e., months where all claims have been paid, usually after the 10th month) claims data should be used with the actuarial data. Therefore after 18 months there should be about 8 months of finished data that can be compared to the original actuarial report. At this point, modifications to accruals should be made only if the actual data reflects a higher percentage of claims than the actuarial percentages. If the actual claims data reflects lower percentages, adjustments should be held off until the end of a 24-month period where there would be approximately 14 months of finished data.

The reports that are needed for analyzing IBNR include the claims lag grid, authorized but unpaid claims, and claims paid by specialty (shows actual, PMPM, and percent of total). All of these reports work together to develop a complete forecasting tool. The older and larger the database, the more reliable the results.

Types of INBR reports include claims aging, cumulative paid claims, actual paid claims, completion ratios, paid as percent of complete, and claims reserve analysis.

The claims lag grid (actual paid claims) is a report of claims recognized in a reporting/accounting period sorted by month of service occurrence. This report is usually illustrated in a matrix that shows the month of service versus month of payment.

This IBNR report is used by MSO fiscal services department on a monthly basis. The key benefits are that claims lag grid reports

1. Are useful analytical tools that provide PMPM cost, utilization, and seasonality analysis

2. Provide an audit of the claims processing functions

3. Can be adjusted to recognize the effects of new contract terms

An important factor in estimating IBNR is a valid and consistent method for estimating the claims outstanding. Information systems that rely on historical utilization experience to generate IBNR lag reports may have shortcomings. In managed care, the assumption that historical events repeat themselves and, therefore, become valid predictors of future performance may lead to inaccurate estimates of potential claim liability. Other factors for consideration when calculating IBNR include[8]

1. *Product design changes.* As benefit packages change, the utilization may increase or decrease, thereby increasing or decreasing the number of claims outstanding. Examples include lower copayments for office visits and increases in mental health coverage

2. *Member mix changes.* Large turnover in membership can either increase or decrease utilization depending on the population case and age/sex mix

3. *Provider contract reimbursement changes.* When providers' contract reimbursement terms are changed, IBNR is affected. If providers are fully capitated, IBNR may be reduced significantly. This is not true where capitation creates leakage (i.e., capitation may lock in the cost of one type of service but increase another type). Changes in provider reimbursement methodology increase the risk of errors in the IBNR calculation. This is because there is usually not a historical track record and providers respond to changes in reimbursement methodology in an unpredictable manner. Also, changes in the size of the provider network will have an effect on IBNR (e.g., increase in specialty panel or addition of new providers who are unfamiliar with network referral procedures)

4. *Claims not recorded in lag tables.* If any claims are handled outside the claims system, it is necessary to include the effects of these costs in the IBNR calculation

5. *Coordination of benefits recovery.* The treatment of coordination of benefits (COB) will affect IBNR calculations. It is important for those preparing the IBNR estimate to know exactly how COB is recorded and how COB affects the lag tables. High COB recovery can reduce IBNR liability

6. *Claims backlog.* MSO claims-processing departments can experience claims payment turnaround times exceeding 120 days or more. In these situations, a backlog in claims not only affects the current IBNR calculation but also distorts lag table information for months and sometimes years. Therefore it is necessary to factor backlog into the IBNR calculations and to adjust historical lag table information once these backlogs are worked off. Typical claims backlog can be broken down as follows:

   a) Claims entered in the system but suspended

REPORT 5
Paid claims and completion report
Claims lag grid

Based on claims paid 11/94 to 6/95

Paid month	11/94	12/94	1/95	2/95
11/94	$6,121	$728,023	$1,914,313	$930,159
	0%	15%	53%	71%
12/94		$2,518	$724,737	$1,729,479
		0%	17%	57%
1/95			$24,580	$726,843
			0%	15%
2/95				$31,720
				1%
3/95				
4/95				
5/95				
6/95				
Total	*$6,121*	*$730,541*	*$2,663,630*	*$3,418,201*

b) Claims not entered in the system but on the claims examiner's desk

c) Claims logged in and awaiting transfer to the claims examiner's desk

d) Claims not logged in yet and awaiting processing in the mailroom

e) Claims not yet submitted by the provider

MONTHLY PHYSICIAN CAPITATION SUMMARY REPORT

This report provides a detailed summary of claims and capitation paid by provider and is useful for contract negotiations. In addition, the reports can be used as a source for profit and loss activity by the medical group, PCP, or hospital. The report shows the amount of business volume directed to each participating IDS provider. On the individual provider

3/95	4/95	5/95	6/95	Totals	Average days
$993,468	$227,076	$96,488	$127,838	$5,023,486	73.7
91%	96%	97%	100%	100%	
$1,272,991	$301,005	$148,419	$155,068	$4,334,217	72.0
86%	93%	96%	100%	100%	
$3,042,352	$565,432	$433,326	$133,908	$4,926,441	64.4
77%	88%	97%	100%	100%	
$2,229,034	$1,860,138	$668,772	$195,589	$4,985,253	54.5
45%	83%	96%	100%	100%	
$37,107	$1,798,869	$2,612,226	$367,527	$4,815,729	54.5
1%	38%	92%	100%	100%	
	$119,817	$1,780,915	$546,079	$2,446,811	43.9
	5%	78%	100%	100%	
		$57,891	$177,104	$234,995	23.4
		25%	100%	100%	
			$166	$166	
			100%	100%	
$7,574,952	*$4,872,337*	*$5,798,037*	*$1,703,279*	*$26,767,098*	*62.9*

level, the report shows the PCP and medical group how much capitation, RBRVS payment, and risk pool surplus was paid to the medical group or PCP based on member volume within a specified time period.

This report is used by MSO fiscal services department and contracting department on a monthly or quarterly basis.

STOP-LOSS REINSURANCE RECOVERY REPORT

HMO stop-loss filing requirements and deadlines make concurrent monitoring of stop-loss thresholds critical. The stop-loss report details year-to-date claims for members exceeding a specific and aggregate stop-loss amount. This report is filed with reinsurers for recovery purposes. Other considerations include

▪ Compare total reinsurance premium paid to amount recovered

REPORT 6
Monthly physician capitation summary report

Physician name	Enrollees	Plan type	Fund enrollment	Retro-spective enrollment	Claims adjust-ments
Chu, Ron, MD	400	Com	$4,800	$480	($960)
	100	Med	$3,600	$120	($480)
	500	Total	$8,400	$600	($1,440)
Smith, David, MD	800	Com	$9,600	$960	($1,920)
	300	Med	$10,800	$360	($1,440)
	1100	Total	$20,400	$1,320	($3,360)
Waterman, Karen, MD	150	Com	$1,800	$180	($360)
	150	Med	$5,400	$180	($720)
	300	Total	$7,200	$360	($1,080)
Sanjay, Raj, MD	526	Com	$6,312	$631	($1,262)
	0	Med	$0	$0	$0
	526	Total	$6,312	$631	($1,262)
Subtotal commercial	*1,876*		*$22,512*	*$2,251*	*($4,502)*
Subtotal Medicare	*550*		*$19,800*	*$660*	*($2,640)*
Total	**2,426**		**$42,312**	**$2,911**	**($7,142)**

REPORT 7
Stop-loss reinsurance recovery report
Claims in excess of $25,000 report

Member ID		Inpatient medical	Outpatient medical	Total
1 member in excess	$25,000.00 total of	$41,262.97	$39,743.00	$81,005.97
1 member in excess	*Subtotal HMO #A*	*$41,262.97*	*$39,743.00*	*$81,005.97*
6 members in excess	*Total all HMO*	*$408,240.00*	*$158,760.00*	*$567,000.00*

Manual adjustments	Withhold amount	Shared risk amount	Net revenue	Net PMPM
$0	($720)	$800	$4,400	$11.00
$0	($360)	$300	$3,180	$31.80
$0	($1,080)	$1,100	$7,580	$15.16
$0	($1,440)	$50	$7,250	$9.06
$0	($1,080)	$75	$8,715	$29.05
$0	($2,520)	$125	$15,965	$14.51
$0	($270)	$800	$2,150	$14.33
$0	($540)	$700	$5,020	$33.47
$0	($810)	$1,500	$7,170	$23.90
$0	($947)	$1,890	$6,624	$12.59
$0	($947)	$1,890	$6,624	$12.59
$0	*($3,377)*	*$3,540*	*$20,424*	*$10.89*
$0	*($1,980)*	*$1,075*	*$16,915*	*$30.75*
$0	**($5,357)**	**$4,615**	**$37,339**	**$15.39**

- Ability to run paid claims data that is relevant for reinsurance recovery (e.g., ensure that all capitated services, nonparticipating provider costs are included). Calculates and determines allowable and nonallowable expenses

- What percent of capitation is paid for reinsurance purposes?

- Can the information system reprice claims experience/encounters according to reinsurance reimbursement amount (e.g., 70 percent of charges)?

This report is used by the MSO fiscal services department, medical management department, and contracting department on a quarterly basis.

REPORT 8
Actual expenses by specialty adjusted by age/sex

Age/Sex	Member months	Total PMPM	Inpatient	Hospital Outpatient outpatient	Outpatient services	ER
<1 M+F						
1–4 M+F	6	$5.99	$1.82	$4.89	$2.70	$0.48
5–19 M+F	76	$29.91	$3.94	$2.45	$2.34	$2.39
20–39 F	399	$83.65	$15.33	$7.47	$5.22	$2.86
20–39 M	461	$44.89	$9.37	$3.75	$2.64	$2.41
40–64 F	301	$127.04	$25.98	$10.59	$7.08	$2.20
40–64 M	316	$94.55	$21.84	$8.28	$4.35	$2.08
65+ F	13	$157.79	$30.67	$18.46	$6.11	$1.36
65+ M						
Total	1,572	$80.50	$16.46	$6.98	$4.51	$2.40

Excludes catastrophic cases greater than $20,000.
Other can include: anesthesiology, neurology, ENT, pharmacy, and cardiology.

ACTUARIAL AGE/SEX REPORT

This report shows the number of claims, encounters, and PMPM by age and sex range. The report can be sorted by payer. The report helps personnel evaluate the distribution of members in various age and sex risk stratas during a reporting period. Useful for explaining the expense and utilization characteristics of the total membership as well as by each HMO payer, medical group, and/or IDS service region. Actual age/sex factors can be compared with budgeted age/sex factors to determine if HMO capitation payments were sufficient given the experience and case mix of the population served.

This report is used by MSO fiscal services and contracting departments on a quarterly basis.

CAPITATION PAYMENT PER MEMBER
RECONCILIATION REPORTS

Reconciling HMO capitation income to membership and negotiated contract terms presents considerable challenges. These challenges include determining the reconciliation period (timing), consistency and accuracy of payment, eligible versus ineligible members, and the com-

Radiology	Surgical	Lab	Ob/GYN	Family practice	Inpatient medicine	Pediatrics	Other
$0.96	$0.22		$0.04	$0.03	$14.50	$3.19	$9.97
$0.64	$2.28	$0.97	$0.30	$1.14	$0.62	$5.01	$7.20
$2.11	$4.71	$6.56	$9.35	$2.75	$5.50	$0.67	$20.31
$1.31	$4.68	$2.47		$2.44	$4.15	$0.03	$11.25
$4.21	$9.49	$8.98	$6.33	$3.51	$10.77	$0.01	$36.05
$2.54	$8.65	$5.15		$3.09	$8.42	$0.01	$28.93
$4.14	$12.33	$10.90	$1.79	$5.00	$9.89		$54.71
$2.30	*$6.33*	*$5.28*	*$3.62*	*$2.80*	*$6.54*	*$0.44*	*$22.01*

plexity of health plan capitation statements. To perform this reconciliation, the information system must integrate enrollment and revenue modules. Secondly, several reports are needed to perform the reconciliation. Determination of retroactive additions and deletions from eligibility is needed as well as the cap amounts for the age/sex of the member. Capitation receivable is estimated and reconciled with actual payment. Variance between estimated payment and actual are audited and followed up for collection action with the HMO payer.

These reports are used by MSO fiscal services and member services department on a monthly basis. The major benefit of capitation payment/member reconciliation reports is the audit of HMO capitation payments to assure payment according to age/sex capitation amounts, membership, and contract terms.

ENROLLMENT AND ELIGIBILITY REPORTS
This report provides a summary of membership enrollment by health plan, contract type (e.g., Medicare, Medicaid, commercial) and by provider (PCP). The report can be used to monitor member counts and member month information. Secondly, MSO personnel can use the

REPORT 9

Capitation payment reconciliation

Effective date	Number of months	Member	Name	Jan–Dec revenue	Health plan Administrative 16.0%	Out of area 1.6%
Jan-94	0	60565	YAA	-	-	-
May-93	8	53957	YAB	2,663.60	426.18	41.29
Jun-93	7	12953	YAC	2,445.10	391.22	37.90
Jan-93	12	33038	YAD	3,870.00	619.20	59.99
Oct-93	3	41498	YAD	998.85	159.82	15.48
May-93	8	16997	YAE	2,794.40	447.10	43.31
Apr-93	9	16740	YAF	2,902.50	464.40	44.99
Apr-93	9	18109	YAG	2,996.55	479.45	46.45
Feb-93	11	17852	YAH	3,842.30	614.77	59.56
Apr-93	9	19221	YAI	2,902.50	464.40	44.99
Dec-93	1	18964	YAJ	332.95	53.27	5.16
Nov-93	2	20333	YAK	698.60	111.78	10.83
Sep-93	4	20076	YAM	1,290.00	206.40	20.00
Sep-93	4	21445	YAN	1,331.80	213.09	20.64
Jun-93	7	21188	YAP	2,445.10	391.22	37.90
Jun-93	7	22557	YAR	2,257.50	361.20	34.99
Jun-93	7	51569	YAS	2,330.65	372.90	36.13
Feb-93	11	22300	YAT	3,842.30	614.77	59.56
May-93	8	23669	YAW	2,580.00	412.80	39.99
May-93	8	23412	ZAM	2,663.60	426.18	41.29
May-93	8	26781	ZBM	2,794.40	447.10	43.31
May-93	8	26524	ZCM	2,580.00	412.80	39.99
Apr-93	9	27893	ZDM	2,996.55	479.45	46.45
Feb-93	11	60561	ZEM	3,842.30	614.77	59.56
Apr-93	9	53951	ZFM	2,902.50	464.40	44.99
Dec-93	1	60304	ZGM	332.95	53.27	5.16
Nov-93	2	61673	ZHM	698.60	111.78	10.83
Sep-93	4	61416	ZIM	1,290.00	206.40	20.00
Sep-93	4	61159	ZJM	1,331.80	213.09	20.64
Total	191			63,957.40	10,233.21	991.38

Notes

Jan–Dec revenue includes beneficiary premium ($10–$45 per month).

Jan–Dec revenue includes age/sex adjustment.

Effective date from eligibility report Feb-94.

Deductions						
Vision $1.45	Rein-surance $2.00	Amount due	Amount paid	Adjusted amount due	Amount due hospital	Amount due physician
-	-	-	-			
11.60	16.00	2,168.53	2,130.88	37.65	20.71	16.94
10.15	14.00	1,991.83	1,864.52	127.31	70.02	57.29
17.40	24.00	3,149.41	3,196.32	(46.91)	(25.80)	(21.11)
4.35	6.00	813.20	838.32	(25.12)	(13.82)	(11.30)
11.60	16.00	2,276.39	2,064.00	212.39	116.81	95.58
13.05	18.00	2,362.06	2,397.24	(35.18)	(19.35)	(15.83)
13.05	18.00	2,439.60	2,397.24	42.36	23.30	19.06
15.95	22.00	3,130.02	3,073.84	56.18	30.90	25.28
13.05	18.00	2,362.06	2,322.00	40.06	22.03	18.03
1.45	2.00	271.07	266.36	4.71	2.59	2.12
2.90	4.00	569.09	532.72	36.37	20.00	16.37
5.80	8.00	1,049.80	1,065.44	(15.64)	(8.60)	(7.04)
5.80	8.00	1,084.27	1,065.44	18.83	10.36	8.47
10.15	14.00	1,991.83	1,956.08	35.75	19.66	16.09
10.15	14.00	1,837.16	1,806.00	31.16	17.14	14.02
10.15	14.00	1,897.47	1,864.52	32.95	18.12	14.83
15.95	22.00	3,130.02	2,929.96	200.06	110.03	90.03
11.60	16.00	2,099.61	2,130.88	(31.27)	(17.20)	(14.07)
11.60	16.00	2,168.53	2,130.88	37.65	20.71	16.94
11.60	16.00	2,276.39	2,130.88	145.51	80.03	65.48
11.60	16.00	2,099.61	2,130.88	(31.27)	(17.20)	(14.07)
13.05	18.00	2,439.60	2,514.96	(75.36)	(41.45)	(33.91)
15.95	22.00	3,130.02	2,838.00	292.02	160.61	131.41
13.05	18.00	2,362.06	2,397.24	(35.18)	(19.35)	(15.83)
1.45	2.00	271.07	266.36	4.71	2.59	2.12
2.90	4.00	569.09	558.88	10.21	5.62	4.59
5.80	8.00	1,049.80	1,032.00	17.80	9.79	8.01
5.80	8.00	1,084.27	1,032.00	52.27	28.75	23.52
276.95	*382.00*	*52,073.86*	*50,933.84*	*1,140.02*	*627.00*	*513.02*

REPORT 10
Enrollment analysis report
Member month enrollment analysis by sex

Payer sort	6/94	7/94	8/94	9/94	10/94	11/94
HMO #1						
F	819	806	803	789	782	785
M	880	858	845	844	852	854
Total	*1,699*	*1,664*	*1,648*	*1,633*	*1,634*	*1,640*
HMO #2						
F	553	541	520	496	490	495
M	649	634	596	573	566	567
Total	*1,045*	*1,021*	*970*	*929*	*918*	*923*
HMO #3						
F	1,482	1,475	1,459	1,455	1,427	1,415
M	1,565	1,585	1,580	1,540	1,556	1,559
Total	*2,650*	*2,664*	*2,643*	*2,604*	*2,594*	*2,586*
Grand total	**5,394**	**5,349**	**5,261**	**5,166**	**5,146**	**5,149**

report to predict utilization based on age/sex of underlying HMO membership. PCP reports are used where on-line eligibility is not available. This report includes new members, terminated members, and current enrollee information.

This report is used by MSO fiscal services, marketing, and contracting departments on a monthly basis.

Summary

Managed care providers are faced with sweeping changes in their financial incentives, partnership structure, and strategic objectives as they migrate toward capitation. Successful management of prepaid risk depends on reengineering the administrative infrastructure and information systems to support the needs of those managing this risk. First steps include developing financial expertise, creating partnership structures in support of mutual strategic goals, developing procedures focused on capitation transactions, and creating intraorganizational

12/94	1/95	2/95	3/95	4/95	5/95	Total member months
794	777	780	754	746	720	9,355
867	850	836	814	798	783	10,082
1,661	*1,627*	*1,616*	*1,569*	*1,544*	*1,503*	*19,437*
499	493	483	480	466	470	5,985
559	552	552	530	534	536	6,846
920	*909*	*900*	*878*	*869*	*875*	*12,831*
1,403	1,408	1,402	1,382	1,374	1,369	17,051
1,557	1,557	1,553	1,507	1,488	1,478	18,524
2,574	*2,578*	*2,569*	*2,512*	*2,489*	*2,475*	*35,575*
5,155	*5,114*	*5,085*	*4,959*	*4,902*	*4,863*	*67,843*

education focused on the implications of capitation on day-to-day operations. Secondly, building an intelligent data system that integrates data from diverse sources in order to provide tracking and performance information is vital for managing capitated risk.

Developing the financial staff, systems, and reports described in this chapter will enable members of an organization to recognize, anticipate, and avoid some of the pitfalls inherent in prepaid risk. This, combined with aggressive negotiation, tight utilization and cost control, comprehensive case management, attention to member satisfaction, and financial incentives tied to performance for all participating providers, should lead to maximizing the potential for success under capitation.

CRITICAL SUCCESS FACTORS

Finally, three critical success factors are crucial for minimizing prepaid risks. Managing information and appropriate financial incentives are the only nonclinical methods for controlling risk.

1. Dedicated personnel with capitation expertise

2. Information system availability to support the capitation process on the front end

3. Education and communication among providers and the MSO constituents

NOTES

1. Larry Bonham, MD, chief medical officer, Physician Venture Management, as cited in Geoffrey Baker, "Tab 600 Integrated Delivery Systems," in *Health Care Capitation and Risk Contracting Manual* (New York: Thompson Publishing Group, 1995), 47.

2. A provider network's performance under at-risk HMO contracts will depend on its ability to assume managed care administrative functions. A fully delegated provider assumes all utilization and quality management, claims and encounter processing, provider payment, and credentialing and panel selection functions from the payer. Empirical evidence in Oregon, California, Arizona, Florida, and New Mexico suggests that the fully delegated model will result initially in some duplication of administrative functions, however, early investments will payoff later. See Baker, "Tab 600," 16–17. *Health Care Capitation and Risk Contracting Manual,* Thompson Publishing Group, 1995, 47.

3. The MSO provides third-party administrative (TPA) and physician group practice services to capitated network providers for an administrative fee. In a fully delegated model, the MSO develops administrative functions that are similar to an HMO. The HMO retains marketing, enrollment, premium billing, benefits management, actuarial, underwriting/reinsurance reserves, and selected member service and provider contracting functions.

4. PODS combine physicians into small groupings of 5 to 20 physicians. Combined results of the physicians within each POD are used to determine risk-sharing and incentive payments.

5. Failure to submit encounter data on a timely basis can impact providers. For example, physician groups may be receiving quarterly risk pool estimates from HMOs in shared risk contracts. Failure to submit encounter data understates actual expenses against the risk pool and may result in an overstatement of surplus funds at year-end.

6. Contribution made by Jim Swoben, Manager of Managed Care Systems, Scripps Health Services, San Diego, California.

7. The source for this section is "Capitation Financial Controls and Reporting for Capitation and Risk Contracting," *Health Care Capitation and Risk Contracting Manual* (Thompson Publishing Group, 1995) chapter 7.

8. Mark Muller, "The Measure of Value: HMOs and Tomorrow's Health Care Systems," (Group Health Association of America Conference, 1991, photocopied).

17

Special issues of ambulatory capitation

William Adamson
Chief Executive Officer
Saint Joseph's Medical Resources
Stockton, California

Mary Schattenberg
Manager
BDC Advisors, Inc.
San Francisco, California

THERE HAS BEEN AN INTENSE focus on the clinical aspects of managed care to achieve economic success for providers. The need for clinically oriented protocols, prospective and concurrent review, and other utilization management functions is generally accepted as a cost control function for managed care systems. Even though these approaches are of proven value, without appropriate managed care financial systems and controls there will be no enduring economic success for any healthcare system.

This chapter deals with the financial issues in ambulatory capitation with a brief section about the relationship between institutional and ambulatory capitation. This focus is for multispecialty groups or individual practice associations (IPAs,) but the principles can be applied to other physician organizations (POs) such as a primary care group contracting with specialists. The distribution of premiums between providers and HMOs will be discussed first, followed by basic reimbursement methodologies for ambulatory providers and linkages of economic incentives to appropriate performances.

The examples in the exhibits are based on commercial populations of working age (under 65) employees and their dependents. The same principles will apply to Medicare members, although the utilization of services will be much higher per member and distribution of services for this population between the types of providers will vary as well.

Determining premium and allocation

PREMIUM

Premium allocation between providers and insurers is the first step to design a financial system, which generally includes an HMO, institutional, ambulatory, and pharmaceutical providers. Vision and dental providers also may be included depending on the plan benefits. The percentage of the premium allocated to an ambulatory provider determines how much any provider—physician or ancillary provider—is reimbursed using a predetermined budget. This reimbursement may be the only source of income to the PO that accepts the risk of providing ambulatory services, although it may receive risk-sharing income from institutional and pharmacy risk pools.

Figure 1 presents a typical distribution of premium between the HMO retention, reinsurance costs, other benefits (e.g., riders such as pharmacy and vision), ambulatory costs, and institutional costs. The level of premium chosen here, $120 per member per month (PMPM), is used for example only. The premium amounts will vary widely across the United States. For example, in California, some systems are producing average premium amounts lower than $100 PMPM for managed care products, while in the eastern United States producing average premiums in excess of $160 PMPM for similar products.

In all, the basic premium should be adjusted for age and sex to account for higher use rates of medical services by different segments of the population (e.g., women of childbearing age, infants, or the elderly). The adjusted premium matches the use of services to provider compensation. The $120 PMPM premium is a weighted average premium blend of all the different population segments. Table 1 represents actuarial weighting of a population with 1.0 being a normative population for utilization of medical services; the premium would be adjusted for a population having an aggregate weighting more than 1.0 (e.g., medical services are higher for individuals at birth and as they age and women of childbearing age have a greater incidence of use). The population in

FIGURE 1
Typical PMPM premium distribution
Risk pool surplus distribution

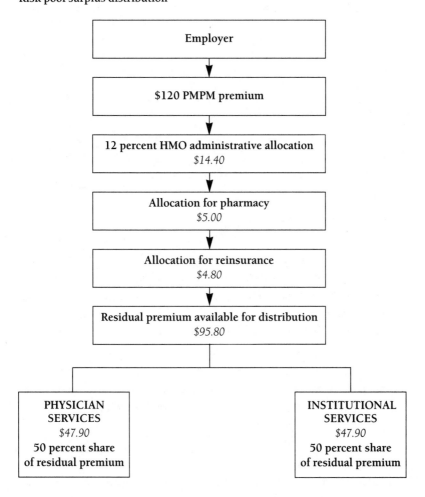

Table 1 has a weight of 105 percent derived by multiplying the weight of each of the age/sex cells by the actual percentage of the population involved and then adding the results together for a total that is compared to the proposed average capitation. The $120 PMPM premium in Figure 1 would be adjusted to $126 PMPM if the premium was adjusted for age and sex by using the weighting multiplier developed in the example in Table 1.

TABLE 1

Representative actual population weighting index

Age/sex category	Actual population distribution	Weight	Weighted population distribution
Child 0–1	2.0%	1.2015	2.4%
Child 2–9	7.6%	0.3858	2.9%
Child 10–17	20.0%	0.4310	8.6%
Female 18–29	9.5%	1.4564	13.8%
Female 30–44	17.0%	1.6385	27.9%
Female 45–64	10.3%	1.7794	18.2%
Female 65+	1.4%	2.0845	3.0%
Male 18–29	10.7%	0.4479	4.8%
Male 30–44	11.1%	0.7448	8.3%
Male 45–64	9.9%	1.4092	14.0%
Male 65+	0.5%	2.4364	1.2%
	100.0%		105.0%

Source: Marin IPA, 1993.

Another factor affecting the premium is the amount of cost borne directly by the patient. This usually takes the form of a noncovered benefit or an advance copayment for office visits, hospitalizations, and in some cases selected procedures (e.g., infertility). The premium for plans with increased patient responsibility will be adjusted lower due to the assumed share of cost borne by the patient. The premium yield will then be decreased by the share of cost for each benefit plan. The ambulatory provider organization (IPA or medical group) should track the utilization in the various categories to determine that the actuarial adjustment made by the HMO is correct.

ALLOCATION

After adjusting the premium for age, sex, and copayment variations, the premium can then be allocated among the HMO and providers. The breakdown shown in Figure 1 reflects a premium typical of advanced managed care systems. The percentage of the premium retained by the HMO varies nationwide. Where not-for-profit health plans have a significant market share (more than 25 percent), such as the Blue Cross Plans in Idaho and Hawaii, HMO retention as a percentage of premiums is as low as 8 percent for all insurance products.

Most HMOs include a drug benefit. Expenditures for pharmaceuticals depend primarily on physician ordering behavior. Thus, there is usually some financial linkage between the pharmacy budget and the ambulatory provider. These amounts can range from $6 PMPM for well-managed systems to $16 PMPM for nonmanaged systems.

RISK AND RISK PROTECTION

HMOs have shifted most risk to the provider organizations, which are usually unwilling to accept risk for events occurring outside of their service area. HMOs have responded to this by covering services provided outside the local service area for slightly lower reimbursement to the PO.

The provider organizations may also desire catastrophic insurance for cases costing more than specified dollar amounts. Such coverage is available from the HMO or can be purchased from a healthcare reinsurance company. While statistical risks are more predictable with larger populations, the risk of one case causing a severe aberration is lowered as the number of enrollees increases. Therefore, reinsurance requirements may be set at lower levels because the population involved is large enough to achieve a normalized risk experience.

Often, there is a coinsurance requirement (i.e., the provider organization bears some part of the risk beyond the first tier of reinsurance as a percentage of cost). Fee-for-service (FFS) payment mechanisms are usually used to measure the cost of service for reinsurance as opposed to some of the interim payment mechanisms referred to later in this chapter. As the covered population grows, tiers may be set at much higher levels. The amount of 4 percent is assumed to be the charge for total reinsurance in Figure 1 ($4.80 PMPM). This expenditure is "net" of reinsurance recoveries (i.e., those funds paid to the PO by the reinsurer for the cost of care over the threshold amount).

The threshold for accepting ambulatory capitation may vary from area to area, but populations of fewer than 5,000 commercial lives or 2,000 Medicare lives are usually considered inadequate to assume most of the risk of covering a population. Additional risk mitigation steps may need to be taken where there is a relatively small population being covered, including FFS fallback payment in the event of substantially higher utilization.

SHARE OF PREMIUM AND SERVICES COVERED

Particular attention should be given to the residual premium after HMO administration, pharmaceuticals, and reinsurance are deducted. The relative share of the residual premium allotted to ambulatory and institutional providers must be determined to define each party's prepaid funding. Residual share distribution and risk-sharing arrangements can be directly negotiated between ambulatory and institutional providers. These "global" capitation arrangements can be a method of working toward integration between these providers by gaining experience with shared revenue and cost structures.

There also must be a delineation of services included in the institutional and ambulatory components of global capitation. A grid such as Table 2 indicates services included in each component. The split between the institutional component and ambulatory component are negotiated in global capitation arrangements. Where there is only an ambulatory capitation agreement between the ambulatory provider and the HMO, a budget for institutional services or shared risk services will be set for risk-sharing opportunities.

Ambulatory capitation may range from 40 to 55 percent of the residual premium after deductions for HMO retention, reinsurance, pharmacy, and other benefits (e.g., mental health or vision). More aggressive managed care systems have demonstrated an ability to negotiate higher proportions of the total premium. As delivery systems become more efficient, the major reduction in costs is achieved in the institutional service area. The absolute dollar amount allocated to ambulatory capitation does not rise, but the institutional component falls both in dollar amount and as a percentage of residual premium. The split used in Figure 1 is 50 percent for ambulatory capitation and 50 percent for institutional services.

Figure 2 shows a similar breakdown of premiums in a health plan. A higher premium assumes a less aggressively managed provider environment or an indemnity provider network. The premium used in this example is $160 PMPM and the pharmacy cost is $15 PMPM. The institutional cost is also higher on an absolute dollar basis due to higher use of institutional services and higher unit pricing.

Distribution of ambulatory capitation

Ambulatory capitation usually includes all of the services listed in Table 2 as indicated under the column head IPA or medical group. Ambulatory providers include primary care physicianss (PCPs), specialty physicians, and allied healthcare providers, which include nonphysician

TABLE 2
Institutional and ambulatory responsibility grid
Full risk environment

Benefits	Responsible party	
	IPA or medical group	*Hospital*
AIDS[1]		
Professional component	■	
Facility component		■
Allergy		
Testing	■	
Serum		■
Ambulance, air or ground		
In area		■
Amniocentesis	■	
Anesthesiology services	■	
Apnea monitor (DME)		■
Artificial insemination	■	
Artificial limbs (DME)		■
Cardiac surgery		
Facility component		■
Professional component	■	
Chemical dependency rehabilitation		
Inpatient facility component		■
Inpatient professional component	■	
Outpatient professional component	■	
Chemotherapy		
Drugs, inpatient[1]		
Drugs, physician's office[1]		
Facility component		■
Professional component	■	
Chiropractic[2]		
Colostomy supplies		
Inpatient and outpatient (DME)		■
Contact lenses		
Intraocular lens (surgically implanted)		■
Incident to cataract surgery		■
Cosmetic surgery (if medically indicated)		
Facility component		■
Professional component	■	
Dental services (for repair of accident or injury only)		
Facility component		■
Professional component	■	
Detox		
Facility component		■
Professional component	■	

TABLE 2 (CONTINUED)

Benefits	Responsible party	
	IPA or medical group	Hospital
Durable medical equipment (DME)		
Surgically implanted		■
Inpatient		■
Outpatient		■
Hearing aids[3]		
Emergency admissions (in area)		
Facility component		■
Professional component	■	
Emergency admissions (out of area)[1]		
Employment physical[3]		
Endoscopic studies		
Inpatient		■
Outpatient	■	
Experimental procedures[3]		
Family planning		
Facility component		■
Professional component	■	
Procedures performed in physician's office	■	
Reversal of sterilization[3]		
Fetal monitoring		
Inpatient		■
Outpatient and physician's office	■	
Genetic testing	■	
Health education	■	
Health evaluation (physical)	■	
Hearing screening	■	
Hemodialysis		
Inpatient		■
Outpatient	■	
Home healthcare		■
Hospice care		
Inpatient		■
Outpatient		■
Hospitalization, inpatient supplies and testing		
In area		■
Immunization and inoculations		
As medically indicated	■	
For work or travel[3]		
Infertility diagnosis and treatment		
Facility component		■
Professional component	■	
Injections and injected substances (outpatient)[2]		

TABLE 2 (CONTINUED)

Benefits	Responsible party	
	IPA or medical group	*Hospital*
Laboratory services		
Inpatient		■
Outpatient	■	
Lithotripsy		
Facility component		■
Professional component	■	
Mammography	■	
Marriage counseling[3]		
Medication		
Inpatient		■
In lieu of hospitalization (IV therapy)	■	
Mental health		
Inpatient facility component		■
Inpatient professional component	■	
Outpatient professional component	■	
Neurosurgery (CNS)		
Facility component		■
Professional component	■	
Nuclear medicine		
Inpatient facility component		■
Inpatient professional component	■	
Outpatient facility component		■
Outpatient professional component	■	
Nutritional and dietetic counseling	■	
Office visit supplies	■	
Organ transplants (nonexperimental)[1]		
Outpatient diagnostic services		
Angiograms	■	
CAT scans	■	
2 D echo	■	
EEG	■	
EKG	■	
EMG	■	
ENG	■	
MRI	■	
Treadmill	■	
Ultrasound	■	
Physician professional services		
Anesthesiology	■	
Audiology	■	
Cardiology	■	
Diagnostic services	■	

TABLE 2 (CONTINUED)

Benefits	Responsible party	
	IPA or medical group	*Hospital*
Physician professional services (cont.)		
Neonatology	■	
Nephrology	■	
Neurology	■	
Pathology	■	
Physical medicine	■	
Pulmonary	■	
Radiology	■	
Radiation oncology	■	
Surgery	■	
Physician visits (any setting)	■	
Podiatry services	■	
Physical therapy		
Inpatient		■
Outpatient	■	
Prosthetic devices		
Surgically implanted		■
Outpatient		■
Rehabilitation (short term)		
Inpatient facility component		■
Inpatient professional component	■	
Outpatient facility component		■
Outpatient professional component	■	
Skilled nursing facility		■
Social services (medical)	■	
Surgical supplies		
Inpatient		■
Outpatient facility		■
Outpatient physician office	■	
TPA and AZT		■
Vision screening	■	
Vision care (medically necessary)	■	

1. Covered by the plan. Financial responsibility for AIDS, chemotherapy drugs, and organ transplants is usually covered by stop-loss insurance.

2. If covered by the plan.

3. Not a covered service.

Source: BDC Advisors' Analysis.

FIGURE 2
PMPM premium distribution
Less aggressively managed system

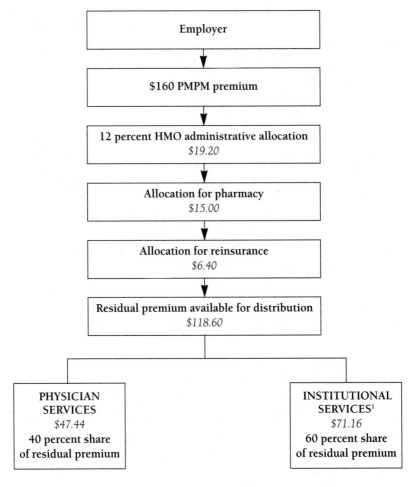

1. Assumes 300 bed days per 1,000 members per year.

mental health providers, physical and occupational therapists, dietitians, and podiatrists. Ambulatory services usually cover physician and ancillary provider professional services as well as outpatient diagnostic services such as clinical laboratory and outpatient radiology services.

The distribution of ambulatory capitation can be based on a simple FFS compensation basis for all physicians and ancillary providers. This may work for a period of time, as long as the fee schedule is set low enough not to overspend the ambulatory capitation. Fee schedules can be modified (e.g., withholds) to provide incentives to providers.

Managed care systems often initially offer PCPs reimbursement for the most common office visits above the normal fee schedule amounts to attract the PCP to the system. These visits typically make up the majority of the revenue of a primary care practice while being a small part of the revenue of specialty care providers.

FEE SCHEDULES

Fee schedules assign either a unit value or an actual monetary amount to a particular procedure. Where a unit value is used, a monetary conversion factor (MCF) is assigned to the unit value. The product of the two is the total fee for the procedure. Procedures are defined by the five-digit value code and two-digit modifier assigned to it in the current procedural terminology (CPT) system, which is in its fourth version, now referred to as CPT-4 codes. The following fee schedule systems are in common use in the current environment.

Resource-based relative value study

The resource-based relative value study (RBRVS), first introduced by the Health Care Financing Administration (HCFA) in 1992, is increasingly favored by payers. The RBRVS was developed to appropriately reward providers of care and to correct perceived inequities in historically based fee systems. RBRVS implementation is expected in 1996. This system is a departure from prior studies in that it attempts to weigh all types of physician services with a common unit value. Other studies have separate weighting systems for medical, surgical, pathology, radiology, and anesthesia services.

Historical fee systems have been driven primarily by market forces. The public perception has been that invasive procedures have more value than cognitive care (i.e., thinking through problems, diagnosing them, and then creating an appropriate treatment plan). Fee schedules therefore tended to favor interventions. This perception has been particularly true in the era of advancing technology. Most historical schedules did not reflect the cost efficiencies once a price had been set because there was a loss of revenue to the provider setting the fee once the price was lowered. On the other hand, if a new procedure required additional expertise or cost, the fees for those procedures were substantially increased over historical alternatives.

Managed care argues that cognitive treatment has proven to be as successful in producing favorable outcomes as interventions. The thoughtful evaluation of a problem, and patience, often allow the substitution of another less costly intervention or the resolution of the problem. However, in the current FFS environment, the lack of financial incentive to perform cognitive care creates a situation where procedures are favored. Managed care organizations have attempted to treat cognitive and procedural services with parity.

Generally, a common weighting system was felt to be necessary to insure parity in the providers' payment. Otherwise, the reimbursement for surgical and diagnostic procedures would have retained its historical bias.

The RBRVS is being revised yearly even though those changes are not always adopted by HCFA. Some integrated delivery systems (IDSs) have taken a transitional approach to adopting the RBRVS. This has taken the form of adopting different MCFs for different tiers of CPT4 codes reflecting some of the historical bias in fees for those systems. A representative fee schedule using a nonadjusted RBRVS weighting is contained in Table 3.

McGraw-Hill Relative Value Study

The McGraw-Hill Relative Value Study also has a different weighting system for medical, surgical, radiology, pathology, and anesthesia services but is updated periodically as is the CPT system. This is crucial when dealing with the payment for services, including modern procedures.

Many of the historical payment inequities can be adjusted by using the appropriate MCFs for each code class. Some systems tier the McGraw-Hill study in similar fashion to the RBRVS to blend in historical payment patterns over time. Both studies have been adjusted for current technological developments so costs are adjusted to reflect efficiencies.

For example, the use of a modern robotic blood chemistry analyzer substantially decreases the amount of labor associated with the tests and this reduction in labor costs is reflected in the decreased unit values for these procedures.

TABLE 3
Comparison of select CPT code reimbursement rates

Monetary conversion factors
RBRVS	$40.00
McGraw-Hill medicine	$6.00
McGraw-Hill surgery	$100.00
McGraw-Hill radiology	$25.00

CPT code	Description	RBRVS units 1995	McGraw-Hill units 1995	RBRVS fee	McGraw-Hill fee
Medicine:					
Monetary conversion factor				$40.00	$6.00
90935	Hemodialysis, one evaluation	2.81	20.00	$112	$120
90937	Hemodialysis, repeat evaluation	4.94	45.00	198	270
93000	Electrocardiogram, complete	0.80	7.80	32	47
93015	Cardiovascular stress test	3.30	37.00	132	222
93307	Echocardiography, complete	5.82	59.00	233	354
93325	Doppler color flow	3.12	31.50	125	189
94010	Breathing capacity test; Spirometry	0.90	10.50	36	63
96425	Chemotherapy, infusion	1.45	5.70[1]	58	34
99201	Office visit, new patient, 10 minutes	0.79	6.50	32	39
99202	Office visit, new patient, 20 minutes	1.25	9.50	50	57
99203	Office visit, new patient, 30 minutes	1.72	14.00	69	84
99204	Office visit, new patient, 45 minutes	2.57	20.00	103	120
99205	Office visit, new patient, 60 minutes	3.22	26.00	129	156
99211	Office visit, established patient, 5 minutes	0.38	3.50	15	21
99212	Office visit, established patient, 10 minutes	0.68	6.00	27	36
99213	Office visit, established patient, 15 minutes	0.96	9.00	38	54
99214	Office visit, established patient, 25 minutes	1.48	13.50	59	81
99215	Office visit, established patient, 45 minutes	2.34	19.50	94	117
99217	Observation care discharge	1.65	9.00	66	54
99222	Initial hospital care	2.97	22.00	119	132
99243	Office consultation, 40 minutes	2.54	22.00	102	132

TABLE 3 (CONTINUED)

CPT code	Description	RBRVS units 1995	McGraw-Hill units 1995	RBRVS fee	McGraw-Hill fee
Surgery:					
Monetary conversion factor				$40.00	$100.00
10040	Acne surgery	1.69	0.50	68	50
11440	Removal of skin lesion, face	1.85	1.20	74	120
11600	Removal of skin lesion	2.59	1.50	104	150
19180	Mastectomy, simple	14.93	10.40	597	1,040
19200	Mastectomy, radical	26.60	19.00	1,064	1,900
30520	Septoplasty	13.64	11.00	546	1,100
45330	Flexible sigmoidoscopy	2.31	1.30	92	130
45378	Diagnostic colonoscopy	8.22	5.10	329	510
55700	Prostate biopsy	3.22	2.00	129	200
55845	Extensive prostate surgery	54.27	35.00	2,171	3,500
57545	Colposcopy	1.78	2.30	71	230
58940	Removal of ovary(s)	14.36	11.00	574	1,100
60100	Thyroid biopsy, needle	2.14	1.50	86	150
63001	Removal of spinal lamina	36.47	35.00	1,459	3,500
66840	Removal of lens material	17.66	18.00	706	1,800
67017	Repair detached retina	33.00	28.00	1,320	2,800
Radiology:					
Monetary conversion factor				$40.00	$25.00
70480	Computerized axial tomography	6.73	23.80	269	595
71020	X-ray of chest	0.96	3.20	38	80
73110	X-ray exam of wrist	0.80	2.70	32	68
73610	X-ray exam of ankle	0.80	2.80	32	70
78306	Bone scan	5.64	17.00	226	425

1. Indicates a per hour basis.

A sample of fees determined using the McGraw-Hill study with separate conversion factors is presented in Table 3. The MCF for each subset of the ambulatory provider system is indicated in the table.

Usual and customary rates

A fee schedule developed by tracking the fees charged in the local medical community and adjusting for fees outside the norm is referred to as a usual and customary rate (UCR). Such fee schedules are usually developed only by payers in the geographic area, primarily due to anti-price-fixing legislation that keeps providers from sharing fee schedules direct-ly. Payers may discount the historical fee or limit its growth over time.

Such fee schedules are not being adjusted for new procedures. Pricing is market driven and therefore arbitrary. There is little basis for compar-ing UCR fee schedules to other systems such as McGraw-Hill or RBRVS since historical data replaces the formal weighting system. There is a decreased use of such UCR schedules due to their arbitrary nature and the difficulty with which new codes are added.

BUDGETARY PAYMENT SYSTEMS

Fee schedule distribution of ambulatory capitation can work as long as the fee schedule is set low enough to guarantee against overspending. This is usually accomplished by implementing a fee schedule and then withholding a portion of the payment to insure against overspending. The PO adopts budget parameters and sets its withhold rate accordingly, usually as a common percentage by all risk-sharing providers. The with-hold is then returned to the extent the capitation is not overspent. The use of fee schedules as the only mechanism to distribute ambulatory cap-itation usually can cause financial difficulties in that all providers of care are encouraged to overutilize as long as a FFS mechanism is used.

Most POs are moving beyond fee schedules and evaluating the share of capitation going to each ambulatory subcontractor even if no budgetary parameters are set. One of the most common types of reports used to assist the management of ambulatory capitation, a PMPM Cost Report, is presented in Table 4. There may be a differential return of withhold based on performance or the fee schedule may be set low enough to provide a surplus that may be used to reward providers who perform under bud-get. There may also be a penalty for overspending in addition to the for-feiture of a withhold.

Budgetary information that is developed locally and based on local experience is of limited value. Comparing inefficiencies of local spend-ing patterns by specialty to local historical trends does not indicate where fundamental changes should be made in the delivery system to make it more competitive while retaining appropriate quality levels. Comparisons of local data with regional and national managed care data is a necessary step to indicate budgetary shares for each component of the delivery system.

TABLE 4
PMPM cost report by specialty area

Activity	Costs PMPM	Budget PMPM	Variance (over) or under budget
Primary care	$ 13.30	$ 13.60	$ 0.30
Psychology	0.72	0.60	(0.12)
Nutrition	0.04	0.00	(0.04)
Physical therapy	1.16	1.00	(0.16)
Clinical laboratory	2.03	1.37	(0.66)
Podiatry	0.83	0.40	(0.43)
Allergy	0.54	0.30	(0.24)
Anesthesiology	2.05	2.00	(0.05)
Cardiology	1.05	0.80	(0.25)
Cardiac surgery	0.05	0.20	0.15
Dermatology	1.49	1.10	(0.39)
Endocrinology	0.16	0.20	0.04
Gastroenterology	0.93	0.70	(0.23)
General surgery	1.27	1.40	0.13
Infectious disease	0.05	0.10	0.05
Neurology	0.21	0.10	(0.11)
Nephrology	0.04	0.16	0.12
Neurosurgery	0.83	0.50	(0.33)
Obstetrics and gynecology	3.90	3.50	(0.40)
Hematology/oncology	0.85	0.04	(0.81)
Ophthalmology	1.26	1.10	(0.16)
Orthopedics	1.42	1.55	0.13
ENT	0.60	0.70	0.10
Plastic surgery	0.46	0.90	0.44
Pulmonary medicine	0.45	0.20	(0.25)
Radiology	3.97	4.00	0.03
Rheumatology	0.22	0.15	(0.07)
Urology	0.80	0.65	(0.15)
Other	2.76	3.40	0.64
	$ 43.44	$ 40.72	$ (2.72)

Source: Sample data—BDC Advisors, Inc.

SUBCAPITATION

Managed care systems are now moving to allocate capitation between ambulatory providers on a budgetary basis and to align economic incentives in order to ensure financial viability. The payment mechanisms move from rewarding any service in any setting to budget-based and prospective payment systems. As providers of care gain experience in the consequences of accepting risk, they may choose to manage the risk of their respective portion of the continuum of care directly. Subcapitation is the process by which a group of providers accepts risk for its portion of the continuum of care by taking a prospective payment for it.

In order for a group of providers to accept risk, they must know which services are their responsibility, defining the scope of services provided under the contract. The definition of services includes both clinical and procedural aspects. The relative responsibilities of a PCP for cardiac care are shown in Figure 3. Clinical boundaries may exist between specialties as well as between primary and specialty care (e.g., back care delivered either by an orthopedist or neurosurgeon).

Subcapitation rates are determined by using the frequency of procedures for each specialty area and multiplying them by the reimbursement rate per procedure. Since utilization rates are variable across the country, POs often transition to standards for frequency rates based on national managed care standards. An example of comparison of utilization rates is shown in Table 5, showing the frequency-of-use rates for certain outpatient procedures in a local service area compared to regional and national standards. The amount of work performed is usually referenced to a fee schedule per procedure using either the RBRVS or McGraw-Hill study and appropriate conversion factors.

An adequate population size is also necessary to assume the risk for a component of care. All of the comments made about risk assumption earlier in the chapter apply to the area of subcapitation. The frequency rate of procedures for a given specialty (e.g., infectious disease or neurosurgery) may argue against accepting subcapitated risk until the population is of large size. The low rate of frequency will cause minimal financial impact even if FFS payment methodology is used.

Techniques such as receiving FFS compensation for frequency rates of selected procedures above the norm can be used to mitigate adverse risk assumed by the provider. Thus, if the standard frequency rate for a procedure such as balloon angioplasty is two per 1,000 persons per year, and the experience for a large population is three procedures per 1,000 per year, additional subcapitation funding for the extra procedure per 1,000 would be considered provided all procedures were considered appropriate. Mitigation of adverse risk can also be accomplished by having reinsurance proceeds augment the compensation of specialty providers when frequency exceeds certain rates.

FIGURE 3
Primary care responsibility

Cardiology

1. Evaluate chest pain, murmurs, and palpitations and recognize significant heart disease by history, examination, electrocardiogram, echocardiogram, and stress testing including stress electrocardiogram, echocardiogram, or nuclear scan
2. Evaluate and treat coronary risk factors including smoking, hyperlipidemia, diabetes, and hypertension
3. Treat hypertension, non-life-threatening arrhythmias, congestive heart failure, and stable angina
4. Treat angina medically with nitrates, beta-blockers, calcium channel blockers, and other medication as appropriate. Evaluate noninvasively those who may need catheterization
5. Determine whether syncope is cardiac (i.e., valvular or arrhythmic) by history, examination, electrocardiogram, ambulatory monitoring, and echocardiogram
6. Diagnose and hospitalize patients with acute myocardial infarctions. Manage their inpatient course, discharge, and follow-up care. Obtain consultation for candidates for thrombolysis, stress testing, catheterization, angioplasty, or surgery and for patients with life-threatening arrhythmias or hemodynamic complications requiring invasive monitoring
7. Consult for
   a) unstable angina post-MI
   b) post-subendocardial MO with or without angina
   c) angina despite maximal medical therapy with maximally tolerated doses of nitrates, beta-blockers and calcium channel blockers
   d) intractable heart failure and arrhythmias
   e) pericardial effusion
   f) congenital or valvular disease. Consult only for diagnosis, noninvasive studies, and to define appropriate follow-up

Source: Miliman and Robertson, January 1994.

Since managed care performance depends on appropriate management of care, capitated providers increasingly depend on the PCP to act as a manager of patient care. These responsibilities may include expanding the historical clinical role to perform procedures previously performed by a specialist as well as managing care to produce a better overall economic result. It is prudent to allow utilization decreases derived from better management to occur prior to the system setting frequency rates for subcapitation purposes. The frequency rate based on a nonmanaged system will be too high and thus the budgeted amount may be excessive for each specialty. POs tend to compensate PCPs through a variety of mechanisms as they mature in managed care performance.

TABLE 5
Stockton Metropolitian Service Area (MSA)
Use rate comparisons (procedures per 1,000)

Procedure Group	MSA		PAC region		Benchmark	
	Total	*Outpatient*	*Total*	*Outpatient*	*Total*	*Outpatient*
Bronchoscopy	0.00	0.00	2.02	0.34	3.45	0.75
Cardiac catheterization	22.05	0.00	16.51	4.23	15.69	5.75
Colonoscopy	6.87	0.00	15.32	9.42	19.05	13.09
Transurethral cystoscopy	0.00	0.00	4.89	1.71	4.86	1.41
Laparoscopic cholecystoctomy	0.00	0.00	2.41	0.39	2.12	0.49
Endoscopy	20.61	10.48	19.11	8.73	21.00	10.65
Injection of chemotherapeutic agent	7.23	0.00	4.70	1.13	3.23	1.02
Coronary angiography	42.30	4.34	30.66	8.20	30.73	11.45
Total	*99.06*	*14.82*	*95.62*	*34.15*	*100.13*	*44.61*

Source: *The Outpatient Utilization Profile,* 1994, HCH and Arthur Andersen.

PRIMARY CARE COMPENSATION

As IDSs move into more aggressive managed care markets, more services are performed proportionally by PCPs. The reasons for this phenomenon are twofold.

First, PCPs have less procedural conflict in that they are not economically motivated to perform procedures, and, presumably, are more able to make appropriate decisions to manage the care of their patients.

Second, historical FFS reimbursement mechanisms do not reward PCPs to extend treatment beyond simple evaluation and referral to an appropriate specialist. The same services performed by PCPs were reimbursed at a lower rate than for specialty providers, if at all. Managed care systems typically correct this deficiency by increasing the compensation to PCPs on the assumption that the cost is lower than in the specialty setting. As managed care systems mature, PCPs may enhance their clinical skill in patient care activities that are particularly well compensated, such as office surgeries and chronic disease management. These compensation mechanisms usually place a value on both scope of skills and patient management.

The scope of services performed is important because the use of a PCP is usually less costly than the use of a specialist. Often the additional services previously performed by a specialist can be performed at the time

FIGURE 4
PCP capitation

Primary care covered services—CPT codes

99201–99215	Office visits
99050–99058	After-hours services
99000–99002	Specimen handling
36413	Venipuncture
10120	Simple foreign body removal
10060	Simple abscess drainage
10140–10160	Simple hematoma drainage
99341–99353	Home services
99221–99292	Critical care visits
99301–99333	Rest home visits
99381–99429	Preventive care
99432–94333	Well newborn care
99281–99285	PCP emergency room visit
99371–99373	Telephone consultation
99070	Supplies
99070 and 99078	Education of patient
69210	Removal of cerumen
90701–90749	Immunizations
90780–90799	Injections
11200–11201	Removal of skin tags
81000–81003	Urinalysis
82270	Stool for occult blood
86580–86585	TB testing

of initial access. The value of a PCP as an effective manger of patient care improves overall financial performance in the cost of patient care and can also improve clinical outcomes.

The scope of services performed is defined both by the types of procedures performed, as shown in Figure 4, and by clinical responsibility sets for each specialty area. A sample of the clinical responsibility in the area of cardiology is shown in Figure 3. These types of clinical responsibility for PCPs define the clinical boundary between primary and specialty care. This boundary needs to be defined in order to set compensation rates for both the primary and specialty care providers.

The lowest common denominator of service must be used in setting primary care capitation rates in an IPA setting. There are wide differences in the scope of service provided by fragmented PCPs. Primary care groups are better positioned to accept an enhanced scope of services due to the specialized skills of individual physicians, thus allowing the group to resolve a wider range of patient health problems without an out-of-group referral.

Primary care services are the most predictable of all services for purposes of assuming financial risk. Typically, commercial patients access a
healthcare system 2.5 to 3.5 times per year. Those visits tend to vary in
intensity (e.g., office visit versus emergency room visit) but can be
accounted for by setting capitation rates at different levels for different
PCP specialties.

Primary care capitation as a payment mechanism has been proven to
be difficult in less-controlled situations such as an IPA. IPAs have difficulty adopting common practice protocols since the member physicians
practice at different locations. There is a tendency to avoid treatment at
the primary care level and dump the required care on a specialist provider if the PCP is capitated, largely because the PCP receives no additional compensation under capitation. Where there is a common treatment protocol (as is usually present in groups, as well as an understanding of costs "downstream" from the PCPs), there is less concern about
dumping because the medical group is able to maintain a common
boundary set for each specialty area.

Less-controlled POs retain FFS payment mechanisms for PCPs in
order to ensure that there is a direct financial incentive to perform the
maximum amount of services at the primary care level. The added
responsibilities of a PCP are often compensated by augmenting the FFS
payments with a patient management fee that is described in the next
paragraph.

Initially, PCPs are often not willing to assume the risk of capitation.
POs may elect initially to base compensation with a FFS payment as well
as a case management or patient management fee PMPM. This fee is
intended to cover the cost to the physician for the extra work of managing patients under capitation. It is usually based on an absolute dollar
amount PMPM and ranges from $1 to $3 in different markets.

Besides the basic primary care compensation, compensation from risk
sharing is a necessary component of primary care compensation. This
will be covered in the risk-sharing section of this chapter.

SPECIALTY COMPENSATION

The range of payment mechanisms for specialty care physicians varies
from FFS payments, to budgeted FFS payments, and to subcapitation.
Determining the responsibility of the PCP in each specialty area bears
directly on the setting of budget or subcapitation rates. These boundaries define the actual work involved.

The number of specialty providers in each area will dictate the PCP services the specialists wish to perform. A specialty panel with limited numbers will usually want to focus on the work of the specialty to maximize reimbursement. There will be increased incentive to educate PCP members to minimize the amount of work performed in the area as well as to refer patients to the specialty provider in a more organized fashion.

ANCILLARY SERVICE COMPENSATION

Ancillary services covered by ambulatory capitation include outpatient laboratory, radiology, physical therapy, diagnostic services, mental health, and relatively small expenditures for other items such as medical social services. Each of these areas has specific guidelines, but they can all be biased if a physician has a financial interest in any particular area.

Laboratory

Laboratory services have often been physician owned. There has also been a problem with fee schedules not reflecting the cost efficiencies of advancing technology. As a result, pricing in the market may be high on a per unit basis during the initial onset of managed care. Most provider networks will gradually convert their own laboratory services to a commercial laboratory fee schedule over time, once the pricing differential is achieved.

Most physician-operated laboratories cannot operate at the same efficiency level as large commercial laboratories and will abandon the economic activity over time. When this occurs a capitation contract with a large commercial laboratory usually produces the lowest-cost service at the highest-quality level.

Radiology

Radiology services are very much site dependent. Members of the typical primary care office will want the immediate diagnostic tools, such as plain film. Certain specialists may also wish to use diagnostic tools as components of their practice (e.g., plain bone films for orthopedics and ultrasound for obstetrics). Those services should be carved out of any subcapitation arrangement since they need to be performed at the orthopedic office. The rest of radiology can be capitated to a radiology group or paid at a fee schedule.

Mental health

Mental health is usually a limited benefit under managed care. The patient share of cost is usually higher than for other services. The clinical definition of the benefit may also apply only to crisis situations and have a limitation such as a maximum of 20 visits per year. The patients involved often continue their care on a self-pay basis after the benefit has expired.

The use of nonphysician mental health professionals, such as nurses, social workers, and psychologists, is common throughout the country. These nonphysician providers typically provide care at a much lower cost. The level of benefits involved and the composition of the provider panel must be considered when setting capitation rates.

Physical therapy

The appropriate use of physical therapy usually requires some oversight from an orthopedic consultant. As a result, subcapitated arrangements may be "rolled up" into an orthopedic subcapitation arrangement. A FFS arrangement in this area is usually paid on a standard charge per visit instead of a tiered service level.

Since ancillary providers depend on physician referral for most of their business, the physician group or IPA usually is able to procure pricing at rates below cost for these services under contract. An open request for a competitive proposal will usually lead to appropriate pricing for most of these services.

Risk sharing and risk pools

POs that start out using only fee schedules usually encounter economic difficulty because there is no economic incentive for the individual provider to control utilization. Usually, an additional component of compensation based on economic performance is necessary to produce fundamental changes in utilization patterns. The use of risk sharing based on utilization targets is a common vehicle for motivating physicians to adopt acceptable utilization rates. Sharing surpluses and deficits gives incentives to individual providers to control utilization and plays a key part in successfully managing ambulatory capitation.

RISK POOLS

HMOs and systems accepting global capitation are usually greatly concerned with institutional costs due to the share of budget attributed to them. These costs lie outside the boundaries of ambulatory capitation. Since physicians exert great influence over these costs, risk-sharing opportunities are usually offered to POs accepting ambulatory capitation. Additionally, there may be risk-sharing opportunities provided within the boundaries of the services provided under ambulatory capitation. For example, both primary care and specialty care physicians usually share in savings and deficits produced by underspending or overspending specialty care budgets. Such risk pools are usually described as specialty risk pools.

Risk-sharing opportunities usually come in the form of a pool of services covered by a budget or target utilization amount. In the event there is lower utilization than budgeted, a portion of the surplus is paid to providers who influence the costs associated with the pool. These pools of services are referred to generically as risk pools. Specific types of pools may be referred to as institutional risk pools (for inpatient/outpatient facility charges) or specialty risk pools (for the professional services of specialty care providers). The movement to subcapitation will eliminate risk pools internal to ambulatory capitation because the providers involved accept direct risk at predetermined utilization levels.

INSTITUTIONAL SHARED RISK POOL DEVELOPMENT

In an institutional shared risk pool, the division of financial responsibility is as follows

Institutional pool

Inpatient hospital services

Outpatient surgery

Skilled nursing services

Ambulance services in area

Emergency room facility component

Home health services

Dialysis services

Ambulatory capitation

Professional services—inpatient

Professional services—outpatient

Outpatient diagnostic tests

Durable medical equipment

ER professional component

Office-based lab and x-ray

Immunizations

Health plan portion

Reinsurance or stop-loss

Out-of-area emergency

Outpatient drugs

The institutional pool has been historically acknowledged by HMOs to be the biggest source of potential risk pool dollars available to physicians. While the ambulatory capitation amount is relatively close to actual costs, there is an inherent (and sometimes explicit) margin in the institutional pool. This is due to the services covered by the pool, particularly inpatient stays, being the highest per unit cost of any service covered by the premium dollar. Usually, in a nonmanaged care environment, admission rates, unit costs, and lengths of stay compound each other to create an inflated institutional cost (see Figure 5 for premium levels and corresponding hospital days variations nationally).

The experience of provider networks on the West Coast in controlling premium costs, for example, demonstrates the efficacy of establishing a pool of funds for potential savings to providers. Those systems have established risk-sharing arrangements for physician groups creating an incentive for them to exercise control over costs in the institutional pool.

Numerous types of methodologies have been developed by health plans and insurance companies to identify and distribute institutional

FIGURE 5
Premium and days per 1,000 correlation

Hospital days per 1,000

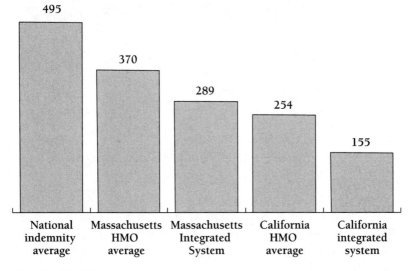

| National indemnity average | Massachusetts HMO average | Massachusetts Integrated System | California HMO average | California integrated system |

Premium PMPM

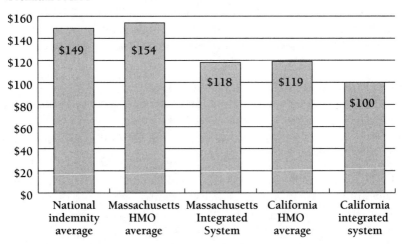

| National indemnity average | Massachusetts HMO average | Massachusetts Integrated System | California HMO average | California integrated system |

Source: The Advisory Board, *The Grand Alliance—Vertical Integration Strategies for Physicians and Health Systems*, 1993.

risk pool savings. As physician groups integrate with institutional providers, the integrated organization may accept full risk contracts. A shared institutional pool is still usually created to enhance the financial performance of the overall system by controlling inpatient utilization.

FIGURE 6
Institutional risk pool participation
Levels of risk assumed

LOW PROVIDER RISK			HIGH PROVIDER RISK	
Plan alone	Physicians and plan	Physicians and plan equal	Physicians, plan, and hospital	Physicians and hospital
	Upside only	*Upside and downside*	*Various proportions Upside and downside*	*Full risk*

Some payers may not wish to transfer such a high level of risk to providers (such as full risk contacts to integrated entities) since this limits the payer participation in risk pools and retention rates over time. There is a continuum of risk assumed and risk pool participation that payers usually provide, as shown in Figure 6.

Figure 6 indicates that in certain situations, the physician group has no deficit-sharing or "downside" risk but has a risk-sharing result only in the event of a surplus. The proportions of deficit or surplus sharing assumed by the payer, PO, and the institutional provider may vary at different stages of managed care growth. As systems mature in managed care performance, there is a tendency to assume greater levels of risk in these pools in order to take advantage of internally generated utilization savings.

This evolution of risk taking is solidly founded on the premise that it is the physician, not the hospital, who truly affects hospital utilization. In the lowest levels of risk, the plan will offer complete downside protection to the PO in return for a sizable portion of the upside savings. These risk arrangements can be offered in a number of different formats: days saved, percentage of savings, and utilization cost containment.

Days saved from target: Tracks actual inpatient utilization and compares it to a target budget. Each day under budget (day saved) is multiplied by a price based on a portion of the total cost, and that amount is returned to the physicians. This methodology is limited because it only uses a measure of inpatient stays to compute the risk-sharing amounts. Total costs involve inpatient stays as well as all of the other services in the institutional pool such as outpatient surgery. There is a significant potential in these situations for the PO to "game" the system by aggressively shifting care to settings other than inpatient. The PO does not gain overall institutional pool management experience because it is not responsible for managing all of the costs associated with the pool.

Percent of savings: If the actual institutional cost is under budget, the physicians receive a percentage of the total PMPM amount saved. These amounts can range from 20 percent of the savings from the budget to as much as 75 percent.

Utilization/cost combination: Physicians receive a payment for beating both utilization targets (days per 1,000 members, usually) and a percentage of the overall savings from the institutional budget. This formula offers the highest incentive.

A significant opportunity and risk exists for the party who is willing to participate early in the evolving managed care marketplace. Once formulas are established and data shared, the providers excluded from these arrangements will rally to be included in the formula. Successful health plans will not relinquish any risk-sharing opportunity, while others will gladly include the physicians to safeguard performance. Hospitals that were not willing to take risk initially in California during the mid- to late 1980s often found themselves shut out of the competitive game. However, once the hospital enters the risk-sharing equation, the combined leverage usually results in a continual erosion of the portion held by the health plan over time.

INSTITUTIONAL RISK POOL PRICING

To effectively manage costs, unit pricing to the institutional pool should be understood by risk pool participants. Charges refer to this actual charge or retail pricing level available to any party and percentage of charges refers to a discounted FFS arrangement. Per diem payment arrangements consist of setting the payment at a certain amount per day of occupancy. No additional charge is allowed for incidental supplies or diagnostic studies under these arrangements. Setting different per diems for different types of stays (e.g., intensive care unit, neonatal intensive care unit, medical bed or surgical bed) is referred to as a "tiered per diem" arrangement. A unified per diem that is the same for all levels of service is an "all-inclusive per diem."

Using the institutional pool structure and the unit pricing definitions above, various pricing arrangements are described in Table 6 for each component of the institutional risk pool. They are arranged with those least effective in controlling cost and utilization on the left to those used by advanced managed care systems on the right.

SPECIALIST AND ANCILLARY RISK POOLS

Development

Incentive pools can also be used for specialist and ancillary services. A PCP-driven system will often capitate PCPs and put them at-risk for up to 50 percent of the surplus or deficit remaining in the specialist fund (see Figure 7) with the remainder of the risk shared with specialty and institutional providers. Specialist-oriented systems will allow PCPs limited

TABLE 6
Payment mechanisms for components of institutional risk pools

Inpatient hospital

Charges	Percent of charges (discount)	Payment by DRGs	Tiered per diems	All-inclusive per diem

Outpatient surgery

Charges	Percent of charges (discount)	Percent of charges Cap at $ _____	Ambulatory service groups (ASGs) rates	Fee schedule negotiation

Skilled nursing facility

Charges	Percent of charges (discount)	Tiered per diems ancillaries* at cost	Tiered per diems ancillaries* included	All-inclusive per diems

Ambulance

Charges	Percent of charges	Separate trip rates for 911 and non-911 cases		Capitation

Emergency room

Charges	Percent of charges	Severity adjusted case rate	Visit rate	Capitation

Home health and dialysis

Charges	Percent of charges	Tier per visit rate		Capitation

*Ancillaries include, but are not limited to: physical, speech, and occupational therapy, lab, x-ray, and pharmacy.

risk in specialist risk pool participation. Participation in the specialty risk pools usually takes one of the following forms:

By specialty: With accurate actuarial data or significant prepaid experience, budgets can be developed by specialty, allowing only those specialists within the specialty to participate in risk sharing for only that component of care.

Global: In this case, the entire specialist population and in some cases the primary care population is eligible for risk sharing within a common pool. An aggregate budget is set and surpluses and deficits are shared on a common basis.

Once a pool or negative surplus of funds is identified by either of the above methods, the terms of distribution are employed. Providers are becoming increasingly creative in the allocation of risk pool dollars (positive and negative), using weighted factors such as

- Productivity

- PMPM costs

- Cost per case

- Utilization management, as measured by an equal combination of length of stay, days per 1,000 members, use of generic drugs, referral patterns, and in-group versus out-of-group activity

- Score on annual patient satisfaction surveys

- Stewardship, as rated by the medical director or compensation committee, to include committee participation, marketing efforts, specialization in a particular aspect of one's specialty (e.g., hand surgery, diabetic treatment), call coverage, and any other behaviors deemed valuable to the group

It is critical that the terms developed above are quantifiable, measurable, objective, aligned with the PO's goals, and have been approved by the general membership. They should also be reviewed annually to ensure that they are still relevant.

As a general rule of thumb, a component service must be relatively costly to warrant attention as a potential risk-pool-sharing opportunity. The two ancillary services most conducive to risk sharing are laboratory services and radiology services. These risk-sharing opportunities are usually eliminated early on as IPAs and medical groups move to subcapitate these areas.

Specialty risk pool pricing

The pricing of services in the specialty pool is usually accomplished by a fee schedule such as McGraw-Hill or RBRVS on an interim basis. If there is a withhold on the posted fee schedule, it is returned before surpluses are calculated. Portions of withholds may be retained to cover deficits.

As providers agree to accept subcapitaton for an area (e.g., allergy, dermatology, or mental health), that area is usually excluded from risk pools since the providers of care are accepting direct risk. It is therefore important to set subcapitation rates using optimal utilization assumptions from an agreed upon unit-pricing arrangement.

Pharmacy risk pool. Outpatient pharmaceutical costs are most controllable by PCPs since the majority of prescriptions are generated by them. Specialty physicians also prescribe drugs, but the incidence is far lower. Pharmacists are sometimes able to control costs by feeding back to physicians acceptable cost-saving alternatives. Occasionally retail dispensing organizations accept subcapitation, in which case there is no pharmacy risk pool.

The steps taken by physicians to control utilization are listed below. These are specific physician behaviors that impact both the per unit costs and the frequency of use of prescribed drugs.

- *Formulary usage.* The use of a workbook that describes alternatives and their relative cost

- *Generic substitution.* The use of less costly "non-brand" drugs for prescriptions

- *Over the counter alternatives.* Often, over the counter drugs are available as an equally efficacious alternative at no cost to the provider system

SHARING RISK AND RESIDUAL PREMIUM SHARE

Those sharing risk in each pool should be those having some influence over the costs generated in that pool (e.g., it would not be appropriate for a hospital to share in a specialty risk pool). A diagram of a typical two-risk pool structure is presented in Figure 7. The PCPs involved are assumed to be taking primary care capitation. There is a risk pool for both primary care and specialty physicians at the specialty or ancillary level and a pool for primary care and specialty physicians along with the hospital at the institutional level. This is a fairly common model for multispecialty POs. Primary care controlled systems may take all of the

FIGURE 7
Two-risk pool configurations: specialty and institutional risk pools

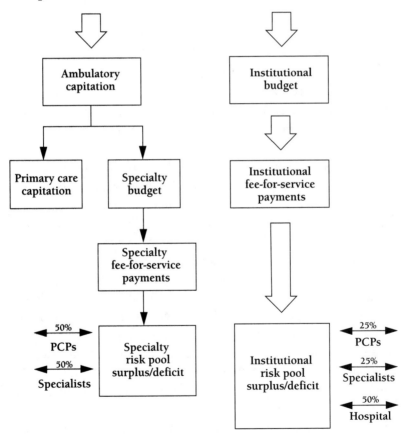

TABLE 7
Typical risk pool splits in various managed care settings

	Loosely managed system	Moderately managed system	Well- managed system
Institutional pool			
Primary care	10%	10%	25%
Specialists	40%	40%	25%
Hospital	0%	16%	50%
Health plan	50%	33%	
Specialist/ancillary pool			
Primary care	33%	50%	100%
Specialists	0%	50%	0%
Health plan	67%	0%	0%
Pharmacy pool			
Primary care	0%	40%	100%
Specialty care	0%	10%	0%
Health plan	100%	50%	0%

participation indicated for specialists included in Figure 7 and substitute PCPs in their place.

Table 7 lists the typical splits in various risk pools for the parties involved in those pools under a variety of managed care settings.

Earlier in the chapter, Figure 2 showed a system that had a $160 PMPM premium example where the share of residual premium after HMO retention, pharmacy costs, and reinsurance going to the PO was 40 percent. The physicians' share of premium usually goes up as managed care systems mature. Typically, advanced managed care systems allocate up to 55 percent of residual premium to ambulatory capitation.

Figure 8 illustrates how risk sharing can transition the share of premium from nonmanaged care to managed care standards through appropriate utilization. The example in Figure 2 of $160 PMPM was predicated on 300 bed days per 1,000 members per year. The same premium configuration is assumed in Figure 8 but the PO has entered a risk-sharing arrangement and has cut utilization by 50 days per 1,000 members per year, thus creating a $12 PMPM surplus in the institutional risk pool. The physician share of the surplus is $6 PMPM which, when added to the ambulatory capitation of $47, causes the physician share of residual premium to rise from 40 to 45 percent. Further drops in institutional utilization will increase the physician share of residual premium.

FIGURE 8
PMPM premium distribution
Risk pool surplus distribution

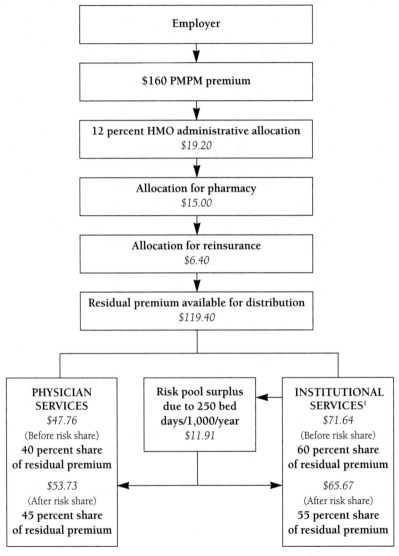

1. Assumes 300 bed days per 1,000 members per year.

These mechanisms must be used with the knowledge that they will change over time. The best approach for each community will be based on the medical standards and the relative supply of physicians and facilities for that community. The advancement of managed care systems may not occur in some areas to the extent reported in the examples here. Prudent financial management of capitation dictates that financial incentives be appropriately matched to each provider system.

Conclusion

In summary, the premium must be allocated into its components in order to understand the development of ambulatory capitation. Costs associated with primary, specialty, and institutional services must be defined as completely as possible. One must understand the interplay between each of these three areas in order to attempt to control costs. The alignment of incentives using risk-sharing models is a useful technique in controlling the overall utilization of services.

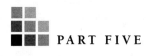

PART FIVE

RESOURCE MANAGEMENT

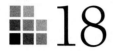

18

Measuring hospital resource consumption

Thomas F. McNulty
Senior Vice President and Chief Financial Officer

Jennifer Elston Lafata, PhD
Staff Investigator, Center for Clinical Effectiveness
Henry Ford Health System
Detroit, Michigan

COST CONTAINMENT CONTINUES TO DOMINATE the nation's healthcare agenda. This is reflected in local healthcare markets where capitated payments are gaining market share and providers are continually being pushed to reduce costs. Surprisingly, this focus on cost containment has lead to relatively few initiatives to measure costs accurately. The result is that healthcare executives and administrators remain forced to rely on flawed cost informaton at a time when the need for accurate cost data could not be more acute.

As managed care and capitation become more widespread, knowledge of underlying product costs becomes imperative. Successful contract negotiating requires product costs be known and understood and that data be available to support claims made. Such data must include accurate information on the unit costs of activities used to produce each hospital stay, as well as the ability to link such accurate cost data to clinical outcomes. It is only when such cost information is available that healthcare provider organizations can have leverage in contract negotiations.

Furthermore, to remain price competitive, administrators must understand their facility's cost behavior and how to improve their efficiency and effectiveness. This information, combined with variance analysis or the identification of costs that deviate substantially from standard or budgeted amounts, can lead to improved financial management, including improved cost allocation accuracy.

To facilitate the availability of cost data, many facilities are implementing elaborate cost-accounting systems. Yet those implementing them often overlook one fundamental premise—each system is only as good as its data. While many of these systems are designed to reflect unit costs and offer great flexibility in their analyses and reporting capabilities, many also rely on charge or charge-based data that do not reflect true costs.[1] Not until accurate cost data are available will the real benefits of these systems be realized.

Finally, because of the reliance on cost-to-charge ratios, many systems fail to cost items beyond those that are currently billable. Yet many other aspects of care can have a profound effect on both patient outcomes and costs. These activities, such as special nursing or dietary procedures, need to be identified and tracked, and their costs need to be appropriately applied to products.

Drawing on principles of financial management and quality planning, this chapter first lays the conceptual foundation for developing the resource consumption unit (RCU), a mechanism for accurately tracking costs in the hospital setting. The chapter then describes a pilot project at Henry Ford Health System in Detroit, Michigan, to evaluate the feasibility of developing such a mechanism.

As envisioned, the RCU would serve both the internal management and external policy needs of the industry. By addressing the combined needs of both these groups of decision makers, the RCU may begin to provide the information necessary to move the hospital industry toward efficient and effective production processes.

Background

While resource consumption tracking and productivity management are standard practices in most industries, such cost management remains in its infancy in the healthcare sector. Historically, hospitals (and other healthcare providers) were reimbursed retrospectively on a "cost-plus" basis. Under such cost-based reimbursement, a hospital's long-term financial security depended almost entirely upon its leadership's ability to manage revenues. This was done by ensuring a constant stream of patients and by maximizing allowable costs. Hospital accounting and information systems that were geared to reimbursement management then evolved. One outgrowth of such a practice is charge schedules that have little, if any, relation to production costs. Yet, the vast majority of hospitals continue to use cost-to-charge ratios to establish a standard cost for each procedure or service rendered.[2] Such top-down costing starts with the charge amount and assumes a consistent relationship between overall charges and overall costs. Although such a methodology is relatively inexpensive to implement, it also is inaccurate.[3]

With the advent of Medicare's Prospective Payment System (PPS) in 1983, the hospital environment began to change drastically. Since PPS, hospitals have seen marked increases in the use of capitated (or fixed) payments—regardless of their costs or charges—from virtually all third-party payers. These reimbursement changes have led to a dramatic shift in economic risks. No longer are patients and third-party payers the primary risk holders. Instead, the vast majority of economic risk is borne by providers of care. Providers, therefore, can no longer depend on revenue management for success and must focus their efforts on understanding and managing their costs. This transition has not come easily.

Healthcare providers in general, and hospitals in particular, often face difficulties in defining exactly what constitutes their end products. Although it is now possible to construct statistically homogenous groups of patients that, at least theoretically, consume similar resources and correspond to products (e.g., diagnostic-related groups, DRGs), the ability to associate a cost with these processes has yet to be resolved. There are literally hundreds of thousands of factors (or inputs) that go into their production. These inputs not only include numerous direct resources (e.g., labor and supplies) but also often include complex layers of overhead (e.g., education and research) that must be allocated.

Because of this overwhelming complexity, few efforts to develop industry mechanisms or standards for tracking resource use have emerged. A notable exception is the process called microcosting. Microcosting attempts to adapt basic principles of industrial engineering and operations research that have been used successfully in other industries to determine product costs in the hospital setting.

Although microcosting is fundamentally sound, it has had difficulty gaining widespread use. It is dependent on the use of resource-intense time and work-sampling studies to develop underlying relative value scales (RVS). In the healthcare industry, this quickly translates not only into exorbitant developmental costs but also extremely high costs of maintenance and updating. In fact, many of the facilities that originally developed information and accounting systems to implement such microcosting methodologies in the early 1980s today cannot justify the costs of maintaining them.

The resource consumption unit

Two of the most pervasive hurdles hindering accurate resource tracking in the hospital sector are the number and diversity of activities in which hospitals are engaged and the lack of accounting and process standardization both within and between hospital facilities. If any mechanism is to become widely used, it must address both these issues. The RCU is designed around two fundamental criteria: the need to limit the number of activities for which resources are tracked in detail and the need for a mechanism that allows for both intra- and interfacility comparisons.

The first is achieved by using the Pareto Principle, or 80-20 rule. This principle was first applied to management by Juran, a pioneer in the field of quality planning.[4] He believed that 80 percent of the trouble comes from 20 percent of the problems and used this principle to urge management to sort out the "vital few" from the "trivial many." Applying this principle to hospital finance implies that a small number of activities in a hospital account for a large percentage of its costs.

Once these high-cost activities are identified, resource consumption tracking efforts can focus on them. The remaining costs can then be allocated to the "residual," relatively low-cost, activities, thereby limiting the number of activities for which detailed cost data are needed.

The second criterion, the need for intra- and interfacility comparisons, can be achieved by focusing primarily on direct costs or those costs that can be directly traced to and associated with a unit of production. In so doing, problems of comparison attributable to layers of overhead are eliminated. By focusing on direct resources such as direct labor, supplies, and equipment, the RCU focuses on costs that are controllable and comparable not only among departments within a facility but among different facilities.

While this approach ensures that resource tracking remains relatively simple, it is not a sufficient foundation for tracking resource consumption. Beyond simplicity, the RCU must be

- Financially and administratively feasible to develop and maintain

- Credible and understandable to users

- A valid and reliable indicator of resource consumption that has clinical and administrative relevance

- Easily adjusted to account for changes in input factor costs, patient activity levels, and technology

- Incorporated into continual, timely monitoring of daily operations

Ultimately, the goal is to track costs along a product (or service) line (e.g., an inpatient stay or diagnostic related group). The problem is that, despite most hospital products crossing department lines, the natural unit of aggregation for staffing and other operational purposes in the hospital remains the department. Information and accounting systems therefore exist to track costs within departments. Ignoring this fact negates one of the few sources of accurate cost data available within hospitals and therefore would severely hinder the feasibility of developing a valid resource consumption-tracking mechanism.

Yet, to be useful, any costing mechanism must be activity based or refer to what organizations do. For example, as part of a hospital's routine operations, lab tests are conducted, nursing care is provided, surgical operations are performed, and reimbursement claims are processed. It is these activities in which hospital staff are engaged on a day-to-day basis, which have clinical relevance, and which administrators must manage to control resource consumption. The RCU, therefore, is designed to be compatible with an activity-based costing system.

While the RCU builds on the current ability to track resources accurately within cost centers (or departments), its main focus is the relatively small number of activities within each department that account for the majority of costs incurred. Although relatively precise resource tracking remains imperative for these high-cost activities, it is not justified for the relatively low-cost ones. Thus, the challenge is to identify high-cost activities for which it is practical and feasible to construct detailed resource consumption measures.

Derivation of the resource consumption unit

The derivation of the RCU can be summarized in six steps (Table 1). First, the activities in which the department is engaged must be identified and defined. Lists of billable services from each cost center may serve as a valuable starting point in the identification of activities. However, it must be remembered that such lists may be incomplete for cost centers that routinely bill for their activities and obviously are nonexistent for those departments that do not currently bill for their services.

As part of the definition, the parameters or boundaries for each activity must be clearly articulated. One approach is to identify departmental outputs and consider the work being done to produce these outputs. It is important to identify the underlying work performed, but it is not necessary to specify all the individual tasks involved in performing that work. Similar activities should be grouped because there is no need to spend time and money tracking resources for multiple similar processes.

Once an exhaustive list of the activities in which the department is engaged is compiled, the Pareto rule can be used to identify the high-cost activities (or groups of activities) within each department (step 2). When identifying high-cost activities, it is important to consider both the activities that in and of themselves are high cost and those that, although they may be relatively low cost to perform because of volume, represent a large percentage of a department's resource use.

Next, the total direct departmental costs must be identified (step 3). These costs can be identified from the statement of revenue and expense. At a minimum, these should be identified by four resource categories: labor, equipment, materials and supplies, and direct support overhead. It is, however, preferable to have more expense detail. For example, the labor expense in a respiratory therapy department could include line-item expenses for each of the main labor categories (e.g., director, manager,

TABLE 1
Deriving the resource consumption unit

1. Identify and define activities
2. Select high-cost activities
3. Identify direct departmental costs
4. Estimate relative resources consumed for high-cost activities
5. Calculate direct unit costs per resource unit
6. Allocate remaining department costs to residual activities

therapist, technician, and pulmonary technician). Where substantial detail is available, decisions regarding whether and how to combine line items may need to be made. Regardless of the level of detail, these costs ideally should represent the controllable costs within the department.

To calculate the Pareto expenses, each of the line-item expense totals are multiplied by either 80 percent or by the proportion of the line-item costs for which the high-cost activities in aggregate are estimated to represent. Although the proportion would likely remain constant across line-items within an expense category (e.g., labor, materials and supplies, and equipment), there may be occassions where it is more appropriate to allow the proportion to vary within and between categories. For example, in radiology the high-cost activities may in aggregate reflect 80 percent of the technicians' time but only 10 percent of the managers' time.

Because the proportion of total direct costs for which these high-cost activities account is an estimate, it is subject to error. The magnitude of this error can be evaluated via methods of validation as described in the evaluation section. Once the magnitude of the error (or bias) is known, adjustments to the estimates can be made as appropriate.

Individual interviews with department directors and managers and facilitated group sessions with department employees can be used to solicit the information necessary to complete steps 1, 2, and 3.

The fourth step consists of estimating the quantity of inputs used to produce each of the high-cost activities. It is often at this stage that industrial engineers and others perform detailed microcosting studies. While such studies can provide valuable information, they are often not justifiable given the time and cost required to conduct them. Instead, departmental work groups—whose members represent all stages of the high-cost activities—should be used to estimate resource use.

For each of the high-cost activities identified in step 2, these facilitated work groups identify two pieces of information for each of the line-item expense categories: the percentage of the time the high-cost activity is performed in which any of the line items is consumed; and when the line item is consumed, the average number of units of the line item that are consumed. Table 2 presents an example for two high-cost activities within a department of radiology. By multiplying the percentage of time the line item is used (column A) and the average number of units consumed (column B), a weighted resource use measure is derived (column C).

TABLE 2
Step 4: Estimated labor use

Head without IV contrast
Departmental frequency: 2,540

Labor class	A Percent use	B Average unit use	C Resource units
1. Supervisor	0.00	0	0.00
2. CAT scan technician	90.00	40	36.00
3. Radiology technician I	0.00	0	0.00
4. Radiology technician II	0.00	0	0.00
5. Radiology technician specialist	10.00	40	4.00
6. Radiology/mammography technician	0.00	0	0.00
7. Darkroom attendant	0.00	0	0.00

Chest, 2 views
Departmental frequency: 18,792

Labor class	A Percent use	B Average unit use	C Resource units
1. Supervisor	5.00	12	0.60
2. CAT scan technician	0.00	0	0.00
3. Radiology technician I	55.00	12	6.60
4. Radiology technician II	10.00	12	1.20
5. Radiology technician specialist	10.00	12	1.20
6. Radiology/mammography technician	22.00	12	2.64
7. Darkroom attendant	100.00	3	3.00

After the quantity of resource units consumed per activity are estimated, the costs per unit must be calculated (step 5). This can be done by consulting with departmental managers to identify one additional piece of information: the frequency with which each of the high-cost activities was performed. Table 3 presents an example of the unit cost calculation for labor for the two high-cost radiology activities identified in Table 2.

As Table 3 illustrates, the resource units (as derived in step 4 and depicted in column A, lines 1–7 and 9–15) are multiplied by the departmental frequency of performance to yield the total number of labor resource units consumed by the department in producing each of the high-cost activities (column B, lines 1–7 and 9–15). Summing these line-item resource totals over each of the high-cost activities yields the estimated grand total of labor units consumed by the department in the specified time period (column A, lines 17–23). Dividing these resource use numbers into their corresponding line-item Pareto expense amounts

TABLE 3
Step 5: Direct labor cost per unit calculations

CAT, Head without IV contrast
Departmental frequency: 2,540

Labor class	A Resource units used per activity	B Total resource units used	C Activity cost
1. Supervisor	0.00	0	$0.00
2. CAT scan technician	36.00	91,440	$27.36
3. Radiology technician I	0.00	0	$0.00
4. Radiology technician II	0.00	0	$0.00
5. Radiology technician specialist	4.00	10,160	$2.96
6. Radiology/mammography technician	0.00	0	$0.00
7. Darkroom attendant	0.00	0	$0.00
8. *Direct labor cost per activity*			*$30.32*

Chest, 2 views
Departmental frequency: 18,792

Labor class	A Resource units per activity	B Total resource units used	C Activity cost
9. Supervisor	0.60	11,275	$0.73
10. CAT scan technician	0.00	0	$0.00
11. Radiology technician I	6.60	124,027	$4.36
12. Radiology technician II	1.20	22,550	$0.78
13. Radiology technician specialist	1.20	22,550	$0.89
14. Radiology/mammography technician	2.64	49,611	$1.87
15. Darkroom attendant	3.00	56,376	$1.29
16. *Direct labor cost per activity*			*$9.92*

Total departmental use

Labor class	A Grand total activity use	B Pareto expense	C Cost per unit
17. Supervisor	11,275	$13,643	$1.21
18. CAT scan technician	91,440	$69,494	$0.76
19. Radiology technician I	124,027	$81,858	$0.66
20. Radiology technician II	22,550	$14,658	$0.65
21. Radiology technician specialist	10,160	$7,518	$0.74
22. Radiology/mammography technician	49,611	$35,224	$0.71
23. Darkroom attendant	56,376	$24,242	$0.43

(column B, lines 17–23) yields an estimated direct labor cost per unit (in this case, per minute) for each line item expense (column C, lines 17–23). At this point, both the total labor resource units consumed (column A, lines 1–7 and 9–15) and their associated unit costs (column C, lines 17–23) are known, thus enabling the calculation of the activity costs for each line-item expense (column C, lines 1–7 and 9–15). Summing these line-item costs for each activity yields an estimated direct labor cost (column C, lines 8 and 16). The process is repeated for both materials and supplies and equipment and adapted for direct support to generate similar estimates of their associated direct costs per activity.

Taking the estimated labor cost for each activity as derived in Table 3 and adding to it the similar estimates for materials and supplies, equipment, and direct support generates the direct RCU for each of the high-cost activities. Table 4 illustrates such a calculation for the two high-cost radiology activities.

Mathematically, the RCU for each of the high-cost activities is simply the sum of each of the estimated average resource units consumed multiplied by the associated per unit "hiring cost" or

Direct RCU $\quad = \Sigma wL + \Sigma uS + \Sigma vK = \Sigma tD$

Direct RCU	= Resource consumption unit: direct cost only
w	= Per unit wage cost
L	= Direct labor resource units
u	= Per unit supply and material cost
S	= Direct supply and material resource units
v	= Per unit equipment or capital cost
K	= Direct equipment or capital resource units
t	= Per unit direct support cost
D	= Direct support resource units

TABLE 4
Direct RCU calculation

Activity code	Activity description	Labor	Supplies	Equipment	Support	Direct RCU
70150	CAT, head no IV contrast	$30.32	$11.76	$16.31	$16.24	$74.63
71020	Chest, two views	$9.92	$6.17	$2.07	$2.08	$20.24

The final step, step 6, is to calculate the direct RCU for the residual, or low-cost, activities. This is done by allocating the remaining direct department costs (i.e., approximately 20 percent of total direct departmental costs) to the low-cost activities performed by each department. In its simplest form, an average cost could be assigned to each of these remaining activities. However, when possible, a method that is based on the resource intensity of each remaining activity should be used, and the method of allocation should be tailored to each department.

Once step 6 has been completed for every department in the hospital, the result will be estimated direct costs for all the activities (or groups of activities) performed by every department (i.e., a direct RCU for every activity of the hospital). Total direct departmental costs for a given time period therefore are equal to the sum of the direct RCU for each specified activity multiplied by the count or number of times the activity was performed during the specified time period. This calculation is shown in Table 5.

However, to comprehensively track resource use, support activities (e.g., the activities of hospital finance, and medical education) must be charged to their appropriate service activities. Once this is done, a full-cost RCU can be calculated for each of the service activities.

For simplicity, departments can be divided into those whose primary functions are patient-centered (or service) activities (e.g., radiology, pathology, operating room, or nursing) and those whose functions are more supportive in nature (e.g., purchasing, medical education, and human resources). Specific direct RCUs for the support activities can then be charged to the patient-centered activities in the service departments. In total, these charges effectively represent a fixed cost allowance (FCA).

Thus, if a full-cost RCU is desired, a seventh step is needed: charge support activity RCUs to patient-centered departments and then allocate

TABLE 5
Direct departmental cost calculations

Activity code	Activity description	Frequency	Direct RCU	Total costs
70150	CAT, head no IV contrast	2,540	$74.63	$189,560
71020	Chest, two views	18,792	$20.24	$380,350
	Department total			*$569,910*

these charges to each of the direct RCUs. Following the principles of activity-based costing, these assignments should be based on the causes of cost. Therefore, if a support activity is done in support of only one service department (or activity), the full cost of that support activity should be charged directly to that one department (or patient-centered activity) and not allocated over a wide range of departments (or activities). If direct charging is not possible, then allocation based on the level of support service provided is appropriate.

Mathematically, the full-cost RCU can be written as

Full-cost RCU   = direct RCU + FCA

    Full-cost RCU   = resource consumption unit: full cost
    Direct RCU   = resource consumption unit: direct cost only
    FCA   = fixed-cost allowance

For example, in the radiology scenario presented in Tables 2 and 3, a FCA of $61.46 for the CAT scan and $7.55 for the chest x-ray could be added to the direct RCU, generating full-cost RCUs of $136.09 and $27.95, respectively.

At this point, service activities and their corresponding costs (either direct or full) can be charged to product lines (e.g., DRGs). Because of the separate direct cost RCU, interfacility comparisons of both activities and product lines can be made. This allows for comparisons of like activities and services without introducing variation in costs due to factors such as accounting practices, facility age, educational activities, and corporate structure. Yet, FCAs can easily be added when full costing is needed for things like capitated contract negotiations. It should be noted that by costing the major activities of all departments—not just the service ones—interfacility comparisons of supportive and service activities can be made.

To ensure the continued validity of both the direct and full-cost RCUs it will be necessary to update them continually. The frequency with which updating occurs needs to balance the costs of updating with the benefits more accurate data can provide. In general, routine updates can be done on an annual basis. However, a series of threshold volume and cost triggers should be established to ensure that updates occur more frequently if needed. The magnitude of these thresholds should vary by the nature of the individual activity.

The pilot project

The fundamental premise of the RCU approach to tracking resources is that valid RCUs can be developed that span facilities and do not require microcosting. To test the RCU methodology, the Henry Ford Health System is conducting a pilot project in a number of departments across three of its acute general hospitals. Initially, RCUs are being constructed for a number of direct service departments (i.e., pharmacy, nursing, radiology, pathology, and respiratory therapy) and one support department (i.e., building services).

The initial step in the pilot project is for members of the pilot project team to meet with directors and managers from each of the selected departments. At this time, the goals of the demonstration project are outlined and the assistance of the directors and their staffs solicited. Directors and managers are then asked to compile a list of all the activities in which their department is engaged and to identify which of these activities represent the high-cost ones. They are instructed to solicit the help of key departmental staff members as they see appropriate.

Once the high-cost activities are identified, facilitated work groups are established within each of the pilot departments. Departmental employees are selected to participate in a manner that ensures that all phases of the work processes that constitute the high-cost activities are represented. Initially, work group participants are asked to review the list of high-cost activities and once the group agrees that the appropriate activities have been identified, a modified Delphi process is used to reach consensus regarding resource use by line-item expense category in producing each of the activities. Participation by all work group members is crucial to the success of the Delphi process. Each individual enhances the understanding of the work processes involved in conducting each activity, thereby allowing the RCU methodology to accommodate unique features of each department. These work groups, which are facilitated by members of the pilot project team, are also being asked to gauge what volume range they believe their estimates to be applicable. Such information will be critical to establishing volume triggers to recalibrate the RCU estimates.

Once the work groups have quantified the resources consumed in producing each of the high-cost activities, the pilot test team uses the direct departmental line-item expenses from the statement of revenue and expense to calculate an estimated per unit cost for each of the resource categories. By combining the quantity of resource units with the estimated unit cost and summing overall expense categories, a direct RCU is derived for each high-cost activity. Total departmental costs associated with the provision of these high-cost activities can be calculated by incorporating data on the number of times each activity is performed. Subtracting the department's high-cost activity total from the total departmental costs results in the department's residual costs. It is these residual costs that must be allocated to the other relatively low-cost activities in which the department is engaged. Interviews with departmental managers and work groups are conducted to ensure that appropriate methods of allocation are used to perform this step.

Evaluation and validation

Because the development and implementation of the RCU remains in the preliminary stages, it is important that both the process of developing the RCU and the resulting RCU calculations be continually evaluated throughout the pilot project. One measure of the success of the pilot test is the ease with which

1. Managers and work groups can identify the activities in which their departments are engaged and which of these activities represent the high-cost activities

2. Departmental work groups can estimate relative resource units consumed

3. Departmental work groups can identify an appropriate allocation basis for direct departmental overhead

The pilot test team also uses brief exit interviews to measure the perceived difficulty of these tasks. The team also keeps detailed records of the time required to complete these tasks. Such information will allow estimates to be made of the costs of developing the RCUs. These cost estimates can then be viewed in light of the perceived benefits of the RCUs.

Perhaps more important than the success of the process used to develop the RCUs is whether the RCUs developed are valid indicators of resource use. This is particularly important because of the likely sensitivity of the RCU estimates to the proportion of total direct costs attributed to them. In step 3, it is assumed that the high-cost activities account for 80 percent of direct departmental costs in each of the four categories. But if this assumption is incorrect, the per unit cost derived in step 5 may be biased and may over- or underestimate actual costs incurred.

The validity of the RCUs developed during the pilot project is being assessed by comparing them with existing relative value unit (RVU) scales and with results from existing microcosting studies (e.g., machine manufacturer guidelines and studies conducted by Henry Ford Health System's Department of Management Services). New microcosting studies are also being conducted to ensure that sufficient benchmarks exist to validate the RCUs. Thus, the extent of the bias can be determined and the RCU estimates can be adjusted as needed. Because the RCUs are being developed at each of Henry Ford's three short-term general hospitals, comparisons among results at each of the three facilities can also be made for common activities.

Extensions of the model

As currently outlined, the RCU is designed to measure actual resource use. That is, it is composed of an estimate of the average quantity of resources used and the actual unit costs of these resources. However, the RCU methodology can be easily adapted to reflect either budgeted or standard quantities, unit costs, or both. The use of budgeted amounts allows the comparison of actual quantities and costs to expected ones, while the use of standard quantities and costs allows the comparison of current activities to what the output should cost in an efficient and effective healthcare provider. By expanding the scope of the RCU to include actual, budgeted, and standard amounts, comparisons between actual, planned, and ideal resource use can be made and divergences can be identified and evaluated.

Conclusions

As capitated payments become more prevalent in the hospital industry, the challenge is not only to develop and implement a mechanism to track resource use but to maintain the mechanism and translate the data provided into meaningful information. This means balancing the level of detail and complexity inherent with any comprehensive resource tracking mechanism in the hospital sector with the required ease of use and maintenance necessary to ensure continued acceptance. Although a handful of organizations have begun to meet this challenge, the costs of such mechanisms have hindered widespread industry acceptance and use.[5]

The RCU greatly simplifies the task of resource tracking by acknowledging that a relatively small number of activities account for the bulk of the industry's costs. By greatly reducing the number of activities for which actual resource consumption must be tracked and by separately tracking direct and indirect costs, the RCU transforms an insurmountable task to a manageable one. It also begins to pave the road for widespread acceptance of a standard mechanism for resource tracking in the healthcare industry.

Because the RCU includes separate resource and cost components and a separate direct and indirect cost component, it can be a powerful management tool. With continual comparisons of actual and expected (standard) resource use and costs, managers can identify deviations from the norm. These variations can then be investigated to pinpoint their causes (e.g., cost, volume, or intensity variations).

Identification of these variations and their causes will enable managers to improve efficiency of their operations. For example, with continual monitoring, staffing levels can be adjusted to reflect changes in activity levels and interdepartmental and interorganizational comparisons can be made to identify the least costly setting in which to produce a particular service or procedure. Furthermore, once managers know how much it costs to perform an activity, they can accurately evaluate make-buy decisions.

Once resources can be tracked accurately at the activity level within each department, they can be integrated with critical pathways or clinical practice guidelines. Such paths or guidelines delineate the daily components (i.e., procedures and services) of an inpatient episode under usual care circumstances. In combination with RCUs, these paths and guidelines can be used to calculate both expected and actual resource use (i.e., cost) per day of an inpatient stay or of an entire length of stay. As such, actual care can be concurrently costed, compared to protocol, and compared to capitated payments. Once this is achieved, unusual variations in care patterns can be quickly identified by comparing actual and expected resource use.

An RCU can also become a part of routine patient ledgers. These ledgers or clinical summaries can be prepared instantaneously from automated billing records. Costs can be compared "to date" against the protocol, empirical averages, or anticipated revenues, making it possible to estimate profit or loss on an individual patient during his or her stay.

Tying actual resource use to clinical episodes also lays the foundation for an outcomes-oriented approach to quality assurance. Once such a resource tracking mechanism is in place, differences in patient outcomes relative to resources consumed can be evaluated. This is the type of information needed for outcomes management that ensures the effective and efficient use of healthcare resources.

NOTES

1. S. A. Flinker, "The Distinction Between Cost and Charges," *Annals of Internal Medicine* 196 (1982):102–9.

2. T. M. Orloff, et al., "Hospital Cost Accounting: Who's Doing What and Why," *Health Care Management Review* 15, no. 4 (1990):73–78.

3. Flinker, "Cost and Charges"; E. Gardner, "Trying to Make Sense of Hospital Charges," *Modern Healthcare* 17 (1990):24; and J. Nemes, "Tight Margins Lead Hospitals to Cost Accounting Systems," *Modern Healthcare* 17 (1990):23, 25–30.

4. J. M. Juran and F. M. Gryna, *Juran's Quality Control Handbook*, 4th ed. (New York: McGraw-Hill, 1988).

5. J. Ashby, *The Accuracy of Cost Measures Derived from Medicare Cost Report Data*, prepared for Prospective Payment Assessment Commission (Washington, DC: GPO, 1993), Intramural Report 1-93-01.

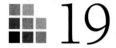 19

Managing hospital capitation

Francine Chapman
Director of Managed Care Programs
UCLA Medical Center
Los Angeles, California

O**VER THE PAST DECADE**, the progressive shift of financial risk to healthcare providers has been an integral part of the growth of managed care. One of the key elements of care management is motivating healthcare providers to watch and conserve resources. Since hospitals consume the greatest percentage of dollars paid for healthcare services, they have naturally been the focus of many different attempts to motivate cost-conservative behavior. Medicare diagnostic-related group (DRG) payments shifted the risk for the overall cost of an inpatient stay to the hospital, and per diem payments (i.e., flat payment per day of stay) shifted the risk for the cost of a day of stay. Other global payments, such as fixed price per surgical case, both inpatient and outpatient, also shifted the burden of hospital resource management directly from the payer to the hospital.

Although capitation is also a risk-shifting methodology, it differs significantly from these other methods. It moves the focus from a single incidence of care for a single patient to population-based responsibility for multiple processes and sites of care. The management of capitated populations requires a broader perspective than the single episode of care. Hospitals entering capitated arrangements for the first time must develop new information and operational systems, new accounting procedures, care review and management protocols, and new relationships with other providers of care in order to succeed financially and clinically in the assumption of population-based risk.

While the activities of managing capitated contracts is similar between physician groups and hospitals, the overall complexity of hospital organizations makes it important to focus on the most important operational activities during the early stages of implementation. Experience in California has shown that hospitals incorrectly assumed that many essential functions to successfully implementing capitated agreements were similar enough to other management and clinical activities to be absorbed without special attention. Initial risk pool settlements reflected substantial losses. This clearly indicated that a different approach to managing the capitated contracts must be put into place.

This chapter presents a brief primer on four management activities that are key to successfully managing capitated enrollment

1. Creating an organizational infrastructure

2. Establishing regular financial and performance reporting

3. Managing and maximizing revenue

4. Establishing comprehensive population-based case management

Organization requirements

Hospitals are accustomed to payment forms such as DRG reimbursement, global case rates, and flat daily rates that place the hospital at financial risk—both positively and negatively—for significant variances between the cost of an episode of care and the payment. Capitation places the risk higher. For example, per case financial risk can be compared to management of the cost of each meal for each member of the family, while capitated reimbursement can be compared to managing the entire family budget, where food expenses are placed in the larger context of income and other significant family expenses. While carefully monitoring the cost of meals is one way to control the family budget, it does not complete the job.

Similarly, under a capitated arrangement, it is necessary to conserve resources on each individual patient stay or incidence of care, as is presently done under DRGs and per diem payments. However, this alone will not lead to financial and clinical success in capitated arrangements.

To comprehensively manage its at-risk responsibilities, the hospital must develop a new set of activities and processes, many of which are not needed under other payment and care arrangements.

DELEGATED RESPONSIBILITIES

When a hospital becomes a capitated healthcare provider, it must move beyond the realm of providing specific care services and seeking payment; it must perform many functions that in fee-for-service (FFS) are performed by insurers and health plans themselves. In FFS, hospitals seek authorization to admit a patient, perhaps to perform a surgical procedure, and are given a length of stay target for the hospital admission by the insurer or health plan. Under capitation, the hospital must determine these service targets when care is given inside its doors. It also must have a process to provide utilization review guidelines to other organizations with whom it contracts for services, and it must have a process to receive claims from these organizations, adjudicate them, and make payments. Most hospitals do not have such staff capabilities and are even less likely to have information systems to support the tracking and analysis needs of external case management as well as claims adjudication and payment.

Because the hospital and its subcontractors will not be billing the health plans, most health plans require overall statistical and patient-specific reporting from the hospital to support their own information needs. This reporting typically includes information on the subcontractors and subcontracts that the hospital holds, detailed billing-type information on all episodes of care the patients receive, and aggregate statistics on services used by the enrolled population.

CUSTOMER AND PLAN LIAISON

Health plan members covered under a hospital's capitation agreement will generate administrative issues that must be handled (e.g., they may receive bills from providers of care for which the hospital is responsible, or question a denial of a service or the specifics of their benefit coverage). Under FFS arrangements, these questions are referred to the health plan, whereas under capitated contracts, the hospital generally is required to address these issues. A responsive, patient-friendly customer service function must be developed, with knowledgeable staff trained in the details of capitation.

As the ultimate guarantor of the cost of care and quality of service, health plans will maintain an oversight function. A well-established contact person within the hospital must be able to work with the health plan representatives on issues regarding financial responsibilities, oversight of quality assurance, customer service, and claims processing, as well as resolve enrollee issues and contractual complications. Initially, this function could be performed by one well-trained individual who works in customer service and knows the details of the contractual arrangement. When capitated enrollment is a significant portion of the hospital's activity, perhaps greater than 15 percent, it is advisable to separate the functions into three areas: enrollee service; claims, financial management, and data; and contractual issues and subcontracting. The ability to develop a positive daily working relationship with the contracting health plan is a key success factor to manage the capitated relationship.

Under a full risk contract, a hospital will receive capitation payments that typically cover all acute hospital services, many hospital-related services, and some services considered alternatives to hospitalization (i.e., skilled nursing and subacute care, ambulatory surgery centers, emergency room services, ambulatory centers for dialysis and chemotherapy, home healthcare and home infusion services, and emergency transportation). Many hospitals do not have such a full array of services under their licenses or their organizational structure. It is necessary to establish subcontracts for those services the organization cannot provide. This requires development of a contracting function as a provider and as a buyer of services. An infrastructure to track and monitor these contracts is required as well as a quality assurance function to assure that the subcontractors meet the licensing and quality standards the health plan, employer, and the physician group find acceptable. The hospital, as payer of claims, will want to structure financial arrangements to create the proper incentives for the subcontracted provider. Creative payment arrangements that further align incentives with the subcontractor can be developed (e.g., subcapitation or development of a financial pool), but the hospital's claims-processing function (or vendor) must be able to administer them.

FINANCIAL MANAGEMENT

It is important to consider changes in financial management activities that must occur under capitated arrangements. Accounting policies for capitated revenue, expense, and contractual allowances have an impact on the hospital's monthly bottom line. The organization's external auditors can be consulted for guidance on acceptable accounting methods for booking capitated revenue and writing off expenses against the capitation revenue. Since most capitated contracts call for some sort of year-end settlement, the method of accounting for the expected year-end transfer of funds to or from the hospital's accounts should be carefully scrutinized, as well as reserving for unpaid purchased service claims that the hospital may receive in the future.

PHYSICIAN-HOSPITAL RELATIONSHIP

The last organizational issue, to develop a structure to manage capitated business, is the most critical in the long run. This is finding an appropriate way to build the necessary working relationship with physicians treating the capitated population. This relationship can make the difference between a positive strategy for both hospital and physicians or a battle over large and small issues. The theory that capitation aligns incentives holds true only to the degree that the physician group and hospital develop an understanding of the basis for the split of capitation, the abilities of one another to influence the overall outcome, and an equitable way to share financial responsibility to the benefit of both parties. This relationship is delineated, to some extent, in the physician and hospital contracts. It is important to evaluate the contractual capitation structure to consider the effects of various provisions on these working relationships. For example, is it better for the hospital to accept the financial responsibility for outpatient imaging or the physician group? If the hospital does not accept that responsibility, some volume and revenue may be lost. On the other hand, if the physicians do not control utilization, the hospital will encounter the financial consequences. Another common issue affecting both the contractual provisions, as well as the ongoing relationship, is which party—hospital, physician group, or health plan—will authorize inpatient admissions and determine the target length of stay?

Once the contracts are developed, establishing a clear framework for decision making, problem resolution and ongoing communication helps alleviate the tensions that inevitably arise. A joint operations committee is a good start to cultivate the information flow for an effective business relationship. This group includes representatives from the hospital, medical group, and the contracting health plan. Appropriate attendance might include management and medical leadership from each organization, as well as representatives of the functions of provider relations, case management, finance, marketing, and other areas when appropriate. The chair could be rotated, an agenda prepared, and minutes kept. Voting authority may also be designated. Membership growth trends, utilization indicators, financial performance issues, subcontractor selection and performance, and coordination of daily activities such as discharge planning, claims authorization and payment, process for completion of the year-end settlement, and management of enrollee grievances or complaints may be appropriate topics for the group.

Regular reporting

Managing capitated enrollment requires different data and measurements than the FFS patient base. The cost to provide care within the institution is a common element to monitor, but under capitation the base of revenue against which the cost of that care is measured is population based, not patient based. Because success in managing capitated enrollment depends on maintaining a population orientation, and a patient-member viewpoint, this requires aggregating individual patient information across multiple sites of care and creating reporting mechanisms that currently do not exist.

On a daily basis, the hospital should know which members are receiving inpatient care at the capitated hospital, as well as other basic information such as the discharge plan and the targeted length of stay. It is important to maintain focus on acute inpatient services at the capitated hospital because they comprise the largest component of the cost of caring for the population. In addition, the hospital must track patients receiving care in other facilities, including acute care, skilled nursing and subacute facilities, outpatient surgery centers, or home or hospice care for which the hospital is financially responsible, to monitor the case management of those patients.

On a monthly basis, it is possible to estimate the ongoing financial status of the contract overall. Basic activity indicators should be totaled, including inpatient stays and days by level of care, separating the units provided by the hospital from those purchased from outside contractors and any provided by noncontracted organizations.

The revenue received should be compared to the known cost of all care provided for which the hospital is financially responsible. This should include the inpatient care at the capitated facility, an estimate of the cost to be incurred from all outside purchased care and an estimate for as yet unknown claims (incurred but not reported claims, or IBNR). By developing a flexible, comprehensive claims-tracking system, the hospital can build the database necessary to fine-tune the estimated costs of outside claims based on what was authorized in advance and what was eventually received and paid.

On a monthly and year-to-date basis, the hospital should estimate any revenue that will come in or be distributed as a result of a risk-sharing provision in the contract. Many financial officers inexperienced in capitation have monitored the profitability of a capitated agreement by comparing revenues and expenses on a monthly basis and found at year-end that a large distribution was due to the health plan or physician group as a result of a contractually determined surplus in the hospital risk-sharing fund. During the month the distribution is paid, it adversely affects the hospital bottom line. Samples of data elements for the monthly revenue summary, activity summary, and contract performance report are shown in Exhibits 1, 2, and 3.

Through the use of benchmark measures, the hospital and medical groups can compare themselves to other providers of care in similar capitation arrangements. The most common benchmarks are admissions per 1,000 enrollees and acute inpatient days per 1,000 enrollees. While these measures are undoubtedly useful, they do not fully encompass all of the important indicators of the way care is managed nor the overall cost of hospital-related care. Additional indices include ambulatory surgeries per 1,000, skilled nursing admissions and days per 1,000 enrollees, emergency room visits per 1,000, and case mix index of inpatient stays. These are crude indicators but would serve as basic guidepoints to compare different populations and to develop better performance indicators for the particular situation. Most health plans can provide planwide benchmarks as a starting point and actuarial studies for similar populations are also available to use as general comparisons.

Data compiled by the hospital should be shared regularly with the physician group. Physicians' clinical practices in caring for patients are the most important factor determining the success of the capitated arrangement. The hospital and physicians should jointly develop goals to improve performance against the basic benchmarks, as well as more focused measures as performance indicates. For example, if emergency department utilization is high against comparative information then the physician group and hospital may want to undertake a further analysis of the types of patient problems presenting in the emergency room, the times of day the patients are being seen, and the admission rate emanating from the visits, to begin to further understand the problem and potential solutions.

Revenue management

One element of a capitated payment scheme is particularly appealing to healthcare providers—the regular flow of cash without the expense and delay of billings and collections. While this is certainly one of the major benefits of a capitated arrangement, it should not be implied that the revenue side of the capitation equation can be taken for granted. There are many opportunities for errors in capitation payments. Likewise, opportunities to augment capitated revenues are present through careful management of individual patient accounts and overall management of the revenue stream.

CAPITATION PAYMENT

Typically, the capitation payment is calculated in one of three ways: a percentage of the premium that the health plan receives for each member (e.g., 38 percent of net employer premium receipts); a flat fixed amount per member enrolled (e.g., $38.00 per enrolled member per month); or a payment for each member based on a table of age/sex demographic cells (e.g., age/sex adjusted capitation), which is illustrated in Table 1.

Under any of these three formulas, however, the hospital evaluates its budget each month based on the total membership in its capitated pool. When it prepares its capitation payments to providers, the health plan counts the number of members for which it is paying and displays this

TABLE 1
Sample capitation payment based on demographic factors

Member sex and age	Capitation payment
Male age 0–1	$90.00
Female age 0–1	$90.00
Male age 2–5	$30.00
Female age 2–5	$30.00
.	.
.	.
.	.
Male age 15–25	$27.75
Female age 15–44	$42.50
Male age 26–44	$21.00

in a statement along with the amount being paid. After receiving a capitation check, the first thing to do is to scrutinize the number of enrollees shown on the capitation statement. If the number varies dramatically from the expected, the variance should be investigated immediately. It may be a computing error or perhaps a large employer was added to or terminated from the insurer's rolls. In any case, the more time that passes before these discrepancies are investigated, the more difficult it becomes to resolve them. The health plan's enrollment files are quite dynamic, with eligibility of particular individual members changing daily.

Many retroactive changes occur to membership in capitated health plans—health plan and employer negotiations take longer than anticipated and a premium adjustment is made retroactively a few months later; a large employer changes health plans and the enrollment process is fraught with computer problems. COBRA enrollment can occur 60 days retroactive. In the case of Medicare plans, HCFA periodically cleans its Medicare eligibility file. In any of these circumstances, the health plan may find that it owed the capitated hospital more or less than it actually paid for a previous month. Generally, the contract would allow the health plan to make those adjustments on a subsequent capitation payment. These adjustments may be easy or difficult to detect on a capitation statement, but for the purposes of good monitoring, it is essential to scrutinize the capitation statement for these types of adjustments. If the contract with the health plan puts a limit on the length of time allowable for retroactivity, the hospital should be diligent in assuring that changes, especially deductions, were not taken after the deadline.

Another reason for careful scrutiny of the capitation statement is to detect retroactive disenrollments of members. If care was provided to a member, the patient account was written off as a capitation adjustment. If the member later is found to be retroactively ineligible, the hospital should pursue the patient for another payment source, either the subsequent health plan in which the patient enrolled, or even the patient directly.

Periodically, hospitals should request an audit of the health plan's capitation calculation system, to be sure that systems are working properly to accurately calculate and pay capitaton. A sample of a health plan's capitation statement is shown in Exhibit 4.

OTHER REVENUE SOURCES

In considering the profitability of capitated arrangements, other funding sources should be considered. As with any insurance arrangement, patients may have other sources available for covering costs of care (e.g., coordination of benefits). It is common for a patient to be receiving care from the capitated plan and also have an indemnity or preferred provider organization (PPO) option as a secondary or primary source of coverage. If a third party, such as an auto insurer, is liable for the care for an injury, for example, the auto insurer can be pursued. If the hospital paid for care from another provider through its capitation, it can also pursue the third party for reimbursement for that care unless the contract specifies otherwise. Insurance carriers often use an outside firm to identify and pursue third-party liability claims, and if the hospital has sufficient capitated enrollment, this is also a strategy to be considered.

MANAGING PATIENT ACCOUNTS

While receivables management is generally absent in capitation, managing of patient accounts remains an important function. As mentioned earlier, retroactive changes in capitated membership do occur. Before an account is written off to a capitation adjustment, a final check of eligibility with the health plan is recommended. If a retroactive ineligibility is found several months later, it may be difficult to locate another source of payment. Beyond eligibility verification, it is important to determine if the specific services the patient received are the hospital's financial responsibility. Most plans develop a list or matrix of services with the financially responsible party—hospital, physician group, or health plan—identified for each service. A sample of this type of matrix is shown in Exhibit 5. A service provided by a hospital (e.g., certain out-patient diagnostic tests) to a hospital-capitated enrollee may not be the responsibility of the hospital, but the medical group's responsibility. The account should not be written off to the capitation adjustment, but billed to the medical group. Capitation account write-off should be delegated to individuals who can properly interpret the services provided against the hospital's designated responsibility listing. An automated approach to screening services on the patient's account against the responsibility listing can also be developed. However, implementing this strategy requires a sizable investment that is probably justifiable only when more than half the hospital's revenues are capitated. Finally, account write-offs should be handled with caution. In the FFS environment, if a bill is submitted to a health plan and the patient is not eligible or the service provided is not a covered benefit, the hospital will receive a denial notice from the company billed. Under capitated arrangements, if a mistake in eligibility or covered benefits is made, an entire account may be written off to a capitation allowance without the error every having been discovered. Therefore, the financial threshold for supervisor oversight of write-offs should be considered, since erroneously writing off and closing a $5,000 inpatient account is a more grievous error than writing off $5,000 instead of $4,000 on an inpatient account of $20,000. Errors in eligibility, financial responsibility, and even identification of the appropriate patients within the capitated program can lead to errors costing thousands of dollars per account.

CLAIMS MANAGEMENT

Depending on the size and breadth of the services available through the capitated hospital, between 10 and 25 percent of all services for capitated patients are purchased from another provider or vendor. The importance of maintaining a system to adequately manage these claims cannot be overemphasized. When enrollment is small (particularly when Medicare patients are not involved) and the claim volume is low, hospitals new to managing capitated contracts generally believe a full-blown claims management system involves more expense than can be justified. They often develop a simple database for tracking of claims. This certainly is the least costly approach, but such a system must be carefully thought out and even more carefully administered. Every variable's function and relationship to other data contained in the database should be considered in the development. Because it is likely that different individuals will enter information over time, it is essential that firm rules be developed for names of providers (e.g., Sun Air Hospital versus Sunair Convalescent), for identification of duplicate claims (e.g., durable medical equipment versus wheelchair), and for strict application of patient identifiers (e.g., St. Clair, James versus St. Clair, J. B.). If the integrity of these identifying fields is not maintained, it will be difficult or impossible to properly administer claims and, further, to aggregate information in accurate and useful ways by individual enrollees and by types of care providers. The information contained in the claims file should be able to be merged with hospital financial records and case management information, so all elements of service and cost for a single enrollee can be aggregated. This is important in analyzing high-dollar cases, filing stop-loss claims, and evaluating care protocols which include multiple sites of care.

If Medicare enrollees are a part of the capitated contract, claims volume will be much greater. Thus, serious consideration should be given to a system with more traditional claims adjudication and processing functions. Consideration should also be given to retaining an outside agency, such as a third-party administrator or management services organization, to process claims and provide the attendant information to the hospital and the health plan.

ESTABLISHING COMPREHENSIVE CASE MANAGEMENT

Successfully managing capitation contracts is dependent on the ability to "outsmart" the financial constraint of fixed revenue and provide the right care for the population's needs. This includes thoughtfully constructed treatment protocols for identified conditions and avoiding episodes of illness through intervention programs developed and implemented by the physician group and the hospital.

Over the past decade, hospitals have adapted to payer-driven managed care initiatives. The first was controlling the length of inpatient stays. Utilization review attempted to trim unnecessary days from inpatient cases. This effort effectively reduced average lengths of stay dramatically in markets with high managed care penetration. Some hospital resources were saved in avoiding patient days altogether, but the use of resources per case did not drop in proportion to the length of stay.

Resource use on a per case basis became more evident as a result of DRG and other fixed per case reimbursement methods.

The effort to monitor hospital days and to control the cost of each case is essential to managing a capitated population. However, the major financial savings under capitation can only be achieved by integrating these two tactics with the goal of avoiding hospitalizations altogether. This tactic is unfamiliar to many hospital utilization review and case management departments because the referral for hospital care has traditionally been the precipitating event which initiates case management. Capitation introduces the financial incentive for hospitals to look beyond their doors to the larger medical and social issues facing their particular capitated populations. In other words, hospitals must begin to work with the capitated physician group in a cooperative effort to avoid the most expensive forms of medical care by jointly developing programs that target avoidable hospitalizations and surgical procedures.

The essential elements of a comprehensive population-based case management program for capitated hospitals include the following:

- Admission and length of stay review

- Care pathways for all common hospital admissions

- Discharge planning which begins, at the latest, on the day of admission

- Authorization for and monitoring of all admissions to hospital, skilled nursing facilities, and home health programs outside the hospital

- Prehospitalization discharge planning for all scheduled major surgical procedures that may include home assessment visits

- Ongoing monitoring of emergency room utilization, to identify frequent users without true emergencies, frequent users with emergencies that can be avoided with proper intervention, and physician convenience referrals to the emergency room

- Community case managers for capitated members (particularly effective for seniors) to address social and environmental issues (e.g., lack of home support, transportation problems, medication compliance, or inappropriate food supply) that contribute to exacerbation of illness or inappropriate use of services

- Ongoing analyses of hospital data to develop the following information: individual physician trends, overall benchmarks for admission rates for particular diagnoses, readmission rates and reasons for readmissions, use of resources per case type, adherence to care pathways, use of alternative methods of service, and other measures that would provide trends on the overall effectiveness of hospital and hospital-related care provided to the population

The first two tactics—admission and length of stay review and care pathways for common admissions—are familiar to most hospitals. They constitute standard managed care practice for commercially insured patients and are also necessary to provide care efficiently to Medicare and Medicaid members. The remaining six tactics, however, may not be well developed and spell the difference between marginal capitated performance and medically effective and profitable capitation contracts.

A common question that arises in implementing such tactics is dividing or sharing case management responsibility with the physician group. In physician organizations with many years of capitated experience, staff are commonly assigned to some or all of the functions cited above. For example, most organized managed care physician groups have staff dedicated to hospital utilization review. Generally, this has been a reaction to fill a need that was not fulfilled elsewhere. However, physician organizations are often willing to share staff costs or share responsibility for the case management functions if this sharing imparts a better-functioning service and a better outcome. Where both physicians and hospitals are capitating for the first time, each organization has an opportunity to demonstrate how it can positively influence the desired outcome with the most efficient use of staff. A genuine opportunity for cost efficiency results.

Hospitals have an advantage in fulfilling case management functions (e.g., early discharge planning, review of care in outside facilities, and data analysis) because they have access to a larger staff that can provide more timely responses, can cover vacations and illnesses, and can rely on a more sophisticated data analysis infrastructure and capability for generating valuable information.

The importance of a strong daily working relationship with the physician organization treating the capitated population cannot be overemphasized. Early in the implementation of a capitated contract communication channels must be established, problem-solving approaches developed, and contractual terms clarified. Agreement must be reached on the selection of subcontracted providers and vendors. The mechanisms for authorizing purchased care and communicating these authorizations among the parties must be resolved. Even with a well-functioning team, installing a new contract dictates some adjustments to accommodate the new health plan's requirements and style. Until communication channels are well established, it is likely that necessary activities will be overlooked. The first high-dollar case that presents itself is an opportunity to focus on coordination between the physician group and hospital and explore ways the team can work together. If this does not happen, then this case can be the situation that causes all parties to question if they can or even should make themselves into a team. The joint operations meetings are the place to infuse the energy of the common goal on the team effort. Opportunities to review total performance often overcome the discussion of the one event gone wrong and serve to turn attention on large issues that can yield the maximum improvement, such as care standardization for common diagnoses and community case management.

In California, experience has shown that it is important for hospitals to provide a tangible improvement in managing healthcare expenses to attract more capitation contracts. Both physician organizations and health plans have benefited financially from ratcheting down hospital reimbursement in managed care contracts paid on per diem or case rates. However, as premiums continue to fall to employer purchasing clout and increasing competition among providers, physician organizations and payers have allowed hospitals to participate in capitation agreements on the theory that some marginal improvement in overall performance will result. Because straightforward tactics such as utilization review have already yielded significant reductions in the overall healthcare expense, the challenge of continuing to lower overall costs, while maintaining and improving service and satisfaction, is much greater now than a few years ago.

One of the challenges hospitals face when entering into capitated contracts for the first time is making organizational and behavioral changes to manage what may initially be a very small percentage of the institution's business. Establishing an elaborate case management structure to monitor emergency service use, visit outside skilled nursing facilities, and provide presurgical home visits, for example, is quite costly at low enrollment levels. Establishing authorization-tracking and claims-processing capabilities is also daunting for a small number of covered lives.

Hospitals that see their future tied to rapid growth of capitated membership may see the expense in building an information and staff infrastructure as a worthwhile investment. Hospitals with sufficient resources will have an opportunity to learn how to competently run capitation systems while the volume of activity and dollars being managed through them is still relatively small.

Organizations that are not persuaded that capitation will be a dominant form of payment may be reluctant to commit major capital and human resources before the approach has shown promise within their institutions. In this situation, it is important to cultivate a small, expert team of staff, dedicated to understanding the essential capitation management activities, and assure their complete and thorough performance to prove the concept. This will probably result in several key departments carving out the activities related to the capitated population and handing them off to the expert team. An example would be the area of patient accounts, which in many hospitals divide responsibility by patient last name, for example. All patient accounts assumed to be covered under the capitated agreements are transferred to a single individual or small group that understands the financial responsibility matrix, the need for scrutiny before write-off, and the paperwork processing requirements of the contracts. Similar designation of patients might happen in case management, so a capitated patient would be managed by a small team, regardless of the patient's diagnostic category. While this approach has been successful, there is still a need at some point to convert information systems from the simple, start-up systems to more complex and sophisticated products, efficient in managing larger populations. Also, it is important to continually train staff for all functions as the capitated enrollment grows. Eventually, a fundamentally different management approach is needed that recognizes capitation as an essential book of business and in which all employees are conversant.

The following outline summarizes the minimal management activities that must be assured to manage a capitated hospital agreement. The activities are broken into three broad categories: contractual (C), financial (F), and operational (O).

1. Distribute a detailed listing of financial responsibilities under the agreement, so all parties agree on which organization (i.e., hospital, physician group, or health plan) will arrange for and pay for all services covered under the enrollees' benefit plan or plans (C, F, O)

2. Arrange all needed subcontracts for services the hospital does not provide but for which it is financially responsible (C)

3. Assign an individual to be the liaison with the health plan for contractual issues (C)

4. Designate someone to receive the capitation check and be responsible for follow-up if it is not received. Estimate expected revenue and compare to actual (F)

5. Arrange a process to receive claims from outside subcontractors, price them at the contracted amount, process the payment, and track all necessary information on the activity. Pay attention to a common identifier for patients between the hospital information system and the outside claims tracking system (F)

6. Scrutinize the hospital eligibility screening process, making sure the hospital does not bill capitated patients, write off accounts of non-capitated patients, or bill either the health plan or the medical group for services for which the hospital is not financially responsible under the distribution of responsibilities (F)

7. Design a regular reporting system with sufficient data elements to monitor the status of the contract (F, O)

8. Agree on accounting methodologies to handle revenue booking, contractual write-offs, allowances for expected claims generated by purchased services, and reserves for risk pool or contractual transfers of funds at the time of the annual settlement (F)

9. Assign an individual to be the liaison with the physician group for case management and utilization issues, contractual issues, and joint problem solving (O)

10. Organize the case management function to be responsible for utilization management, discharge planning, and oversight and coordination of precare, aftercare, and community case management (O)

11. Arrange for a care and payment authorization process for purchased services, such as skilled nursing, durable medical equipment, and home healthcare for patients (O)

12. Organize the system through which the health plan will receive its encounter information for both hospital-provided services as well as those purchased (O)

13. Coordinate a process with the physician group to notify the hospital of capitated patients authorized for service (preferably before they arrive) so they can be followed appropriately (O)

14. Assign an individual to be the liaison to the enrolled individuals for resolving issues related to billing, benefits, and authorizations (O)

EXHIBIT 1
Expense summary

HMO plan: _____

Period: _____

Hospital-based expenses
A. Inpatient care

Type of care	Days	Charges	Cost	Chargeable expense to the pool
Intensive care	_____	$ _____	$ _____	$ _____
Medical and surgical care	_____	$ _____	$ _____	$ _____
Obstetrics	_____	$ _____	$ _____	$ _____
Pediatrics	_____	$ _____	$ _____	$ _____
Neonatal care	_____	$ _____	$ _____	$ _____
Total acute care	_____	$ _____	$ _____	$ _____
Subacute care	_____	$ _____	$ _____	$ _____
Total inpatient care	_____	$ _____	$ _____	$ _____

B. Outpatient Care

Type of care	Number of visits	Charges	Cost	Chargeable expense to the pool
Ambulatory surgery	_____	$ _____	$ _____	$ _____
Outpatient diagnostic	_____	$ _____	$ _____	$ _____
Emergency room	_____	$ _____	$ _____	$ _____
Home health	_____	$ _____	$ _____	$ _____
Total outpatient care	_____	$ _____	$ _____	$ _____

EXHIBIT 1 (CONTINUED)

Purchased services

	Days or visits	Cost	Cost per day or visit	Cost per member per month (PMPM)
Acute inpatient services	_____	$_____	$_____	$_____
Skilled nursing	_____	$_____	$_____	$_____
Emergency services	_____	$_____	$_____	$_____
Home health— authorized visits	_____	$_____	$_____	$_____
Skilled nursing	_____	$_____	$_____	$_____
Home health aide	_____	$_____	$_____	$_____
Physical therapy	_____	$_____	$_____	$_____
Occupational therapy	_____	$_____	$_____	$_____
Speech therapy	_____	$_____	$_____	$_____
Social work	_____	$_____	$_____	$_____
Infusion services	_____	$_____	$_____	$_____
Durable medical equipment	_____	$_____	$_____	$_____
Ambulance	_____	$_____	$_____	$_____
IBNR (incurred but not reported)	_____	$_____	$_____	$_____
Total purchased services	_____	$_____	$_____	$_____

Hospital-based and purchased services

	Total cost	Cost PMPM
Total expenses	$_____	$_____

EXHIBIT 2
Revenue summary

HMO plan: _____
Period: _____

Gross revenue	$ _____
Members capitated (paid) this month _____ members	
Gross revenue PMPM $ _____ PMPM	
Retroactive adjustments:	
Capitated dollars	$ _____
Membership adjustment	$ _____
Deductions:	
Stop-loss	($_____)
Claims paid	($_____)
Other	($_____)
Net capitation payment (reconciles to capitation check amount)	$ _____
Net revenue PMPM	$ _____

EXHIBIT 3
Performance summary

HMO plan: _____

Period: _____

Plan activity

Enrollment for the month _____ Members

Disenrollment for the month _____ Members

	Days or visits	Days or visits per 1,000 annualized
Inpatient hospitalizations		
Inpatient acute days (in hospital)	_____	_____
Inpatient acute days (other providers)	_____	_____
Total acute inpatient days	_____	_____
Subacute days	_____	_____
Skilled nursing days	_____	_____
Total subacute and skilled nursing days	_____	_____
Outpatient services		
Outpatient surgeries	_____	_____
Home health visits	_____	_____
Emergency room visits	_____	_____
Emergency transport trips	_____	_____

Risk pool summary

Total net revenue		$_____
Expenses		
Inpatient care	$_____	
Outpatient care	$_____	
Emergency services	$_____	
Other expenses	$_____	
Total contractual expenses		($_____)
Total surplus/(deficit)		$_____
Hospital retention		($_____)
Medical group payable/(receivable)		$_____

EXHIBIT 4
Sample capitation payment statement

HEALTH PLAN, INC.
American Hospital senior plan capitation statement
August 1995

HCFA capitation calculation

June 1995 Reconciliation

A. Actuals:	Actual membership	5,162	
	Actual rate	$527.64	
	Actual HCFA revenue		$2,723,678
B. Estimates:	Estimated membership	5,166	
	Estimated rate	$529.77	
	Estimated HCFA revenue		$2,736,792
C. Net adjustment			($13,114)

August 1995 estimates

A. Estimated enrollment	5,161	
Estimated rate	$527.64	
Estimated HCFA revenue		$2,723,150
Retroactive transfers	$0	
Reversal of June revenue adjustment		$91,317
Retroactive additions—see attached list		$13,478
Adjusted current month's revenue		$2,632,197

American Hospital payment:	
Current month's revenue × 42.25 percent	$1,112,103
Less: IBNR withhold at 7.5 percent	($83,408)
IBNR adjustment	($120,772)
Total senior capitation payment	$907,923

EXHIBIT 5
Sample responsibility matrix

Division of financial responsibility
Hospital capitation agreement

	IPA	Hospital	Plan
Professional services	∎		
Administration of anesthesia	∎		
Allergy testing and treatment	∎		
Alpha fetoprotein	∎		
Biofeedback (Medicare approved)	∎		
Chemotherapy (not inpatient)		∎	
Chiropractic care (Medicare approved)	∎		
Consultations	∎(*)		
Hepatitis B	∎		
Injectables—human growth hormones if provided outpatient	∎		
Injections and immunizations	∎		
Office visits	∎		
Outpatient hemodialysis		∎	
Outpatient physical, speech therapy	∎		
Outpatient radiation therapy		∎	
Outpatient x-ray and lab		∎(*)	
Patient health education	∎		
Periodic health evaluations	∎		
Physician examinations	∎		
Physician's visit to hospital or skilled nursing facility	∎		
Physician's visit to home	∎		
Podiatry service (Medicare approved, requires medical group authorization)	∎		
Preadmit, x-ray and lab	∎(*)		
Preexisting pregnancy	∎		
Sterilization (Medicare approved)	∎		
Total obstetrical care, pre- and postnatal	∎		

	IPA	Hospital	Plan
Hospital services			
Ancillary hospital services:			
Use of hospital equipment		∎	
Surgical and anesthetic supplies		∎	
Physical, speech, and occupational rehabilitation		∎	
Oxygen, drugs, and medications		∎	
Laboratory examinations		∎	
X-ray examinations		∎	
Appliances		∎	
Implantable devices and appliances		∎	
Professional charges for x-ray and lab if part of inpatient, outpatient surgery, or emergency service		∎	
Take-home drugs		∎	

EXHIBIT 5 (CONTINUED)

	IPA	Hospital	Plan
Hospital services (cont.)			
Institutional and facility services			
Inpatient hospital services		▪	
Injectables—human growth hormones (inpatient)		▪	
Medical social services		▪	
Home health			
Home health nursing, physical and occupational therapy		▪	
Medical social services		▪	
Subacute and skilled nursing facility			
Subacute facility services		▪	
Skilled nursing facility services		▪	
Professional charges for x-ray and lab if part of skilled nursing care		▪	
Emergency/urgently needed services			
Emergency room (in area)			
Professional services, initial treatment		▪	
Professional services, consultations	▪		
Facility		▪	
Emergency room (out of area)			
Professional			▪
Facility			▪
Urgent care services (out of area)			
Professional			▪
Facility			▪
Alcohol and drug rehabilitation			
Outpatient substance abuse rehabilitation	▪		
Professional services for alcohol and drug	▪		
Institutional/facility services			
Inpatient hospital including alcohol and drug		▪	
Inpatient substance abuse rehabilitation		▪	
Other services			
AIDS			
Professional	▪		
Facility		▪	
Alternative birth centers		▪	
Ambulance		▪	
Autologous blood (not covered)			
Chemotherapy (inpatient)			
Professional		▪	
Drugs		▪	
Cosmetic surgery (Medicare approved)			
Professional	▪		
Facility		▪	

EXHIBIT 5 (CONTINUED)

	IPA	Hospital	Plan
Other services (cont.)			
Dental care (Medicare approved, surgery of the jaw and related structures due to accident or injury only			
Professional	▪		
Facility		▪	
Durable medical equipment	▪ (OP)	▪ (IP)	
Lithotripsy			
Professional	▪		
Facility		▪	
Organ transplants (Medicare approved)			
Professional	▪		
Facility		▪	
Outpatient surgery center			
Professional	▪ (*)		
Facility		▪	
Prosthetic devices	▪ (OP)	▪ (IP)	
O/P prescription drugs (for members with benefit)			▪
Vision care			
Vision exams	▪		
Vision care (non-cataract-related lenses and frames)			▪

(*) See hospital benefit matrix.

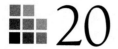20

Clinic-based utilization management

Debra Carpenter
Director of Utilization Management
Blue Plus of Minnesota
St. Paul, Minnesota

I N 1974 BLUE CROSS and Blue Shield of Minnesota established Blue Plus, a mixed model HMO and point-of-service
plan. Today the plan has approximately 325,000 members and contracts
with many primary care clinics (PCCs) throughout the state. The state's
physicians practice predominantly in groups, the average clinic compris-
ing between 8 and 10 physicians although some large clinics may have as
many as 200 physicians; there are few solo practitioners in Minnesota.

Blue Plus generally reimburses a contracting PCC on a fee-for-service
(FFS) basis with a withhold adjusted to reflect that clinic's past performance. The withhold may vary from 0 to 30 percent. Each contracting
PCC has an age/sex adjusted financial goal based on its membership
composition. While this goal may be considered a "pseudocapitation"
since it includes costs for all aspects of care except mental health and
chemical dependency, each PCC assumes responsibility for managing
care provided, including outpatient, inpatient, skilled nursing facility
stays, home healthcare services, and prescription drugs. Blue Plus also
pays each PCC $1.00 per member per month (PMPM) for case man-
agement and quality improvement. This capitation rate includes indirect patient costs such as quality improvement and care management
activities (e.g., referral management, inpatient review, and catastrophic
care management).

A stop-loss provision for each PCC creates a maximum liability protection and allows them to still meet performance goals despite a

catastrophic case. The current maximum is $22,000 per patient per year (an initial threshold of $15,000 plus 20 percent risk up to $50,000).

In the past, utilization management has posed many challenges to Blue Plus in urban and rural areas. Large urban clinics with high Blue Plus enrollment have an incentive to manage utilization effectively but may not have appropriate tools or effective approaches. Many clinics in rural areas have had much less experience with managed care, and participation in Blue Plus may be their first exposure to working within managed care requirements. Moreover, where there are relatively small numbers of Blue Plus enrollees in a specific clinic, those clinic physicians may have limited incentives to reconsider their utilization patterns.

In response to these concerns, Blue Plus decided in 1989 that effective utilization management should be a shared responsibility between itself and its contracting PCCs rather than an oversight function of Blue Plus. Blue Plus tested several approaches to foster increased PCC res-ponsibility for utilization management. The approach regarded as most effective was one to help individual clinics develop utilization management programs tailored to specific aspects of care management. In 1990 the Blue Plus Clinic-Based Utilization Management Program was developed to meet that need.

In the Clinic-Based Utilization Management Program, Blue Plus utilization management staff serve as consultants to the PCCs to help them develop and implement their managed care processes. This chapter provides an overview of the initial creation and operation of that program and then discusses the program's evolution over time, including the introduction and refinement of bonus programs. It will include the process used to select those PCCs with which Blue Plus will contract as well as the process used.

Initial program development

In 1989, Blue Plus found that many of its clinics were struggling and questioning their ability to meet their utilization goals—a prerequisite for receiving their withhold. Blue Plus intended to move more business into its evolving managed care products and realized clinics would need more assistance to learn how to better manage care.

USE OF DATA

Although the Clinic-Based Utilization Management Program initally focused entirely on clinics with performance problems or high PMPM costs, Blue Plus selected three clinics to pilot its new clinic-based approach. The three targeted clinics were all considerably above PMPM goals. As a first step, Blue Plus staff arranged a site visit to each clinic and, during that site visit, presented clinic-specific data on common components of care such as office visits, laboratory, radiology, surgical procedures, emergency room, inpatient days, and number of admissions.

These data summarized the target clinic's performance, expressed in utilization per member and in dollars PMPM for each component of care. Separating volume from cost is important since not all cost variation is driven by volume. At times, higher office visit costs occur even though the volume of services is comparable to the network average. This could reflect either upcoding or more visits to specialists (which may be either new patient visits or more comprehensive consultations). Clinics also received data comparing their current performance with their performance for the same period of time in the previous year.

In addition to clinic-specific data, comparative benchmarks of similar clinics and network averages provided the clinic's physicians and staff with an important analytic tool. Typically, Blue Plus staff selected as benchmarks two clinics similar in geographic location, composition of physicians, and number of members. The Minneapolis–St. Paul metropolitan service averages also served as a benchmark since this area has both the majority of Blue Plus membership and the highest managed care penetration rates in the state. The combination of individual clinic data and comparative data help to distinguish which factors actually drive the variation observed in a given clinic. Understanding the causes of high costs and utilization in a clinic helps to develop actions.

CLINIC SITE VISITS

Initially the Blue Plus team, made up of a Blue Plus medical director, a utilization management coordinator, and a provider relations representative, conducted the clinic site visit. This team approach has proven very effective. The plan medical director as part of the team enhances the clinic's responsiveness, and as many clinic physicians and administrative staff (such as referral or managed care coordinators) as possible are encouraged to attend. Besides assessing the clinic, the site visit also creates a good networking opportunity between Blue Plus and clinic staff, opening opportunity for future collaboration.

The input of the Blue Plus provider relations representative is also very important in the site visit. The representative's past experience with the clinic is useful during the meeting, offering informaton and key factors about the clinic that may affect performance (e.g., whether physicians are paid a portion of the laboratory and x-ray revenues based on the volume of services they order). The representative also knows the physicians in the group and knows which physicians are most influential and which may be most skeptical of the need to actively manage utilization.

KEY FACTORS

Three key factors contribute to the success of these clinic site visits: advance preparation, the nature and presentation of the data, and the participation of a Blue Plus medical director.

Advance preparation

The site visit team discusses all relevant factors during a preparatory meeting, typically held about one week before the visit. In this meeting, the site visitors analyze the clinic-specific data in advance and determine if any additional data may be useful. The preparatory meeting also helps the team decide specific issues to be discussed. In addition, the site visit team agrees on the utilization management approach(es) to be suggested to the clinic, the desired course of action to be taken, the anticipated outcome, and the potential follow-up.

Nature and presentation of data

The validity of the data and use of peer clinic benchmarks are very important to the presentation of the data. Clinic members are likely to respond if they feel the data are accurate and if they believe benchmarks are useful. Since the time available with the clinic staff is relatively short, the information needs to be conveyed in a concise, easily understood format. Bar graphs were selected by Blue Plus staff for visual ease to display the comparative data. Figures 1 and 2 depict more current versions of the information provided to a clinic in a site visit.

FIGURE 1
1994 medical clinic office utilization

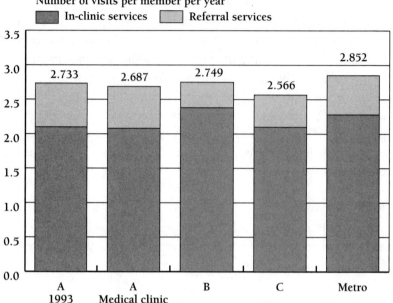

Number of visits per member per year

In-clinic services   Referral services

Participation of Blue Plus medical director

As indicated previously, the presence of the plan medical director is of vital importance. The plan medical director's participation increases the clinic's awareness of the Blue Plus commitment to work with that clinic and underscores the plan's intent to use clinic-specific data as a means to improve care.

SITE VISIT FOLLOW-UP

The Blue Plus physician and the utilization management staff share joint responsibility for site visit follow-up. The Blue Plus team sends a written summary of the site visit to the clinic, documenting the actions the plan and the clinic will take as a result of their meeting and discussions. This written summary is helpful to prevent misunderstandings about the next steps, and clarifies the use of a tracking form that specifies elements of the follow-up plan and helps Blue Plus and clinic staff periodically evaluate progress.

FIGURE 2
1994 medical clinic office utilization

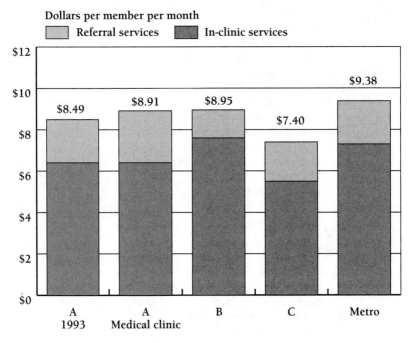

Dollars per member per month

■ Referral services   ■ In-clinic services

Blue Plus also uses a continuous quality improvement (CQI) approach to help the clinics create and implement its utilization improvement plans. This CQI approach is critical since it focuses the clinic on incremental improvement and also reinforces the clinic's interest to reach a "best practice" standard. Since standards are still evolving, Blue Plus utilization management staff needs to continually review best practice standards.

Blue Plus's ability to report data at diagnostic- patient- or service-specific detail level is essential to make the information actionable for clinics. For example, if a clinic with a higher than expected use of chest x-rays adopts a guideline on indications for chest x-rays, it will want to establish a baseline rate to measure subsequent improvement. Thus, the clinic may need a detailed listing of patients who received chest x-rays, first to establish its baseline rate, and then to determine if the adopted guidelines have resulted in improvement. Tables 1 and 2 present sample detailed reports that focus on emergency room usage by enrollees of a

TABLE 1
Medical clinic
Blue Plus emergency report
January–December 1994

Total number of visits: 349
Total number of patients: 311

Top 10 diagnoses by settlement

		ICD9	Dollars
1.	786	Symptoms involving respiratory system/other chest symptoms	$3,797.74
2.	923	Contusion of upper limb	$3,184.86
3.	873	Other open wound of head	$2,031.06
4.	789	Other symptoms involving abdomen/pelvis	$1,936.53
5.	431	Intracerebral hemorrhage	$1,421.73
6.	427	Cardiac dysrhythmias	$1,209.98
7.	590	Infections of kidney	$999.73
8.	592	Calculus of kidney/ureter	$981.31
9.	558	Other noninfectious gastroenteritis/colitis	$931.92
10.	883	Open wound of finger(s)	$931.59

Top 10 diagnoses by number of visits

		ICD9	Visits
1.	873	Other open wound of head	23
2.	786	Symptoms involving respiratory system/other chest symptoms	15
3.	789	Other symptoms involving abdomen/pelvis	13
4.	883	Open wound of finger(s)	11
5.	780	General symptoms	10
6.	924	Contusion of lower limb and of other and unspecified sites	8
7.	382	Suppurative/unspecified otitis media	8
8.	842	Sprains/strains of wrist/hand	8
9.	462	Acute pharyngitis	8
10.	923	Contusion of upper limb	7

Top 10 providers

		Percent of settlement	Number of patients
1.	Hospital A	73.7%	247
2.	Hospital B	8.0%	5
3.	Hospital C	3.0%	1
4.	Hospital D	2.0%	8
5.	Hospital E	1.4%	4
6.	Hospital F	0.9%	3
7.	Hospital G	0.7%	3
8.	Hospital H	0.7%	1
9.	Hospital I	0.7%	2
10.	Hospital J	0.5%	2

Total settlement: $38,799.12

specific clinic. This level of detail enables the clinic to pinpoint areas of concern by diagnosis, number of visits, provider, and patient, thus helping the clinic structure appropriate interventions.

During or after the site visit, the Blue Plus utilization management staff responsible for follow-up consultation and guidance may also provide the clinic with appropriate industry literature and protocols, such as the preventive service guidelines or the Agency for Health Care Policy and Research's guidelines. Information on utilization improvement projects conducted by other clinics can also assist the target clinic to evaluate its practice and design improvement activities.

TABLE 2
Medical report
Blue Plus emergency report
January–December 1994

Top 10 patients by settlement amount

	Age	Name	Diagnosis	Dollars	Visits
1.	40	J. Doe	923.00	$2,951.50	1
2.	78	J. Doe	431	$1,421.73	1
3.	77	J. Doe	786.50	$1,248.14	1
4.	18	J. Doe	590.8	$1,147.00	2
5.	50	J. Doe	592.1	$934.00	1
6.	35	J. Doe	644.03	$761.07	1
7.	40	J. Doe	786.50	$698.56	1
8.	62	J. Doe	427.50	$638.70	1
9.	43	J. Doe	786.50	$582.14	1
10.	54	J. Doe	427.5	$571.28	1

Top 10 patients by number of visits

	Age	Name	Diagnosis	Dollars	Visits
1.	41	J. Doe	346.90	$324.39	5
2.	38	J. Doe	844.0	$149.58	3
3.	24	J. Doe	883.0	$189.33	3
4.	37	J. Doe	789.0	$468.41	3
5.	1	J. Doe	780.3	$147.53	2
6.	3	J. Doe	462	$162.76	2
7.	11	J. Doe	466.0	$147.79	2
8.	44	J. Doe	782.1	$71.49	2
9.	0	J. Doe	569.3	$306.55	2
10.	17	J. Doe	789.02	$155.71	2

Program evolution

COMBINED CQI/UM SITE VISITS

Although Blue Plus used to conduct separate site visits for quality improvement (QI) and for utilization management (UM), these site visits are now combined. Plan medical directors (who formerly participated in UM visits) and consulting physicians (physicians from other contracting PCCs who formerly participated in QI site visits) are all cross-trained on CQI/UM, to reduce overlap between the two areas.

Moreover, the combined site visit approach has yielded other benefits. As a peer, the consulting physician can not only identify with a given situation but can also offer a firsthand perspective of what another clinic has done to manage utilization more effectively. The consulting physician can also provide reassurance that utilization management does not compromise quality and may in fact enhance quality.

In addition, the UM data can often be used to develop a CQI project to focus on improving the effectiveness and the efficiency of care delivery. For example, a clinic with high chest x-ray usage chose to adopt a protocol on indications for chest x-rays. The implementation and measurement of that protocol became one of that clinic's quality improvement projects for the year. Each clinic must undertake at least two quality improvement projects per year, projects that the clinic determines will benefit the care management within the clinic. PCCs are also required to participate in planwide projects such as immunization rate increase or mammogram improvement projects. These utilization management data then become a source of information in defining areas for focus for quality improvement.

Combined CQI/UM site visits can also facilitate discussions with a clinic about its practice patterns. Typically, PCCs may have little opportunity to discuss best practices because they focus on delivering services and caring for the day-to-day needs of their enrolled members.

For instance, one clinic's data indicated a chest x-ray rate of 99 percent in the network. During the site visit, the clinic's medical director expressed doubts about the data, believing that no physicians in the group still ordered routine chest x-rays. The utilization management coordinator, however, remarked that there were still physicians ordering routine chest x-rays. This was confirmed by some of the physicians around the table, and the clinic subsequently began a CQI project on indications for chest x-ray use. During a chart review to determine the baseline, it was noticed that some of the charts did not have a chest x-ray order by the physician even though an x-ray had been performed. All such instances were determined to be routine physical exam visits. A subsequent investigation discovered a standing order that was several years old and had been forgotten by everyone except the receptionist. As patients presented for a routine physical, the clinic receptionist sent them to the hospital x-ray department (in an attached building) for a routine chest x-ray. The procedure had outserved its original purpose, but no evaluation process existed to revise or discontinue the procedure.

FOCUS ON LARGE CLINICS

While the Clinic-Based Utilization Management Program initially focused on clinics with performance concerns, it now concentrates primarily on larger clinics—those with the highest volume of Blue Plus members. It became important for Blue Plus to understand how these clinics were delivering care to members. These clinics, for several reasons, represent a good source of information on how systems and processes can succeed in clinics. For instance, one clinic may have a well-developed inpatient care management system, while another may have created an excellent educational process on referrals or emergency care use for all new patients. Focusing on these clinics also yields knowledge about the barriers clinics encounter in improving processes of care (such barriers might include effective education of staff and physicians about changes or development of a new procedure for a particular aspect of care management). This knowledge also is useful because other clinics confront these same issues and Blue Plus can better prepare those clinics to avoid or overcome identified barriers.

REFERRALS AND FEEDBACK

Although the process for referring members to specialists is one with which many clinics have difficulty, communication to members on this process is essential so that members know what to expect should they need a referral. Problems often arise from processes such as a clinic committee to review all referrals; the efficiency of a committee that may only meet once per week can create difficulties. As a clinic examines its referral process, Blue Plus staff can provide the clinic with information on more effective approaches adopted by other clinics, such as clinics' referral structure, physician involvement, and patient communication. Information about key contact person is also provided.

Information sharing by Blue Plus and its clinics not only can lead to clinic-specific changes but also to planwide adjustments in policies and procedures as Blue Plus receives feedback from clinics. Updated information about the impact of plan policies on the PMPM financial goals and risk arrangements allows both parties to reevaluate risk-sharing arrangements of the contracts and to better determine which portion of the costs belongs to the clinic and which to the plan. For example, while analyzing pap smear rates at one site visit a few years ago, a clinic noted that after the plan took a withhold from the fee schedule rates for pap smears, the clinic was unable to cover its laboratory costs. Since this negative financial incentive for pap smears was inconsistent with Blue Plus's emphasis on preventive services, the plan revised its policy. Withholds are no longer taken on pap smears, mammograms, or immunizations, and the costs of these services are not included in the clinic goals, assuring that there are no disincentives for performing these services.

Clinic feedback can also lead to other changes, such as amending a stop-loss provision. One clinic with a ventilator-dependent child was adversely impacted by the cost of the catastrophic care year after year. Today, if a member reaches stop-loss in one year, the costs for that member in subsequent years are totally excluded from the clinic's financial goals. This prevents a chronic case from adversely affecting a clinic's utilization and financial performance over the long term. Another change was made in the financial risk arrangements for high-risk newborns or newborns who remain hospitalized beyond the mother's stay. By state regulation, parents have 60 days to select the PCC for newborns and enroll them. Previously, the newborn's experience was accrued retrospectively to the selected clinic, even though that clinic may not have known about the care the newborn received or that the newborn was a clinic member. Since the clinic may not have had the opportunity to manage that care, that experience no longer accrues to the clinic.

CQI/UM BONUS PROGRAMS

Since the development of the program, the original CQI/UM bonus programs have been expanded to focus more on quality indicators rather than exclusively on utilization. Bonus program components now reward individual clinics for high achievement in four areas: patient satisfaction, CQI results, childhood immunizations, and financial performance.

The patient satisfaction bonus is based on a score the clinic receives in the annual patient satisfaction survey, reflecting a composite of 10 patient satisfaction parameters (see Table 3). Clinics that receive higher scores than the network benchmark receive a retroactive $0.25 PMPM bonus.

Clinics with higher than expected CQI results also receive a bonus. The clinic's CQI program is scored during the annual CQI visit conducted by the plan. The scoring reflects whether the clinic exceeded the expected program requirements on seven components of the clinic's own quality improvement program. Clinics that have all the expected components and have made additional attempts to develop a more comprehensive quality improvement program receive this bonus. Both the patient satisfaction and CQI program bonuses are calculated on a PMPM basis at the end of the year with an established maximum amount for a given clinic.

A bonus program that promotes childhood immunizations is based on the number of fully immunized two-year-old children. Thirty-five dollars is paid for each fully immunized Blue Plus two-year-old member, regardless of whether or not the clinic itself directly immunized the child. To receive the payment, the clinic must verify the complete immunization status of the child. This program encourages clinics to establish tracking systems for immunizations and to accept responsibility for ensuring that all of their members are fully immunized.

TABLE 3
10 patient satisfaction survey items

The following 10 items are scored by patients on a 1 to 5 scale:
- Outcomes
- Physician skills, experience, and training
- Thorough examination, accuracy of diagnosis
- Thoroughness of treatment
- Overall care recieved at the primary care clinic
- Attention to patient description of medical problems
- Physician and staff support of patient
- Ease of access to care
- Personal interest in patient medical complaints
- Time spent with patient by physician and staff

The fourth bonus program rewards good financial performance by providing a financial incentive for clinics to meet their PMPM cost targets. This bonus varies based on the individual PMPM costs and on the extent to which the clinic exceeded its target.

SUCCESS FACTORS

As Blue Plus developed and refined the Clinic-Based Utilization Management Program, the plan has identified several factors required for a successful program. Table 4 summarizes those essential factors.

The site visit should involve not only clinic leaders but other physicians and clinic staff members since they can contribute important information to the discussions. This also allows them to receive information firsthand from the health plan and to ask any questions directly, thereby avoiding any miscommunication in data's meaning.

The plan's provider relations representative plays a vital role to provide input for the meeting and in follow-up with the clinic and consultation as the clinic plans and initiates tailored UM/QI activities. The tracking form, which documents the follow-up plans, is a useful tool for subsequent discussions with the clinic on their progress toward making changes.

Clinic selection

Although not an explicit component of the utilization management program, the process of selecting clinics to participate in the network as PCCs has now been recognized as a critical factor in care management. The importance of careful clinic selection became evident to Blue Plus in the course of an unsuccessful effort to work with a PCC on improving its performance. After several meetings with this clinic, it became apparent that there was no shared philosophy regarding care management. Since

TABLE 4
Keys to successful clinic-based utilization management

- Presite visit meeting to analyze data and focus discussions
- Valid data and meaningful benchmarks
- Presence of the plan and clinic medical directors at the site visit
- A CQI and partnership approach
- Ability to report data at detailed levels
- Provider relations representative's input and follow-up
- Written follow-up of the site visit

the clinic and the plan could not arrive at mutual agreement, the relationship was discontinued.

CLINIC COMMITMENTS

A commitment to working with the Blues in a long-term relationship prompted the development of an explicit set of expectations by Blue Plus of the PCCs it selects as partners. As Table 5 depicts, these expectations fall into three categories: attitudes, programs, and function. These expectations became the basis for a precontract site visit agenda and it also explains a scoring system for choosing potential partners, avoiding long-term relationships that do not meet the needs of either organization.

Evidence of this commitment can include

- *Acceptance of the program components,* including a credentialing process for all clinic physicians and allied health professionals; formal complaint review, logging, categorization, and trending system for any patient or plan complaint; and a designated medical director for CQI and UM, either the same physician or different physicians depending on the clinic's management structure and the physician's interests

- *Medical record standards for documentation,* whereby clinics are expected to randomly review a specific number records for completeness and legibility; are encouraged to have condition-specific chart reviews to improve documentation and provide feedback to clinic staff; and to

TABLE 5
Expectations of a successful PCC

Attitudes
Physician support for combining case manager and patient advocate roles

Programs
Acceptance and implementation of
- Clinic participation expectations
- Patient medical record requirements
- Quality improvement requirements and commitment to CQI
- Utilization management plan
- Preventive services recommendations
- Preterm birth program
- Referral network

Function
- Cohesiveness as a medical group

participate in plan reviews of charts conducted during the initial site visit and at subsequent site visits by plan staff

- *Quality improvement program requirement and commitment to CQI,* including clinic QI meetings, addressing specific quality problems, and performing clinic-specific quality projects as well as plan-determined quality projects. The number of quality projects expected is based on the size of the clinic

- *Clinic participation expectations standards that focus on access to care,* including developing examples of standards for waiting times for different types of appointments

- *Utilization management program requirements,* including preadmission notification, concurrent review, case management, referral management, and review of data and follow-up of any utilization management issues noted by the plan

- *Acceptance of and adherence to preventive service guidelines established by the plan,* whereby guidelines are implemented by the clinic as the minimum set of preventive services

- *Preterm birth program,* whereby the plan and clinic work together to systematically identify high-risk pregnant women and provide education about recognizing signs of preterm labor for these members

- *Adoption and use of the plan's referral network,* whereby the clinic uses network specialists for any necessary referral care, except when the medical needs of the member cannot be appropriately met through use of these network providers

The clinic must also be willing to accept new patients and have adequate capacity to provide primary care for additional members, as determined by a ratio of members to physicians. Blue Plus also evelutes the clinic's ability to provide a full range of primary care services or to have other arrangements in place (which do not inconvenience members) to meet these needs. The assessment should be also to determine if there is a need for this clinic based on the location and the health plan's current capability to provide adequate clinic sites for its membership.

PRECONTRACT SITE VSIT

The balancing of roles is a key discussion topic for the precontract site visit, and all clinic physicians are expected to participate in the dialogue. Blue Plus expects its primary care physicians to balance the roles of gate keeper and patient advocate. Any discomfort regarding this issue can negatively impact the patient-physician relationship. For instance, physicians who feel that the patient should be able to see a specialist and choose which specialist to see (thus bypassing the primary care physician as the manager of care) will be uncomfortable in the care management role Blue Plus expects.

Other clinic commitments, such as UM/QI programs, are discussed in detail to ensure that the prospective partner clinic is aware of its commitments and to allow the clinic to better evaluate its potential fit with the plan.

There are also discussions around clinic processes to support care delivery, including patient satisfaction, effective utilization control practices, and the delivery of high-quality medical care. Clinics demonstrate this by using data to focus quality improvement efforts on aspects of care that have been determined to be good opportunities for improvement. The clinic's quality improvement or utilization data can be gathered in a number of ways, such as patient satisfaction surveys, staff feedback, condition-specific studies, and plan feedback. Clinics that do not currently survey their patients should commit to using the plan's patient survey data to improve care. Once a clinic becomes a contracting PCC in the plan, it receives annual data on its own satisfaction rates as compared to the overall network. Clinics with lower satisfaction rates on a specific variable—such as time spent with patient by physician and staff or ease of access to care—should use that information to determine how best to modify and improve these areas.

Prospective clinics are likewise evaluated to determine whether they have effective utilization control practices in place, which may include a referral committee, an HMO or referral coordinator, a designated UM medical director, a defined referral network in place, and agreement by all physicians about this referral network. Other important elements of utilization control at the clinic level include feedback systems for referral care, systems determining the scope of the referrals and the appropriate point for transitioning care back from specialists to PCCs, and systems to monitor inpatient care and to manage chronic, catastrophic cases.

The cohesiveness of the medical group is also assessed at the precontract site visit. Evidence of cohesiveness would include whether the clinic's physicians feel it is important to discuss how their partners practice and whether structures (such as committees or other types of meetings) exist to facilitate discussions about practice patterns. The site visit team also explores the clinic's ability and willingness to use data. Physicians who indicate a reluctance to use comparative data or who may be reluctant to discuss practice variation within their own group are not likely to engage in evaluating and improving their performance based on plan data and suggestions.

Finally, the precontract site visit also allows the Blue Plus visitors to conduct a firsthand inspection of facilities and medical records. The facilities need to be clean and aesthetically pleasing to members. During a tour of the clinic, a sample of medical records is also reviewed to determine if documentation is appropriate.

Conclusion

While some clinic attributes such as cohesiveness or willingness to use data are not as definable for measurement or scoring purposes, they have been determined to be important attributes of successful clinics. This more structured, interactive system of evaluating clinics provides the foundation for a long-term relationship between Blue Plus and PCCs that are better matched to the plan's expectations and values.

The combination of careful clinic selection plus the clinic-based, CQI-focused approach to improving utilization and quality has proven to be an effective pair of strategies as Blue Plus moves toward its goal of creating an optimally managed health plan.

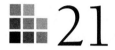

21

Developing and implementing care management programs

James O. Hillman
Executive Director
Unified Medical Group Association
Seal Beach, California

Alan Zwerner, MD, JD
Chief Executive Officer
The Medical Quality Commission
Seal Beach, California

IN ANY MEDICAL PRACTICE, a small percentage of patients can be expected to require a large percentage of the provider's total medical resources. In a fee-for-service (FFS) system, physicians earn a greater percentage of their compensation from services provided to those who are chronically or catastrophically ill or extremely frail and less from patients they see only once a year.

Under capitated systems, the same small percentage requiring more resources can tip the scales toward or away from financial success. Capitated providers who receive a fixed fee per member per month (PMPM), regardless of the amount of care provided, must learn quickly how to manage the care of high-risk, high-utilization patients with strategies that lead to fewer complications and acute episodes.

Successful capitated providers do not count on good luck or favorable risk factors but develop systems, strategies, policies, and controls that bring proven business methodologies, such as data analysis and productivity measurements, into the management of healthcare. They focus heavily on the four mandates of successful capitated healthcare delivery:

increased quality, improved clinical outcomes, decreased utilization, and decreased medical-legal risks.

A crucial step in capitation is to identify the subpopulations most likely to require frequent and costly care and to spend more time on these patients. Though individual unit costs are still important, the overriding goal is to reduce total spending over a long period of time. Too much concern about short-term goals or a monthly capitation will shift that focus and undermine long-term strategies for controlling costs.

Withholding or reducing needed care to save costs is never an answer. Reducing the need for care is. This requires innovative care management programs, geared to the needs of high-utilization patients or groups of patients and drawing on a variety of resources, offered by both the provider and within the community (e.g., patient education classes offered by the provider or nutrition programs offered by a community organization). Some HMOs and providers even arrange low-cost fees at local fitness clubs for their members.

To develop an effective program, the provider group must give its care management staff trust and authority to make educated decisions about providing nonmedical services. The goal must be more than managed costs; it must be managed care.

Case management categories

Case management is a broad term that has most often been used to define the process of managing care of specific hospitalized patients. Its purpose is threefold: to ensure a continuum of care for the patient, to prevent hospitalization of patients who do not require acute care, and to discharge those who no longer require acute care as quickly as possible. While "case management" is sometimes used to describe the management of care within the ambulatory environment, two newer terms—ambulatory care management and ambulatory disease management—are more widely accepted, offering greater definition in the complexities involved.

Ambulatory care management, or ambulatory case management, extends the earlier concept of case management, focusing on the care of specific patients most likely to become high users. Its focus is on an ever-changing subpopulation representing the frail elderly, the chronically or catastrophically ill, and people with multiple medical problems, such as heart and lung diseases or cancer complicated by chronic disease. Care managers, who are generally nurses with experience in case management, shepherd specific patients through the complex medical system, making sure that each patient's care plan is followed to help achieve an optimal outcome. Ambulatory care management extends the time between patient discharge and admission to an acute care facility, not just the time between admission and discharge. Research indicates that between 2 and 6 percent of the nonsenior population may require ambulatory care management at any given time.

Ambulatory disease management addresses the issue of how best to manage populations with specific diseases, considering the natural course of each disease process. It addresses populations suffering from such diseases as asthma, congestive heart failure, chronic lung disease, degenerative neurologic disorders, and AIDS. Disease management focusing on high-volume, high-cost disease categories attempts to implement systems that improve the quality of care and decrease cost. One example is the asthma clinic, established to help asthmatics and their families. Components might include patient and family education, prescription drug monitoring to increase compliance, nurse practitioners and physician assistants who specialize in the problems of the asthmatic, specific telephone "help lines" and literature, and physician education, both formal CME-credited education and informal education.

There is an overlap between ambulatory care and disease management. The former is patient specific, and the latter is disease specific. A particular patient with a common disease is likely to encounter both. Ambulatory disease management and ambulatory care management overlap only in tactics and in the patient groups they serve. Both concepts, however, share the same overall goals:

- Prevent acute exacerbation, prolong intervals between acute exacerbations, and decrease the severity of acute exacerbations

- Improve outcomes and patient satisfaction

- Decrease costs

- Decrease medical-legal risk

They also share the same strategies:

- Education (patient, physician, nurse, physician assistant, or nurse practitioner)

- Increase of patient compliance with physician instructions

- Assurance the care plan is carried out

- A multidisciplinary approach that includes psychosocial, community services, education, transportation, telephone communication, and family involvement

Throughout this chapter, the term care management is used to refer to both programs. Ambulatory disease management and ambulatory care management are used when differentiating one from the other.

Care management is essentially where quality management, utilization management, risk management, and outcomes management come together. Good care management introduces creative, nontraditional approaches to manage chronic and catastrophic health problems, bringing together medical and nonmedical services to meet the needs of specific patients. Its purpose is to simultaneously improve the quality of patient care and achieve greater cost effectiveness. A good care management program looks for ways—both conventional and unconventional—to invest in keeping high-utilization patients as healthy as possible.

Quality management, utilization management, risk management, and outcomes management, all important and separate disciplines, are also essential parts of care management. When these elements work in concert, they complement and support each other, creating value beyond that brought by any one of the disciplines.

Quality, utilization, risk, and outcomes management

QUALITY MANAGEMENT

Quality management (QM), as part of the care management process, should be broad and inclusive, with standards, the delivery process, outcomes, and all the elements of accepted QM programs being considered. A care manager, familiar with the patient's total health and life, may be able to take it one step further.

An example of this occurred at Summit Medical Group in Summit, New Jersey, when an elderly patient was about to be released from the hospital. The patient's care manager, who visited him prior to his scheduled release, knew he was very frail. She also knew that his wife was undergoing chemotherapy for cancer and would not be able to give him the care needed at home. She intervened, got the appropriate insurance authorization, and scheduled him for care at a subacute care facility instead. This decision almost certainly prevented a return to the hospital, which would have been more costly and would have caused extra stress for the patient and his family. This is the kind of uniquely appropriate care that can be provided when one person in the medical group understands every aspect of the patient's situation.

Care management also offers an opportunity to integrate creative, supportive services that enhance the physician's work and meet the individual patient's needs. While many such services will be clinical, others may not be. Some may come from within the medical group, others will be found elsewhere in the community. Most will be covered services, but there will be times when providing uncovered services is cost effective. If a patient is in danger of poor nutrition, it becomes appropriate to make arrangements with the local Meals-on-Wheels program. If a patient has difficulty walking, it may be prudent to provide a cane or walker to help prevent falls. Extended services such as these may not be within the boundaries of traditional medicine but are at the heart of prepaid, managed care. When done thoughtfully and with the patient's welfare in mind, they redefine quality and meet the needs of each patient in a unique and personalized way.

UTILIZATION MANAGEMENT

Utilization management (UM), another essential component of care management, is most often misunderstood by those outside managed care, but it is very advantageous to the patient. UM is not intended to withhold care but to provide patients with several second opinions, at no additional cost, offering them the increased confidence of a medical consensus.

UM seeks to prevent overutilization, underutilization, and misutilization. Its goal is to deliver the right amount of care, in the right way, at the right time. Good capitated healthcare encourages the provider to consider both the patient's medical needs and overall satisfaction. If medical needs are not met in a timely fashion, the cost of care increases. If patient satisfaction is not achieved, patients will move to other provider groups. If the outcome is poor, litigation may ensue.

Problems sometimes arise when the patient's needs and the patient's wants are not the same, but physicians cannot abrogate their responsibility to determine the appropriate course of treatment. Patients do not have appropriate medical training and knowledge, and not all physicians have the social-cultural skills to read the patient's needs. Often, neither patients nor physicians understand the alternative healthcare settings or community resources available. The type and amount of care are properly determined by the physician, in consultation with a fully informed patient, not by a third-party payer or a utilization decision maker who is not closely involved in the case.

Overutilization—unneeded and ineffective care—is a drain on medical resources and has the potential to expose patients to unnecessary risk. When marginally effective therapies, "placebo" treatments, and unnecessarily extended hospitalizations are employed, there is little good done for the patient. In capitated healthcare, overutilization also represents the quickest route to a budgetary crisis. Money spent on inappropriate care for one patient reduces the total remaining budget and causes a serious financial risk for the provider. It is an ineffective, wasteful use of healthcare resources.

Underutilization—the withholding of necessary, or indicated, medical care—is a risky route for any medical organization to take. It results in poor-quality patient care, can lead to increased long-term costs, and multiplies the possibility of malpractice lawsuits. Courts are quick to punish managed care organizations when they suspect that negligent or intentional underutilization may have led to patient injury. Increased exposure to liability risk is a gamble no medical provider should take. Ethical considerations aside, only the shortsighted provider will do less than medically necessary. However, cost considerations can, and should, be taken into account in the choice of treatment options.

Acute care costs more than preventive care, and complications cost more than early intervention. While acute care and complications cannot always be avoided, appropriate preventive and early intervention techniques can delay the need for more costly care and sometimes prevent it altogether.

Misutilization comes in two varieties: doing the "wrong" thing, and doing the "right" thing poorly. Misutilization of resources is misguided and wasteful. Insufficient screening that leads to incorrect referrals and writing a prescription when dietary changes might work just as well are misutilization of resources.

In capitated healthcare, control of underutilization, overutilization, and misutilization means doing the right thing, in the right way, at the right time.

RISK MANAGEMENT

Risk management has become mandatory for any provider group, and care management can be an important part of a risk management plan. The risk of litigation is greatest when one or more of these occurrences are present: the outcome is poor or the outcome is unexpected, the patient is angry, provider-patient communication is poor, or one physician casts doubt about the care of another and tells the patient. While a poor outcome cannot always be prevented, the occurrence of unexpected outcomes and angry patients can be minimized with frequent and accurate communication.

A major responsibility of any care management program is to make sure the patient's care plan is executed to ensure that everything that is supposed to happen does. Effective case managers monitor compliance, making sure appointments are kept, prescriptions are filled, and tests are completed. Appropriate oversight almost always results in improved compliance, and many times it also results in greater patient satisfaction. Patient noncompliance is a frequent cause of complications and poor outcomes. Often it can be legally argued that the provider is at fault even when the patient does not follow instructions.

The real and ever-present risk of litigation, both medical malpractice (i.e., tort) and contract (i.e., insurance bad faith or utilization decision making) requires that capitated provider organizations practice "medical-legal prophylaxis." This means complete and proper oral and written communication along with complete and accurate documentation.

The medical record serves both an evidentiary and a communication function. High utilizers of medical resources are high litigation risks, and poor outcomes are more common in high utilizers. Poor outcomes—especially unexpected poor outcomes—can lead to anger and potential litigation. Only a loose correlation exists between actual negligence causing injury and allegations that negligent care caused injury.

Effective communication between provider and the patient and family before, during, and after medical intervention helps ensure four things: expectations will be reasonable, misunderstandings and unexpected outcomes will not occur, anger will be prevented, and lawsuits will occur less frequently.

Healthcare providers can minimize medical-legal risk in a number of ways:

- Prevent poor outcomes, when possible, by doing the right thing at the right time, and by continuous communication among caregivers

- Sustain effective communication between the physician and the patient and family before the outcome is known (i.e., addressing unreasonable patient expectations in advance)

- Diffuse anger when it occurs by listening to patients and their families, by letting them "vent," and by educating and showing understanding of angry people without becoming defensive or combative

- Mitigate prospectively when anger occurs in order to dissuade patients from suing. Try to find out what the patient or family wants, preventing lawsuits even after a "potential compensable event" has taken place. Consider a settlement, which can be done without admitting negligence. Because angry people talk to their friends, employers, regulatory agencies, the media, and their attorneys, it is always in the provider's interest to decrease or mitigate that anger

- Document effectively to ensure quality evidence of events. The medical record is a reflection of the quality of care rendered in the eyes of a jury. If the medical record is inadequate or incomplete, jurors are more likely to conclude the medical care was also inadequate and incomplete. In addition to this evidentiary function, the medical record has an important communication function, serving as a link between multiple healthcare professionals

OUTCOMES MANAGEMENT

Clinical outcomes of medical intervention play a paramount role in measuring the success of caring for high-risk, high-utilization patients in capitated health plans. For physicians who provide healthcare to senior populations, the need is even more acute.

Outcomes research asks the question, "How are we doing?" It is an absolute prerequisite to the success of the capitated provider group. Providers must do it right the first time in order to be financially successful. Increasingly, they must also be able to demonstrate the quality of their services to payers with hard facts, accurate statistics, and measured outcomes. Practice variation (i.e., utilization of medical services) must be controlled, high-risk populations must be screened and aggressively managed, and clinical and cost outcomes must be monitored to control excess utilization. To the capitated provider, quality must be the first concern. Poor quality increases costs—poor service means fewer patients.

Quality should evolve from definitive, measurable standards that patients can use to evaluate the care they receive and physicians can use to evaluate the care they deliver. One challenge for physicians is to identify "best practices" to minimize unnecessary practice variation and define standards. Another is to demonstrate value, as perceived by both patients and payers, based on cost, quality, and patient satisfaction.

Measurement techniques are becoming more sophisticated and the ability to evaluate outcomes according to accepted standards will continue to increase. Outcomes research need not be expensive, sophisticated, or time consuming. Even without electronic medical records, many important aspects can be measured and must be measured if a capitated provider expects to compete successfully. Satisfaction, utilization, and patient wellness can be measured now. Clinical guidelines can be implemented and monitored for compliance now.

The future will offer even more opportunities to measure, assess, and evaluate what works best. Such data will be useful to negotiate more favorable contracts with managed care organizations and will help prevent medicine from becoming a commodity-based business. In the future, quality, demonstrated by outcomes measurement, will increasingly become the single most important point of differentiation among healthcare providers.

Care management examples

The following illustrates how physician groups associated with Unified Medical Group Association (UMGA), a national organization of prepaid medical groups, have implemented care management. UMGA, located in Seal Beach, California, and its member groups have documented the value care management has offered patients and providers. Many of UMGA's member groups have developed innovative programs to address the needs of high-risk, high-utilization patients. While the largest medical groups may have access to more resources, even small groups have formalized disease management programs that effectively reduce costs and improve overall quality.

While the acute care of episodic illness will always be a necessary and important part of medicine, in a capitated healthcare environment it is especially important to concentrate on reducing the need for acute care. Prevention and early intervention are the first lines of defense in the battle against acute, episodic disease, and injury. It is the responsibility of the care management team to develop strategies to make those lines of defense work. One focus is on high-risk, high-utilization patients whose care is aggressively managed to increase the time between acute exacerbations and to make sure inevitable exacerbations are less severe.

Another part of the first-line defense is an emphasis on education and wellness. While not all HMOs and providers have learned to implement such programs well, the most successful medical groups use patient education programs to their full advantage. For example, they teach expectant mothers how to take care of themselves to produce healthy babies and offer classes to manage arthritis and other chronic diseases. One health plan began an aggressive patient education program along with a change in basic treatment for pediatric asthma patients in an effort to reduce hospital stays.[1] They taught patients how to use inhalers, nebulizers, and peak-flow meters and educated them on the differences among bronchodilators, inhaled steroids, and oral corticosteroids. This intensive program helped decrease hospital days per 1,000 from 17 in 1988 to 5.4 in 1994, saving the HMO about $10 million over a six-year period.

Although many prepaid providers offer no-cost or low-cost programs in such areas as smoking cessation, stress reduction, and weight control, wellness, in the form of diet and lifestyle change, is more difficult. The cost effectiveness of these strategies has not been determined and many potential gains of such intervention are attenuated by the longtime delay in return on investment and the problem of patient turnover.

One UMGA medical group, Med Partners Mullikin-West of Long Beach, California, uses just such an integrated approach to care for its senior patients. Mullikin reaches out to every new Medicare enrollee with personal contact. A case manager contacts and welcomes each of these senior patients, asking about their health, their lifestyle, and any problems they might have. The case manager also tells them about medical group services and community resources that may be of value. This direct contact helps the group identify seniors who can benefit from a care management program, giving them an opportunity to identify potential health problems and to implement steps to prevent or delay those problems. Providers who monitor certain subpopulation groups also have the opportunity to document and evaluate the effectiveness of preventive and early intervention measures over a long period of time.

An integrated approach also helps to enhance communication between patients and providers. Patients do not always tell their physicians about the real problems that exist in their lives, not recognizing how one aspect of their lives affects another. For example, low-income patients may not tell their physicians they can only afford one meal a day and elderly patients may not discuss their loneliness, stress, or depression. In one case, when a Mullikin case manager was talking with a new Medicare enrollee, the patient said she seemed to be falling often. A home visit and conversation revealed that the woman had broken her glasses and had no way to get new ones. The medical group took her for an examination and bought her new glasses, though neither home visits nor glasses were covered services. In this case, the group invested in uncovered services to avoid the use of covered but more costly services at a later date. The cost of new glasses is small compared to the cost of mending a broken hip from a trip or fall. A good care management program is the only way this kind of creative and beneficial solution be found.

Gaining physician acceptance

Establishing a good care management program is a process that requires a strong commitment, thorough planning, and the willingness to make changes. The most critical factor is the commitment of the organization's physicians and management.

Many physicians and other healthcare professionals are reluctant to endorse any kind of case management program, believing they will be relinquishing control over their patients' care. These physicians will accept care management only when they understand that it will not reduce their control.

Some examples of physician concerns include

- Loss of control of the patients' care

- Care managers, not physicians, making medical decisions

- Quality and cost controls

- Recordkeeping capability

- The effect a new department will have on the profitability of the group and individual physician compensation

- How incentive changes will affect physician compensation

Care management enhances the caregiving capabilities of physicians and increases their knowledge of the patient's total lifestyle and health potential. When physicians understand this and "buy into" the program, they are far more likely to cooperate with and use the services of care managers, and the program has a better chance of succeeding.

Provider groups just entering managed care, or those unfamiliar with the role of care management, may need to use a wide range of resources to gain physician support. Physician education is the single most critical factor. If the physicians do not realize the value of care managers, they will not use the program. To address that issue, provider groups will need to bring in statistics, case studies, and outside consultants who can answer their questions and concerns.

To educate physicians, many groups seek out providers already using care management to discuss its advantages and disadvantages. Others take key physicians on site visits to witness care management. UMGA, for example, has demonstrated to many organizations how such a program will help their physicians deliver better care.

Regardless of the basic compensation, a well-structured financial incentive program is an important part of the presentation. It should provide financial rewards to physicians for using the services of care managers effectively. Whatever methods are employed, however, the information must presented with a clear understanding of the physician's point of view. When physicians see the benefits, they are much more likely to embark on a new approach to healthcare. Once in place and supported by the physicians, any investment in case management will be realized many times over in terms of patient satisfaction, quality of care, and cost savings.

Care management staff and systems

DEVELOPING STAFF

An effective, multidisciplinary care management staff is essential to success. To work with providers, patients, families, and other associates, care managers must be good communicators. They need to be effective listeners and should possess exceptional organizational skills to coordinate services from a wide variety of sources. Resourcefulness and creativity will help them find unusual, yet effective, ways to meet a patient's needs. Problem-solving skills are essential for helping patients and their families make critical decisions about care options. All these qualities will prove valuable when case managers are called on to "shepherd" frail, elderly, or catastrophically ill patients through a complex medical system. The lack of any of these skills will reduce the impact of the program.

Typically, care managers implement a patient support system to supplement, and even interrupt, the traditional ambulatory to acute hospital care pattern. Their challenge is to find ways to improve the patient's quality of life and manage finite healthcare resources.

MANAGEMENT INFORMATION SYSTEMS

A good electronic medical records (EMR) system is critical to a case manager's time. It can assess past experience, track events today, and spot problems in advance. It can provide timely information not available in any other way.

The use of EMR is growing and can be expected to leap forward in the next few years. One study showed that in 1993, 17 percent of medical groups had EMR and 75 percent had automated appointment scheduling. Of those without EMR, 43 percent planned to automate during the next two years. Of those without automated scheduling, 58 percent intended to automate in the next two years.[2]

At a minimum, any management information system (MIS) employed as part of a care management program should be able to monitor and analyze experience, utilization patterns, covered and noncovered services, and costs. It should be able to gather information on individual patients and sort it by specific populations or groups of patients. Adaptability to future needs and technology advances is also essential. An effective system can track patient compliance information and will monitor whether appointments are kept, prescriptions are filled, and screenings and checkups are scheduled as instructed. It will contain an electronic library of resources and community services. If kept up-to-date and used effectively, this data will contribute to improved quality, better utilization management, and long-term cost savings. It can present a clear picture of where case management is most valuable and provide insight for future planning.

The most sophisticated MIS is of little value unless it is used to its full capabilities. It is of little benefit to invest in an expensive system and not in the staff training required to use it.

Information is power—when it is accessible, timely, and understandable. A reputable consultant specializing in medical informatics can help providers select the best system for their practice and provide training to make it work to their advantage.

Identifying care management candidates

The selection and assignment of patients for care management can mean the difference between success and failure of a capitated program. If the wrong cases are assigned, the system will be costly and inefficient, and if too many cases are assigned to a single case manager, quality will suffer.

Care management programs should be structured for the most care-intensive and cost-intensive diseases occurring in a medical group's panel of patients. Clearly specifed care pathways, accompanied by patient education and compliance measures, offer the opportunity to reduce exacerbations and prevent recurrent hospitalizations among carefully identified subpopulations. Patients with asthma, congestive heart failure, chronic lung disease, advanced diabetes, and AIDS are among those who benefit most from ambulatory disease management.

Candidates for ambulatory care management may be selected from among many groups of patients, including the chronically and catastrophically ill. Though nearly all senior Medicare patients are appropriate for care management screening, many are healthy and require little medical attention. It is more effective to identify subpopulations from within the over-65 group: those who are frail, those with chronic or terminal illnesses, and those in the oldest age range (i.e., over 85).

Studies estimate that those subpopulations, representing about 6 percent of Medicare patients, account for 60 percent of all Medicare expenditures.[3]

Any three of the following criteria would qualify a patient for care management:[4]

- Multiple active chronic diagnoses (e.g., four or more)

- Multiple medications prescribed on a chronic basis (e.g., four or more)

- Multiple hospitalizations in past 12 months (including skilled nursing facilities in lieu of acute hospitalization), particularly if the rehospitalization is related to the same illness (e.g., two or more)

- 75 years of age or older

- Multiple emergency room visits in past 12 months, particularly if related to the same illness (e.g., two or more)

- Significant impairment in one or more major activities of daily living (e.g., bathing, toileting, dressing, feeding, or ambulating)

- Significant impairment in any of the instrumental activities of daily living (e.g., preparing meals, shopping, transportation, using the telephone, basic housekeeping, and managing finances), particularly when there are no relatives or other support system in the home

One of UMGA's southern California members, Bristol Park Medical Group, relies on its utilization management nurses to identify which patients to assign to a case manager. These registered nurses have the knowledge, managed care experience, and interpersonal skills needed to deal with patients and physicians. Bristol Park typically assigns case managers to senior patients, all inpatient hospitalizations, patients in skilled nursing facilities or requiring durable medical equipment, and those requiring such outpatient therapies as home nursing visits and IV antibiotics. Other groups make similar choices depending on the demographics of their patient base. For example, if a group has an exceptionally large senior population, it may narrow its choices to the frailest seniors or to those over a certain age. If a group has more young families, it may focus its case management heavily on first-time pregnancies.

Program for the terminally ill

The needs for care management differ among provider groups, depending on their size, demographics, and medical specialties. At HealthCare Partners Medical Group in Los Angeles, a study of hospitalized patients revealed that a number of patients were hospitalized repeatedly without corresponding improvements in their medical condition.[5] The group began to search for ways to prevent acute episodes that were leading to hospitalizations and to improve the overall quality of health of the patients involved. The study led to establishing a well-integrated program for terminally ill patients with a very poor quality of life. The group found that many of these patients preferred to remain at home, yet their families often did not know how to care for them. The patients felt they had little control over their care at a time when they needed the most control.

As a result of the study, HealthCare Partners developed a program called Options to give these patients more control. The program provides comprehensive and supportive care and gives patients choices for how their care is rendered during the final stage of life. For its Options program, HealthCare Partners has organized a wide range of resources into a single comprehensive program. It has assembled a dedicated care management team that includes the Options program medical director, the attending physician, the patient and family, and various medical group staff members. Social workers and therapists are included, along with representatives from the clergy and home healthcare organizations. Families are involved so that everything possible is provided to meet a particular patient's needs.

The Options process begins with a referral by the patient's primary care physician or a requested referral from a nonprimary care physician or other ancillary provider who feels the patient can benefit from enrollment in the program. Once a patient is referred to Options, the group's social services department evaluates the patient to see if the patient would be well served by the program. This evaluation takes into account a variety of factors, including home and social environment, access to caregivers, and mental health status.

In evaluating the program, HealthCare Partners found the longer the patient was in the Options program, the lower the risk of hospitalization. In the program's first year, 79 patients were enrolled and only 25 percent needed hospitalization. Of those, most had been enrolled in the program for less than a month. In the second year, only 10 percent required hospitalization. The program has won the support of physicians and the praise of patients and their families and is a tribute to the value of a well-planned ambulatory care management program.

Many times, care management programs such as HealthCare Partners' Options will provide noncovered services, requiring additional expenses to the group. However, the reduction in hospitalization costs tends to reduce all-around, long-term expenditures.

The basic tenet of care management is to look at the big picture: the patient's total health and the long-term management of capitated payments. A small outlay of funds at a crucial time can bring a substantial long-term return.

Benefits for patients and providers

Patients respond very positively to ambulatory disease and care management. They appreciate extra attention when they are in pain, discomfort, or distress and feel comfortable about having a team of specialists to talk to who understand their case and the medical system. Many patients and their families say they feel more secure about their healthcare than ever before.

When a provider group establishes a care management program, it sets up expectations to be met. Patients and families will lose confidence in any group when promises are not kept or personal concerns are not addressed. The care manager becomes the key contact for patients in the program, the person those patients can talk to when their physician is not available, and someone who understands the healthcare system. Patients, particularly those who are frail or catastrophically ill, see their care manager as a friend. That represents a great responsibility, but it also provides great rewards.

Care managers also serve as patient advocates, taking on an ombudsperson role. It is their responsibility to see that everything is done right—coordinating services provided by others, making certain all loopholes are closed, and keeping a close watch on quality. They monitor compliance and make sure their patients take prescriptions correctly and follow dietary and other clinical instructions. Ideally, they work in partnership with their patients' physicians, adding value while freeing physicians for the practice of medicine. All of this benefits the patient.

Under capitated systems, a good care management program is not an expense but an investment. Providers who succeed in the prepaid sector manage their patients' total health, and they look at expenditures in terms of long-term budgeting. The provider who does not understand these basic premises will not be able to adapt to the realities of capitation. If relatively small preventive expenditures this year prevent costly treatments next year, the provider gains. If the provision of a simple, noncovered service decreases the possibility of hospitalization, both the patient and the provider benefit. If taking the time to carefully monitor the progress of the frail elderly helps keep most of that subpopulation healthier, everyone wins. It is a question of value or values. Well-spent dollars and integrated services add up to healthier patients and a better bottom line.

An FHP patient in California, suffering from insulin-dependent diabetes mellitus, endstage cardiomyopathy, and congestive heart failure, had frequent emergency room visits followed by five- to seven-day hospitalizations before being assigned to a care manager. The care manager began contacting her frequently at home to identify potential health problems, educated the patient on the importance of dietary compliance and prompt medical attention, and initiated home-administered diuretics. The result was a 97 percent decrease in hospital utilization, saving FHP an estimated 8 to 14 acute hospital days or $14,000 per month.[6]

Conclusion

Ambulatory disease and ambulatory care management are two programs that merit a place in any medical group's capitation budget. Costs can often be controlled by appropriately shifting care from acute hospitals to skilled nursing facilities or other outpatient settings. Shifting of care is good for the patient; almost any patient is better off outside the hospital if effective and appropriate outpatient care is provided. To reduce costly hospital days is also good for the provider and payer.

Besides costs, care management can increase the level of the quality of care provided. Because cases are considered on an individual basis, patients receive more personal attention and have access to services to meet their particular needs. This same concept gives providers greater flexibility to encourage and reward creative solutions and to pay for non-covered benefits when it makes financial sense in the long run. These extras benefit the provider as well as the patient.

Establishing ambulatory disease management and ambulatory care programs takes an extensive investment of time, talent, and money. It is not an easy task or a quick solution to a provider's financial problems. Disagreements, turf wars, and power struggles can arise, while some degree of physician resistance can be expected. Nevertheless, any provider organization will be better off if the effort is made and an effective care management program is implemented. When the financial incentives are right and an organizationwide commitment is made, the rewards are well worth the effort. A well-planned care and disease management program can lead to improved quality, greater efficiencies, and lower costs. The unexpected benefits may be even more satisfying: improved patient satisfaction and a more rewarding provider-patient relationship.

NOTES

1. P. Wynn, "Patient Education Is Critical For Managing Asthma," *Managed Care: A Guide for Physicians* (May 1995).

2. Marion Merrell Dow, *Marion Merrell Dow Managed Care Digest, Medical Group Practice Edition* (Kansas City, Mo.: Marion Merrell Dow, 1994).

3. J. Beck, ed., *General Principles of Aging: The Demography of Aging, A Core Curriculum in Geriatic Medicine* (New York: American Geriatrics Society, 1991).

4. H. Kirby and C. Beharie, "The Challenge of Managing High-Risk, High-Cost, High-Volume Patients," *The FHP Journal of Clinical Research III* (Fall 1992).

5. United Medical Group Association, *Successful Senior Care: Enhancing Your Medicare HMO Program* (Seal Beach, Calif.: Unified Medical Group Association, 1993).

6. S. Aliotta and A. Zwerner, "FHP Patient Care Management Department Guides Care for the 'Frail Elderly' and Chronically Ill," *The FHP Journal of Clinical Research* (Winter 1994).

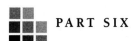

PART SIX

CONTRACT NEGOTIATION PRINCIPLES

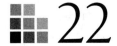

22

Using actuarial cost models to evaluate contracts

Timothy J. Feeser, FSA, MAAA
Consultant
Towers Perrin Integrated HealthSystems Consulting
Minneapolis, Minnesota

A S MANAGED CARE PAYERS CONTINUE to shift increasing amounts of risk to healthcare providers, it becomes increasingly important for those providers to develop a sound contracting strategy. The use of an actuarial cost model as a tool to assist in evaluating managed care contracts is useful to assess their feasibility, as well as providing insight into managing underlying risks.

The key components of the actuarial cost model are the utilization and pricing assumptions. Development of assumptions by detailed service expense categories can be a tool to evaluate managed care contracts. Separate cost models for varying populations also can be developed to evaluate contracts for commercial, Medicare, and Medicaid business.

This chapter discusses issues surrounding the development of model utilization and pricing assumptions, using exhibits to illustrate the formats of a prospective cost model for a commercial population. A demonstration of how the model can be used to evaluate a potential global capitation contract is also provided.

Utilization assumptions

There are several issues to consider when setting utilization assumptions for the actuarial cost model.

First, the intended population to be contracted with has a significant bearing on expected utilization levels. For example, a commercial population will experience different utilization rates than a Medicare population. Hospital days per 1,000 members per year (PMPY) for a commercial population may be in the 250 range, while Medicare days PMPY may be in the 1,200 to 1,600 range. Likewise, commercial physician office visits PMPY may be in the 3,300 range, while the number for the Medicare population may be more in the 6,500 range. Utilization levels for the Medicaid population will also be different from that expected of a commercial population. Hospital days PMPY for the Medicaid population may be in the 600 to 800 range, with physician office visits in the 4,000 range.

Utilization also can be expected to vary by geographical area, due to different demographic characteristics of the population. Varying physician practice patterns across the country also have an effect on utilization. In addition, utilization may vary by an urban versus suburban demographic mix (e.g., an urban population may be older than a suburban population).

An HMO's benefit mix can have an effect on utilization. For example, a high-option HMO plan with low member copayments may be expected to have higher utilization than a low-option HMO where members pay higher copayments. Going from a $0 office visit copayment plan to a $10 office visit copayment plan may reduce utilization by 5 to 10 percent.

Another consideration affecting utilization is the relative reimbursement mechanism used to pay physicians. Expected utilization may be higher under fee-for-service (FFS) reimbursement than under capitation. If providers are capitated, they may have a greater interest in controlling utilization. Therefore, for physician hospital organizations (PHOs) reimbursing providers on a capitated basis, the model could reflect inherently lower utilization assumptions than might be expected under FFS.

Managed care penetration also may have a bearing on expected utilization levels. In a very mature managed care marketplace such as California, a start-up PHO would be expected to deliver services at a utilization level in line with market expectations. Alternatively, in a state such as Arkansas with very low levels of managed care penetration, utilization levels may look more like fee-for-service utilization. To the extent the PHO feels comfortable that the affiliated providers will be successful in managing utilization, the assumptions may be adjusted to incorporate these phenomena. This type of adjustment is highly subjective and should be made by those experienced within the managed care industry.

Data sources

To build an actuarial cost model, it is important to gather necessary information to determine appropriate utilization assumptions. The following summarizes the sources available to PHOs considering developing a cost model.

Publications are an excellent source to determine aggregate utilization measures, such as hospital days per 1,000 and total physician encounters per 1,000. *The Managed Care Digest,* published by Marion Merrel Dow, a manufacturer and marketer of prescription and over-the-counter pharmaceuticals in North America, Europe, and the Pacific Basin, provides per member per month (PMPM) and physician encounter rates for both the commercial and Medicare populations by state. *The HMO Industry Profile,* published by the Group Health Association of America, Washington, DC, provides similar measures of utilization, categorized by major region of the country. *The Guide to the Managed Care Industry,* published by HCIA, a company established in 1985 to provide the healthcare industry with a centralized source of reliable and timely information, provides hospital utilization PMPY, as well as PMPM revenue measures for every HMO in a given state.

Rate filings with the state insurance departments can be useful to provide detailed utilization assumptions for a particular plan. However, the level of detail provided in a rate filing may depend on a state's prescribed rate filing format. For example, states such as New York and Ohio have very stringent requirements regarding the level of detail required to be shown to support premium rates, whereas other states are more lenient about what is required.

At the very least, knowing the actual medical expense PMPM for health plans in a marketplace can be very useful to determine the relative target that a PHO needs to achieve to be competitive in the marketplace.

Existing data specific to providers affiliated with the PHO can also be of use in determining utilization assumptions. While this information may not be the direct source, it can be a helpful secondary source to fine-tune any of the assumptions. In addition to provider-specific data, use of databases contained by some of the actuarial consulting firms may also be of assistance.

In all, there is no perfect data source. It is very important to understand the limitations of the data and how to incorporate subjective adjustments when warranted. Calling upon actuaries for assistance to provide these subjective adjustments can be helpful.

Pricing assumptions

In addition to utilization, the other critical model component is the pricing assumption. A pricing assumption is normally expressed as an average cost per unit of service. For example, for hospital services, the average cost per unit is expressed as an average cost per day or per admisssion. For physician office visits, the pricing assumption reflects an average cost per office visit. The average costs for a grouping of services represent weighted averages based on procedure code.

On the hospital side, it is common for contracts to be negotiated on a per diem or diagnostic-related group (DRG) basis. For the purpose of this discussion, it is assumed that the contracts are on a per diem basis and pricing assumptions for inpatient hospital services are expressed as an average cost per day. For outpatient hospital services, the average cost per unit will be expressed consistent with the service category shown in the model. For example, for same-day surgery facility services, the average cost per unit reflects the average cost for use of the same-day surgery facility. For physician services, the average costs per unit are expressed as weighted averages for current procedural terminology (CPT) code groupings into identifiable expense categories. The individual fees would be based on a negotiated fee schedule.

For physician services, it is becoming very common for PHOs to reimburse physicians on a unit-based fee schedule, such as the Medicare Resource-Based Relative Value Scale (RBRVS) or the McGraw-Hill Relative Value Units (RVUs). Each of these systems creates great flexibility for PHO management to administrate physician reimbursement.

However, there are also several issues to be considered in deciding whether to use Medicare RBRVS or the McGraw-Hill system. The Medicare RBRVS system is widely recognized by physicians but was developed specifically for Medicare. In developing the RBRVS system, Medicare reevaluated the relative value of cognitive- and procedure-based services. Therefore, it is often difficult to convince specialists performing procedure-based services to accept commercial reimbursement under a RBRVS fee schedule. An inconvenience of the Medicare RBRVS system is that approximately 25 percent of procedures require substitute unit values. Medicare excludes coverage for certain services and did not develop unit values for these services. To replace the missing unit values, it is common to use the McGraw-Hill scale as the means to develop substitute values for the RBRVS scale.

The RBRVS relative value units consist of three components weighted by geographic practice cost indices. The three components of the total RVU are the work RVU, the practice expense RVU, and the malpractice insurance expense RVU. These RVU components are weighted by the geographic practice cost indices to determine a total area-specific RVU. RVUs are determined for all procedures by CPT code. The actual fees themselves are created by multiplying the area-specific RVUs by a weighted dollar conversion factor.

The McGraw-Hill unit value system is also widely recognized by physicians. However, it was developed with no specific bias regarding primary care or specialist services. RVUs are developed for all procedures: therefore, there is no need for any replacement unit values to be developed. RVUs in the McGraw-Hill system are not adjusted to be area specific. There are five considerations inherent in each unit value, which consist of the time involved in performing the procedure, the skill required in performing the procedure, the severity of illness, the risk to the patient in performing the procedure, and the risk to the physician in performing the procedure. As with the RBRVS system, actual fees are determined by multiplying the unit values for each CPT code by a weighted dollar conversion factor.

Developing the model

Once the data has been collected and decisions have been made regarding intended reimbursement schemes (e.g., inpatient per diems, same-day surgery case rates, and physician RBRVS), an actuarial cost model can be developed. Ideally, the cost model should coincide with the risk-sharing mechanism of the PHO. The model reflects cost pools for hospital facility, PCP, referral physician, and pharmacy services. Ultimately, the cost pools underlying a model will be specific for a given PHO. An illustration of the hospital budget pool is shown in Table 1.

For hospital services, expense categories are shown that make up the majority of costs. However, to develop an actual cost model, costs can be broken down into further detail for hospital outpatient services. For

TABLE 1
Hospital budget—commercial

Inpatient services	Admissions	ALOS	Days	Per diem	PMPM
Medical/surgical	0.045	4.50	0.203	$1,000.00	$16.92
ICU/CCU	0.009	4.20	0.038	$1,500.00	$4.75
Maternity	0.022	2.10	0.046	$1,250.00	$4.79
Boarder baby	0.002	2.30	0.005	$250.00	$0.10
Mental health	0.002	10.50	0.021	$550.00	$0.96
Substance abuse	0.002	9.50	0.019	$400.00	$0.63
Out of area					$1.41
Total inpatient	*0.082*	*4.05*	*0.332*		*$29.56*

Outpatient services	Utilization	Average cost	PMPM
Same-day surgery	0.0600	$1,200.00	$6.00
Emergency room	0.1300	$200.00	$2.17
Home health	0.0300	$125.00	$0.31
Skilled nursing	0.0050	$300.00	$0.13
Other services	0.4000	$200.00	$6.67
Out of area	0.0100	$250.00	$0.21
Total outpatient			$15.49
Total hospital facility			$45.05
Provision for stop-loss			$2.25
Total hospital budget			*$47.30*

Assumptions:
- Utilization assumptions have been divided by 1,000.
- Inpatient services based on negotiated per diems.
- PMPM cost is derived by multiplying the utilization rate by pricing assumptions and dividing by 12.
- Pricing expressed in average cost per visit.

example, the "other services" category shown in the hospital outpatient section could be broken down into expense categories such as laboratory, x-ray, pharmacy services, rehabilitation, durable medical equipment, blood products, dialysis, and cardiac services. A miscellaneous category may still be shown to include all other low-volume services.

A PCP cost buildup is shown in Table 2. The expense categories illustrated correspond to the PCP services definition in Table 3. The frequency assumptions represent actual visits PMPY. The average cost assumptions are based on weighted average fees by CPT codes sorted into the illustrated service categories.

The specialist physician and pharmacy costs are illustrated in Table 4. The cost buildup for specialist physicians reflects the aggregate cost of all

TABLE 2
Primary care physician budget—commercial

Primary care physician services	Frequency	Average cost	PMPM
Office visits	2.400	$45.00	$9.00
Preventive care	0.225	$75.00	$1.41
Inpatient visits	0.045	$90.00	$0.34
Consultations	0.010	$100.00	$0.08
Vision/hearing screening	0.065	$55.00	$0.30
EKGs and pulmonary services	0.025	$40.00	$0.08
Immunizations and injections	0.400	$20.00	$0.67
Allergy shots	0.180	$15.00	$0.23
Emergency visits	0.010	$100.00	$0.08
Minor office surgery	0.075	$90.00	$0.56
Venipuncture	0.080	$5.00	$0.03
Laboratory services	0.840	$10.00	$0.70
Administrative services			$0.25
Total PCP services			*$13.73*

Assumptions:
- Frequency assumptions represent visits PMPY.
- The average cost assumptions are based on weighted average fees by CPT codes sorted into the illustrated service categories.

TABLE 3
Primary care physician budget—commercial

Service category	CPT codes
Office visits	99201–99215
Hospital visits	99218–99238, 99251–99255
Office consultations	99241–99245, 99256–99275
Emergency services	99281–99285
Skilled nursing visits, home visits	99301–99353
Case management services	99361–99373
Immunizations and injections	90701–90799
EKG services	93000–93010
Hearing screening	92551
Vision screening	92002
Pulmonary services	94101–94160
Allergy shots	95120–95155
Miscellaneous medical services	99000–99080
Preventive medicine	99381–99429
Newborn care	99431–99440
Simple surgery (abscess drainage)	10060, 10120, 10140, 10160
Simple surgery (benign lesions)	11050, 11400–11402
Simple surgery (repair lacerations)	12001–12013
Burn care	16000–16020
Destruction of lesions	17000–17002, 17110, 17200, 17340

TABLE 3 (CONTINUED)

Service category (cont.)	CPT codes
Musculoskeletal system	20600, 20605, 20610
Cauterization of nasal passages	30801–30901
Routine venipuncture	36400, 36410, 36415
Removal of foreign bodies	65205, 65220, 69200, 69210
Urinalysis	81000–81003, 81005
Chemistry	82270
Glucose	82948
Blood tests	85014, 85018
Immunology	86580, 86585
Microbiology	87060, 87070

TABLE 4
Specialist physician budget—commercial

Specialist physician services	Average frequency	Cost	PMPM
Office visits	1.000	$45.00	$3.75
Inpatient visits	0.270	$90.00	$2.03
Consultations	0.100	$100.00	$0.83
Eye exams	0.020	$55.00	$0.09
Hearing exams	0.020	$35.00	$0.06
Skilled nursing and home health care visits	0.005	$60.00	$0.03
Cardiac services	0.095	$60.00	$0.48
Psychiatric services	0.200	$80.00	$1.33
Physical therapy	0.300	$25.00	$0.63
Immunizations and injections	0.050	$10.00	$0.04
Allergy treatments	0.120	$15.00	$0.15
Emergency visits	0.080	$100.00	$0.67
Anesthesia	0.080	$400.00	$2.67
Surgery	0.370	$375.00	$11.56
Venipuncture	0.020	$5.00	$0.01
Normal delivery	0.014	$1400.00	$1.63
Cesarean section	0.006	$1600.00	$0.80
Laboratory services	2.000	$20.00	$3.33
Radiology (total)	0.740	$90.00	$5.55
Miscellaneous services	0.200	$45.00	$0.75
Total specialist physician services			$36.39
Pharmacy	5.200	$30.00	$13.00

Assumptions:
- Frequency assumptions represent visits PMPY.
- The average cost assumptions are based on weighted average fees by CPT codes sorted into the illustrated service categories.

specialist physician services. Note that the radiology services component includes the professional and technical component. Depending on the availability of data, cost buildups by subspecialist physicians could be developed. Cost detail by subspecialty physician provides the necessary information to determine subspecialty capitation budgets.

Table 5 provides a summary of the cost pools. In addition to medical expenses, PHO administrative expenses need to be considered. After payers deduct their administration from the premium dollar, there is not much left for PHO administration. PHOs are currently allocating anywhere from 1 to 2 percent for PHO administration.

Developing a set of average age/sex factors to correspond with the underlying cost model may be beneficial in evaluating prospective contracts. Table 6 provides a set of average age/sex factors intended to approximate the underlying target population of the cost model. The age/sex factors will be useful to determine whether a prospective payer has, on average, a younger or older membership mix.

TABLE 5
Total medical budget—commercial

Expense category	PMPM
Hospital services—medical	$45.05
Hospital services—stop-loss	$2.25
PCP services	$13.73
Specialist physician services	$36.39
Pharmacy	$13.00
PHO administration	$1.25
Total medical budget	*$111.67*

TABLE 6
Normalized age/sex factors

Age category	Sex category	Enrollee mix	Age/sex factors
<20	M and F	36.0%	0.650
20–29	M	8.0%	0.585
20–29	F	10.0%	1.475
30–39	M	9.5%	0.635
30–39	F	11.5%	1.385
40–49	M	6.5%	0.860
40–49	F	7.0%	1.255
50–59	M	4.0%	1.490
50–59	F	4.5%	1.725
60 +	M and F	3.0%	2.355
Composite		*100.0%*	*1.000*

Evaluating prospective capitation contracts

Once a cost model has been developed, it can be a useful tool to evaluate prospective global capitation contracts. This section illustrates how this tool can be used to evaluate a prospective capitation contract from a managed care payer. The following example, as illustrated in Tables 7 through 14, has been simplified; however, the example should illustrate how the model can best be applied.

A summary is provided regarding the preliminary targeted cost for the PHO and a proposed global capitation payment from a managed care payer is illustrated in Table 7.

One of the first things to obtain from managed care payers is their pricing assumptions. In many cases, the managed care payer will not be willing to share this information. However, obtaining rate filings from the state insurance department can provide some insight into the relative underlying costs of the medical expense capitation rate. While getting the actual pricing assumptions may be difficult, the PHO should be able to obtain the payer's benefit design mix as well as the age/sex mix of the membership to be capitated.

The average copayment savings expected from the membership to be capitated can be determined using the benefit mix distribution provided by the managed care payer. Table 8 illustrates how PHO management would evaluate the average copayment to be plugged into the actuarial cost model.

TABLE 7
Total medical budget—commercial

Expense category	PMPM
Hospital services—medical	$45.05
Hospital services—stop-loss	$2.25
PCP services	$13.73
Specialist physician services	$36.39
Pharmacy	$13.00
PHO administration	$1.25
Total medical budget	*$111.67*
Payer's proposed capitation	$107.50

A similar type of analysis can be done for the age/sex demographic mix of the proposed membership to be capitated. Table 9 provides a comparison of the specific payer's enrollment mix applied to the PHO's average age/sex factors.

TABLE 8
Analysis of payer's benefit mix

Coverage category	Benefit plan design			
	High option	*Standard option*	*Low option*	*Average option*
Office visits	$5.00	$10.00	$15.00	$7.25
Consultations	$5.00	$10.00	$15.00	$7.25
Physical therapy	$5.00	$7.00	$10.00	$6.05
Outpatient psychiatric	$10.00	$15.00	$20.00	$12.25
Inpatient psychiatric	20%	20%	20%	20%
Emergency room facility	$25.00	$35.00	$50.00	$30.25
Same-day surgery facility	$0.00	$50.00	$100.00	$22.50
Pharmacy	$5.00	$7.00	$10.00	$6.05
Payer's enrollee distribution	70%	15%	15%	

Note: The weighted average copayments that reflect the average option are derived from the payer's enrollee distribution. For example: $7.25 office visit copay = ($5) (.7) + ($10) (.15) + ($15) (.15).

TABLE 9
Normalized age/sex factors

Age category	Sex category	Enrollee mix	PHO age/sex factors	Payer's enrollee mix	PHO age/sex factors
<20	M and F	36.0%	0.650	38.0%	0.650
20–29	M	8.0%	0.585	9.5%	0.585
20–29	F	10.0%	1.475	10.5%	1.475
30–39	M	9.5%	0.635	10.0%	0.635
30–39	F	11.5%	1.385	10.5%	1.385
40–49	M	6.5%	0.860	5.5%	0.860
40–49	F	7.0%	1.255	6.0%	1.255
50–59	M	4.0%	1.490	3.5%	1.490
50–59	F	4.5%	1.725	4.0%	1.725
60 +	M and F	3.0%	2.355	2.5%	2.355
Composite		*100.0%*	*1.000*	*100.0%*	*0.969*

Note: The PHO's expected average enrollment mix underlying the cost model weights to an average cost factor of 1.000. The weighted average age/sex factor for the specific payer enrollment mix equals .969.

Based on this analysis, the specific payer's enrollment mix is a younger membership mix versus the expected average. Therefore, this membership could be expected to be a lower-cost group. Such information can be used by PHO management in making subjective adjustments to utilization assumptions to account for a potentially healthier patient mix, on average.

In addition to analyzing the benefit mix and demographic mix of the prospective payer, reevaluation of the pricing assumptions may also be warranted. Greater volume of membership being brought to the PHO may warrant steeper discounts by the PHO. For example, Table 10 illustrates the volume versus price discount argument for providers.

For PCPs, granting steeper discounts in exchange for volume is only beneficial if the PCPs are not operating at full capacity. Once an ultimate productivity level is reached, increasing membership and decreasing price results in decreasing income per physician. Additionally, increases in membership would result in increased capacity needs for a network that is already running at full productivity. For hospitals with

TABLE 10
Analysis of volume versus price dynamics

Primary care physicians

Annual membership	5,000	10,000	20,000
PCP office frequency PMPY	2.5	2.5	2.5
Projected annual PCP office visits	12,500	25,000	50,000
Average office visit fee	$45.00	$43.00	$42.00
Projected office visit revenue	$562,500	$1,075,000	$2,100,000
Targeted productivity per PCP	3,500	4,500	4,500
Number of network PCPs	5.00	5.50	11.10
Office revenue per PCP	$112,500	$195,455	$189,189

Inpatient hospital services

Annual membership	5,000	10,000	20,000
Hospital frequency PMPY	0.220	0.220	0.220
Projected annual days	1,100	2,200	4,400
Average per diem	$1,000.00	$950.00	$900.00
Projected revenue	$1,100,000	$2,090,000	$3,960,000

Note: The effect on revenue per physician is analyzed as membership increases and price decreases. Key assumptions are a beginning network staffing of five PCPs and an ultimate productivity level of 4,500 visits per physician per year.

excess capacity, granting steeper discounts in exchange for greater membership volume will be feasible as long as the negotiated per diem covers variable cost.

In addition to reevaluating pricing assumptions, the PHO may also want to consider its ability to renegotiate contracts for services intended to be carved out from the global capitation rate. For example, hospital services, such as transplants, spinal cord injuries, or severe burn cases, may be carved out to tertiary providers to deliver these services at cheaper rates. Also, on both the hospital and physician side, it is common to carve out psychiatric services to specialty providers.

The PHO's ability to implement and succeed at utilization management will also be critical to its success under the capitation arrangement. Success in implementing admission authorization and critical pathway programs will go a long way in achieving utilization targets necessary to be successful in the managed care marketplace. In addition, carefully structured risk-sharing schemes that promote financial incentives while maintaining quality care will facilitate success.

An important factor in the rate of utilization will be the kinds of utilization management systems in place.

A system with a primary care gatekeeper may reduce overall costs 5 to 7 percent. A very aggressive case management system may reduce specialty visits, ancillary services, and hospital days. Systems that use clinical pathways will frequently see reduced hospital bed days. In the most mature of the managed care settings, an actual increase in outpatient costs usually accompanies dramatic reductions in hospital costs. These systems increase the intensity of services in the office, emergency room, and home care settings to achieve their remarkable reduction in hospital bed days.

Tables 11 through 14 illustrate the development of an adjusted global capitation rate. Each table is based on adjustments to the actuarial cost model specific to the proposed membership base. Based on adjustments specific to this payer, it appears as though the proposed capitation rate would be reasonable. While this example has been somewhat simplified, it illustrates how the actuarial cost model can be used in evaluating prospective managed care contracts from specific payers.

TABLE 11
Hospital budget—commercial

Inpatient services	Admissions	ALOS	Days	Per diem	Copay	PMPM
Medical/surgical	0.042	4.40	0.185	$1,000.00		$15.42
ICU/CCU	0.009	4.20	0.038	$1,500.00		$4.75
Maternity	0.022	2.10	0.046	$1,250.00		$4.79
Boarder baby	0.002	2.30	0.005	$250.00		$0.10
Mental health (capitated)	0.002	9.50	0.019	$500.00		$0.79
Substance abuse (cap)	0.002	9.00	0.018	$400.00	$80.00	$0.48
Out of area						$1.37
Total inpatient	*0.079*	*3.94*	*0.311*			*$27.70*

Outpatient services	Utilization	Average cost	Copay	PMPM
Same day surgery	0.0600	$1,200.00	$22.50	$5.89
Emergency room	0.1300	$200.00	$30.25	$1.84
Home health	0.0300	$125.00		$0.31
Skilled nursing	0.0050	$300.00		$0.13
Other services	0.4000	$200.00		$6.67
Out of area	0.0100	$250.00		$0.21
Total outpatient				*$15.05*

Total hospital facility	$42.75
Provision for stop-loss	$2.19
Total hospital budget	*$44.94*

Assumptions:
- Medical/surgical admissions have been decreased to account for a younger age/sex mix and implementation of clinical management strategies.
- Inpatient mental health and substance abuse services have been carved out and capitated to subspecialty providers. The FFS equivalent assumptions underlying the capitations are illustrated.

TABLE 12
Primary care physician budget—commercial

Primary care physician services	Frequency	Average cost	Copay	PMPM
Office visits	2.230	$45.00	$7.25	$7.02
Preventive care	0.225	$75.00		$1.41
Inpatient visits	0.040	$90.00		$0.30
Consultations	0.010	$100.00	$7.25	$0.08
Vision and hearing screening	0.065	$55.00		$0.30
EKGs and pulmonary services	0.025	$40.00		$0.08
Immunizations and injections	0.400	$20.00		$0.67
Allergy shots	0.180	$15.00		$0.23
Emergency visits	0.010	$100.00		$0.08
Minor office surgery	0.075	$90.00		$0.56

TABLE 12 (CONTINUED)

Primary care physician services (cont.)	Frequency	Average cost	Copay	PMPM
Venipuncture	0.080	$5.00		$0.03
Laboratory services	0.781	$10.00		$0.65
Administrative services				$0.25
PCP capitation revenue PMPM				*$11.66*

Assumptions:
- PCPs within the PHO will be capitated so utilization assumptions have been adjusted to reflect the capitated reimbursement strategy.

TABLE 13
Specialist physician budget—commercial

Specialist physician services	Frequency	Average cost	Copay	PMPM
Office visits	0.975	$42.75	$7.25	$2.88
Inpatient visits	0.260	$85.50		$1.85
Consultations	0.095	$95.00		$0.69
Eye exams	0.020	$52.25		$0.09
Hearing exams	0.020	$33.25		$0.06
Skilled nursing and home healthcare visits	0.005	$57.00		$0.02
Cardiac services	0.095	$57.00		$0.45
Psychiatric services (capitated)	0.180	$66.50	$12.25	$0.81
Physical therapy	0.300	$23.75	$6.05	$0.44
Immunizations and injections	0.050	$9.50		$0.04
Allergy treatments	0.120	$14.25		$0.14
Emergency visits	0.080	$95.00		$0.63
Anesthesia	0.070	$380.00		$2.22
Surgery	0.360	$356.25		$10.69
Venipuncture	0.020	$4.75		$0.01
Normal delivery	0.014	$1,330.00		$1.55
Cesarean section	0.006	$1,520.00		$0.76
Laboratory services	1.950	$19.00		$3.09
Radiology (total)	0.740	$85.50		$5.27
Miscellaneous services	0.200	$42.75		$0.71
Total specialist physician services				*$32.40*
Pharmacy	5.200	$30.00	$6.05	$10.38

Assumptions:
- Specialist physician utilization for certain expense categories has been reduced to account for a younger age/sex mix and the implementation of clinical management strategies.
- Outpatient psychiatric services have been carved out and capitated to subspecialty providers.

TABLE 14
Total medical budget—commercial

Expense category	PMPM
Hospital services—medical	$42.75
Hospital services—stop-loss	$2.19
PCP services	$11.66
Specialist physician services	$32.40
Pharmacy	$10.38
PHO administration	$1.25
Total medical budget	*$100.63*
Payer's proposed capitation	$107.50

Capitation allocations among providers

Once the PHO has accepted a global capitation contract, it will be necessary to allocate the capitation dollar among the various medical providers. The PMPM cost allocations for the hospital and pharmacy budgets should be readily available; however, actual reimbursement levels to physicians warrant further considerations.

For PCPs, a distribution scheme needs to be developed to allocate the capitation. To achieve an equitable distribution of the primary care capitation dollar, it is necessary to allocate the capitation on an age/sex basis.

Table 15 provides an illustration of how the primary care capitation rate varies by age and sex, as well as by plan design. Tables 16 through 18 show the determination of the composite capitation rates by plan design, including the development of estimated composite copayment versus PMPM.

If the PHO has sophisticated management information systems (MIS), varying the primary care capitation reimbursement by benefit design and age/sex factor will produce the appropriate reimbursement levels to in-dividual PCPs. Reimbursing the average primary care capitation (i.e., the $7.25 average copay plan) among all PCPs will produce the appropriate reimbursement as long as the membership benefit mix remains constant. If the membership benefit mix changes, then a revised average capitation rate based on the new membership benefit mix should be calculated. Exhibits 1 and 2 at the end of this chapter provide

TABLE 15
Primary care capitation allocations by age/sex

Age category	Sex category	Members	Age/sex factors	PCP option plan	High option plan	Standard option plan	Low average plan
<1	M and F	70	4.892	$59.98	$53.42	$47.65	$57.04
1	M and F	180	2.678	$32.83	$29.24	$26.08	$31.23
02–14	M and F	1,550	0.927	$11.37	$10.12	$9.03	$10.81
15–19	M and F	1,650	0.618	$7.58	$6.75	$6.02	$7.21
20–29	M	650	0.515	$6.31	$5.62	$5.02	$6.00
20–29	F	1,000	0.721	$8.84	$7.87	$7.02	$8.41
30–39	M	950	0.772	$9.46	$8.43	$7.52	$9.00
30–39	F	1,100	0.875	$10.73	$9.56	$8.52	$10.20
40–49	M	700	1.081	$13.25	$11.80	$10.53	$12.60
40–49	F	750	1.287	$15.78	$14.05	$12.54	$15.01
50–59	M	450	1.329	$16.29	$14.51	$12.94	$15.50
50–59	F	500	1.339	$16.42	$14.62	$13.04	$15.61
60+	M	220	2.254	$27.63	$24.61	$21.95	$26.28
60+	F	230	2.094	$25.67	$22.87	$20.40	$24.42
Composite		*10,000*	*1.000*	*$12.26*	*$10.92*	*$9.74*	*$11.66*

TABLE 16
Primary care physician budget—commercial

Primary carephysician services	Frequency	Average cost	Copay	PMPM
Office visits	2.280	$45.00	$5.00	$7.60
Preventive care	0.225	$75.00		$1.41
Inpatient visits	0.040	$90.00		$0.30
Consultations	0.010	$100.00	$5.00	$0.08
Vision and hearing screening	0.065	$55.00		$0.30
EKGs and pulmonary services	0.025	$40.00		$0.08
Immunizations and injections	0.400	$20.00		$0.67
Allergy shots	0.180	$15.00		$0.23
Emergency visits	0.010	$100.00		$0.08
Minor office surgery	0.075	$90.00		$0.56
Venipuncture	0.080	$5.00		$0.03
Laboratory services	0.798	$10.00		$0.67
Administrative services				$0.25
PCP capitation revenue PMPM				$12.26
Copayment revenue Office visits	2.280		$5.00	$0.95
Consultations	0.010		$5.00	$0.00
PCP copayment revenue PMPM				$0.95
Total PCP revenue PMPM				*$13.21*

Note: For simplicity, the effects of increasing copayments on utilization have been ignored.

TABLE 17
Primary care physician budget—commercial

Primary care physician services	Frequency	Average cost	Copay	PMPM
Office visits	2.160	$45.00	$10.00	$6.30
Preventive care	0.225	$75.00		$1.41
Inpatient visits	0.040	$90.00		$0.30
Consultations	0.010	$100.00	$10.00	$0.08
Vision and hearing screening	0.065	$55.00		$0.30
EKGs and pulmonary services	0.025	$40.00		$0.08
Immunizations and injections	0.400	$20.00		$0.67
Allergy shots	0.180	$15.00		$0.23
Emergency visits	0.010	$100.00		$0.08
Minor office surgery	0.075	90.00		0.56
Venipuncture	0.080	$5.00		$0.03
Laboratory services	0.756	$10.00		$0.63
Administrative services				$0.25
PCP capitation revenue PMPM				$10.92
Copayment revenue				
Office visits	2.160		$10.00	$1.80
Consultations	0.010		$10.00	$0.01
PCP copayment revenue PMPM				$1.81
Total PCP revenue PMPM				*$12.73*

TABLE 18
Primary care physician budget—commercial

Primary care physician services	Frequency	Average cost	Copay	PMPM
Office visits	2.064	$45.00	$15.00	$5.16
Preventive care	0.225	$75.00		$1.41
Inpatient visits	0.040	$90.00		$0.30
Consultations	0.010	$100.00	$15.00	$0.07
Vision and hearing screening	0.065	$55.00		$0.30
EKGs and pulmonary services	0.025	$40.00		$0.08
Immunizations and injections	0.400	$20.00		$0.67
Allergy shots	0.180	$15.00		$0.23
Emergency visits	0.010	$100.00		$0.08
Minor office surgery	0.075	$90.00		$0.56
Venipuncture	0.080	$5.00		$0.03
Laboratory services	0.722	$10.00		$0.60
Administrative services				$0.25
PCP capitation revenue PMPM				$9.74
Copayment revenue				
Office visits	2.064		$15.00	$2.58
Consultations	0.010		$15.00	$0.01
PCP copayment revenue PMPM				$2.59
Total PCP revenue PMPM				*$12.33*

a detailed analysis of PCP age/sex reimbursement by individual plan design as well as average plan.

The PCP rates illustrated in the tables and exhibits are net member copayments. The PCP will collect member copayments at the time of the office visit. The actual copayment revenue is dependent upon benefit design of the PCP's members. The composite copayment PMPM could be adjusted by age and sex to better approximate copayment revenue per physician membership panel.

The accepted global capitation budget may have affected the ultimate capitation budget allocated for the specialist physician group. If the specialist capitation budget has changed as a result of steeper fee discounts from the target assumptions, the corresponding fee schedule must also change. Assuming a unit-based fee schedule is the means used to reimburse physicians, this would involve adjusting the conversion factors.

At first glance, it may be tempting to simply discount the conversion factors uniformly by major expense category. It may be more beneficial to consider adjusting conversion factors separately by major expense category. It may also be necessary to discount the conversion factors applicable for medical procedures at a greater level than discounts for surgical procedures. For instance, a key consideration for PHO management is the level of relative discounts distributed among specialist physician services that must be sold to the group. The chosen conversion factors must result in fee levels that, when applied to the target utilization assumptions, produce a PMPM cost consistent with the capitation constraint. Table 19 illustrates the relative differences in conversion factors and RVUs for the RBRVS and McGraw-Hill systems.

TABLE 19
Analysis of unit-based fee schedule modifications

Service category	Major expense category	Weight	Target mean
Office visits	medical	19.64%	$45.00
Preventive care	medical	0.50%	$75.00
Inpatient visits	medical	4.14%	$90.00
Consultations	medical	3.77%	$100.00
Anesthesia	anesthesia	0.30%	$400.00
Surgery	surgery	26.55%	$375.00
Normal delivery	surgery	2.71%	$1,400.00
Laboratory—total	laboratory	7.70%	$20.00
X-ray—total	x-ray	3.17%	$90.00

TABLE 19 (CONTINUED)

Service category (cont.)	RBVS conversion factors	McGraw-Hill conversion factors	Average RBVS unit	Average McGraw-Hill unit
Office visits	38.59	5.37	1.166	10.068
Preventive care	55.56	9.03	1.350	6.828
Inpatient visits	54.91	6.09	1.639	13.586
Consultations	33.40	5.79	2.994	24.037
Anesthesia	37.50	45.01	10.667	9.893
Surgery	62.70	111.88	5.981	4.325
Normal delivery	36.94	118.06	37.899	18.184
Laboratory—total	15.22	13.68	1.314	2.308
X-ray—total	37.47	21.18	2.402	7.323

Model maintenance

As a PHO accepts managed care contracts, it will be important to track utilization expenses to monitor physicians and to update model assumptions. The format in which the data is collected is also important as PHO management will want to produce specific reports useful in managing the managed care business. Specific reports may include costs broken down by age and sex for each payer, utilization reports by physician specialty, inpatient and outpatient hospital utilization reports, and utilization of pharmacy services.

Essentially, as the PHO matures and becomes the primary risk taker within the managed care arrangement, it will be necessary to operate more like a health insuring organization. Unless the PHO begins to contract directly with employers, the primary purpose of the managed care health insuring organization is that of a marketing agency.

As the PHO gathers a sufficient managed care membership base, it will be beneficial to determine PHO-specific age/sex factors based on the PHO's accumulated managed care population. Specific age/sex factors will provide a more realistic base to make the demographic adjustments considered in the earlier example, as well as providing the means to distribute PCP capitations. Tracking the cost information by age and sex on an ongoing basis would put the PHO in a position to develop plan-specific age/sex factors. Table 20 illustrates the process used to calculate age/sex factors.

The age/sex factors determined in Table 20 reflect the cost distribution for total medical services. It will be beneficial to calculate age/sex factors by major medical expense categories such as hospital, PCP, specialty physician, and pharmacy services. Having age/sex factors by major

TABLE 20
Development of age/sex factors

Age category	Sex category	Members	Total incurred claims	PMPM	Age/sex factors
<20	M and F	3,800	$3,100,000	$67.98	0.664
20–29	M	950	$725,000	$63.60	0.621
20–29	F	1,050	$1,800,000	$142.86	1.395
30–39	M	1,000	$1,100,000	$91.67	0.895
30–39	F	1,050	$1,736,000	$137.78	1.345
40–49	M	550	$690,000	$104.55	1.021
40–49	F	600	$873,600	$121.33	1.184
50–59	M	350	$700,000	$166.67	1.627
50–59	F	400	$784,000	$163.33	1.594
60+	M and F	250	$784,000	$261.33	2.551
Composite		*10,000*	*$12,292,600*	*$102.44*	*1.000*

medical expense category allows PHO management to make adjustments for membership demographics under capitated reimbursement schemes to providers.

Finally, the concept of incurred but not reported (IBNR) claims needs to be considered. If the PHO is updating the model utilization assumptions based on the experience of existing membership over a particular period, it will be critical to consider adjustments for IBNR. Table 21 illustrates the consideration of IBNR to determine incurred utilization experience over a calendar year period.

Lag factors illustrated in Table 21 would be developed using historical paid claims information over a multiple-year period. The basic premise to determine lag factors is that incurred claims experience for a given contract period emerges in later months to the ultimate level. A general rule of thumb is that claims could be considered complete in approximately nine months following the end of the contract period. A key factor affecting the development of the fully incurred claims experience is the claims-processing systems that are in place by the PHO.

It will be beneficial to track incurred claims experience by major expense category to develop an internal IBNR reserving mechanism. As illustrated in Table 21, the pattern in which incurred claims experience emerges varies by major expense category. For example, pharmacy incurred claims generally emerge at a more rapid rate than hospital or physician services. This is due to pharmacy claims being submitted and processed at a faster rate than physician claims.

TABLE 21
Incurred claims—emergence of IBNR

	Utilization based on paid claims as of 12/31/95	Utilization based on paid claims as of 3/31/96	Utilization based on paid claims as of 6/30/96	Utilization based on paid claims as of 9/30/96
Pharmacy	5.000	5.200	5.200	5.200
Lag factor	0.962	1.000	1.000	1.000
Inpatient days	0.250	0.310	0.320	0.320
Lag factor	0.781	0.969	1.000	1.000
Physician office visits	2.500	2.800	3.400	3.500
Lag factor	0.714	0.800	0.971	1.000

Note: The successive payments during 1996 are for services incurred in calendar year 1995.

Risk sharing

In addition to evaluating the feasibility of managed care contracts, the cost model can be used to measure performance related to pertinent risk-sharing arrangements. Many PHOs determine risk pools to insulate the organization from adverse claims experience. Budgets are set for each of the risk pools, and actual experience is compared to budget to determine whether a gain or loss has occurred. If gains occur, savings will be distributed among participating providers. Table 22 illustrates the analysis of risk sharing for a hospital risk pool.

There is no magical formula to determine how much of the surplus cash provider groups receive. Issues such as which providers take on the most risk, as well as who takes on the most responsibility for determining hospital utilization experience, play a major role. The greater the role of the PCP in monitoring hospital admissions as well as length-of-stay management, the greater the PCP's share will be in the hospital risk pool. Specialists also have a large role in determining hospital admissions and inpatient activity and may receive a significant portion of the surplus. The hospital exerts the least control over its utilization experience, and in many instances, takes a lesser share than do the physicians.

Some pools may experience a gain while others experience a deficit. Typical practice is that surpluses in a given pool would be used to cover deficits in other pools before distribution to providers. In addition, PHOs may allocate a percentage of the global capitation to a contingency fund to cover deficits, as well as to smooth out experience deviations due

TABLE 22
Analysis of risk sharing—hospital pool

	Admits	ALOS	Days	Per diem	PMPM
Total inpatient—budget	0.082	3.95	0.324	$1,065.93	$28.78
Total inpatient—incurred	0.077	· 3.75	0.289	$1,092.75	$26.32
Gain/(loss) on inpatient hospital					$2.46
Members					10,000
Total pool (PMPM gain × members × 12)					*$295,200*
Risk-sharing allocations:					
Primary care				40%	$118,080
Specialists				40%	$118,080
Hospital				20%	$59,040

Note: Risk-sharing allocations will vary depending upon reimbursement strategies. For example, if the hospital is capitated, the risk-sharing allocations among physicians and the hospital may be a 50-50 split.

to varying IBNR estimates used to approximate incurred claim experience in the short run.

Risk-sharing strategies within PHOs are continuing to evolve as capitation takes a greater role in the marketplace with plans moving away from FFS withholds to strict capitated reimbursement. In developing any risk-sharing strategy, it will be critical to ensure appropriate alignment of incentives among the providers.

Conclusion

As PHOs continue to flourish across the country with increased penetration of managed care, it will be important for these organizations to garner the tools to properly assess risk. The development of a sound actuarial cost model can be of great value to the PHO as it moves forward in accepting capitated contracts within the managed care industry.

In addition to the cost model, an understanding of how implemented clinical management strategies will affect prospective costs is critical. For example, this information tells the health system how to get from 300 hospital days per 1,000 down to 200, while still delivering quality healthcare. Integration of the financial and clinical aspects of managing an integrated health system will be essential to ensure success in the rapidly changing healthcare industry.

EXHIBIT 1

Age/sex distribution of capitation by plan design

Age category	Sex category	Members	PCP age/sex factors	High option members	High option plan
Pediatrician: Dr. Jones					
<1	M and F	42	4.892	30	$59.98
1	M and F	99	2.678	69	$32.83
02–14	M and F	620	0.927	434	$11.37
Composite		761	1.374	533	$16.88
Actual plan mix				70.0%	
Weighted average of individual plans					
Pediatrician: Dr. Casey					
<1	M and F	28	4.892	20	$59.98
1	M and F	81	2.678	57	$32.83
02–14	M and F	930	0.927	650	$11.37
Composite		1039	1.170	727	$14.35
Actual plan mix				70.0%	
Weighted average of individual plans					
Family practitioner: Dr. Rodriguiz					
15–19	M and F	825	0.618	577	$7.58
20–29	M	293	0.515	205	$6.31
20–29	F	300	0.721	210	$8.84
30–39	M	523	0.772	367	$9.46
30–39	F	440	0.875	308	$10.73
40–49	M	280	1.081	196	$13.25
40–49	F	263	1.287	185	$15.78
Composite		2,924	0.789	2,048	$9.67
Actual plan mix				70.0%	
Weighted average of individual plans					
Family Practitioner: Dr. Hanson					
15–19	M and F	825	0.618	578	$7.58
20–29	M	357	0.515	250	$6.31
20–29	F	700	0.721	490	$8.84
30–39	M	427	0.772	299	$9.46
30–39	F	660	0.875	462	$10.73
40–49	M	420	1.081	294	$13.25
40–49	F	487	1.287	341	$15.78
Composite		3,876	0.822	2,714	$10.08
Actual plan mix				70.0%	
Weighted average of individual plans					

Standard option members	Standard option plan	Low option members	Low option plan	Total members	Average plan
6	$53.42	6	$47.65	42	$57.04
15	$29.24	15	$26.08	99	$31.23
93	$10.12	93	$9.03	620	$10.81
114	$14.91	114	$13.31	761	$16.02
15.0%		15.0%			
					$16.05
4	$53.42	4	$47.65	28	$57.04
12	$29.24	12	$26.08	81	$31.23
140	$10.12	140	$9.03	930	$10.81
156	$12.78	156	$11.40	1039	$13.65
15.0%		15.0%			
					$13.67
124	$6.75	124	$6.02	825	$7.21
44	$5.62	44	$5.02	293	$6.00
45	$7.87	45	$7.02	300	$8.41
78	$8.43	78	$7.52	523	$9.00
66	$9.56	66	$8.52	440	$10.20
42	$11.80	42	$10.53	280	$12.60
39	$14.05	39	$12.54	263	$15.01
438	$8.62	438	$7.69	2,924	$9.20
15.0%		15.0%			
					$9.22
124	$6.75	123	$6.02	825	$7.21
53	$5.62	54	$5.02	357	$6.00
105	$7.87	105	$7.02	700	$8.41
64	$8.43	64	$7.52	427	$9.00
99	$9.56	99	$8.52	660	$10.20
63	$11.80	63	$10.53	420	$12.60
73	$14.05	73	$12.54	487	$15.01
581	$8.98	581	$8.01	3,876	$9.59
15.0%		15.0%			
					$9.60

EXHIBIT 1 (CONTINUED)

Age category	Sex category	Members	PCP age/sex factors	High option members	High option plan
Internist: Dr. Frost					
50–59	M	180	1.329	126	$16.29
50–59	F	350	1.339	244	$16.42
60+	M	110	2.254	77	$27.63
60+	F	58	2.094	41	$25.67
Composite		698	1.543	488	$18.93
Actual plan mix				70.0%	
Weighted average of individual plans					
Internist: Dr. Backus					
50–59	M	270	1.329	189	$16.29
50–59	F	150	1.339	106	$16.42
60+	M	110	2.254	77	$27.63
60+	F	172	2.094	120	$25.67
Composite		702	1.664	492	$20.38
Actual plan mix				70.0%	
Weighted average of individual plans					

EXHIBIT 2
Analysis of revenue neutrality

	Patient panel	Revenue based on average plan	Total annual plan	Revenue based on weighted average	Total annual dollars	Difference
Dr. Jones	761	$16.02	$146,276	$16.05	$146,569	($293)
Dr. Casey	1,039	$13.65	$170,161	$13.67	$170,438	($277)
Dr. Rodriguiz	2,924	$9.20	$322,799	$9.22	$323,511	($712)
Dr. Hanson	3,876	$9.59	$445,849	$9.60	$446,515	($666)
Dr. Frost	698	$18.00	$150,728	$18.03	$151,019	($291)
Dr. Backus	702	$19.40	$163,410	$19.42	$163,594	($184)
Composite	*10,000*	*$11.66*	*$1,399,223*	*$11.68*	*$1,401,646*	*($2,423)*

Note: The difference is less than .1 percent.

Standard-option members	Standard-option plan	Low-option members	Low-option plan	Total members	Average plan
27	$14.51	27	$12.94	180	$15.50
53	$14.62	53	$13.04	350	$15.61
16	$24.61	17	$21.95	110	$26.28
9	$22.87	8	$20.40	58	$24.42
105	$16.82	105	$15.02	698	$18.00
15.0%		15.0%			
					$18.03
40	$14.51	41	$12.94	270	$15.50
23	$14.62	21	$13.04	150	$15.61
16	$24.61	17	$21.95	110	$26.28
26	$22.87	26	$20.40	172	$24.42
105	$18.14	105	$16.27	702	$19.40
15.0%		15.0%			
					$19.42

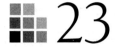

23

Risk-adjusted capitation

Alice F. Rosenblatt
Principal

David Chin, MD
Principal
Coopers & Lybrand LLP
Boston, Massachusetts

Providers and managed care organizations are using capitation as a reimbursement strategy to control healthcare utilization and to develop integrated delivery systems (IDS). What are the implications of this movement for the high-risk segments of the population? This chapter explores these implications and provides some recommendations.

Historical perspective

The start of insured programs for medical insurance can be traced to the 1940s when the Blues plans were the original insurers. These insurance contracts, which were offered to employers, involved the negotiation of discounts or fee schedules with providers. They used community rating, an important concept. As used by these early insurance plans, the rates distinguished between individual versus family plans, area, and plan design, although plan design was much simpler and less varied.

As the commercial carriers entered this market, it became more competitive and risk-selection techniques were used. These techniques made use of underwriting and rating techniques for competitive advantage. It was recognized that in a voluntary insurance market, as carriers expanded marketing to individuals and small employer groups, it was likely that those most in need of healthcare services would be the purchasers. Medical underwriting was used to decline individuals and small groups of higher-than-average expected risk. Carriers, including the Blues plans where allowable by state laws, recognized that to be competitive, community rating would not work. So carriers increased their rating variables from those of community rating to include age, sex, industry, experience, and health status.

In the 1970s, self-insurance by employers became very popular due to the high levels of interest rates and an awareness by employers that they were losing valuable cash flow due to the retrospective rating techniques of the carriers. These retrospective rating techniques would compare the group's premium (which usually included a margin for adverse experience) at the end of the policy period with the actual experience of the particular group. If the group's experience was better than anticipated in the premium, a retrospective settlement was paid to the employer; whereas if the group's experience was worse than expected, a deficit was created, which was often carried forward to future years' accountings by the carrier. This accounting often involved credibility and pooling of large claims. Thus, if the employer was not large enough for one year's experience to be credible, its actual experience was weighted with the expected experience of similar groups in the calculation. It was also recognized that a given group would experience a deficit in any year in which a catastrophic claim occurred. Thus the carrier used a pooling technique, where claims above a given size were not charged to the experience of the group, but instead an average charge was assessed (similar to a reinsurance premium).

In effect, other than the protection afforded by the pooling of catastrophic claims, the employers were absorbing the insurance risk and often suffering from a cash flow perspective as they funded premiums up front and received refunds several months after the close of the accounting period. This led to the demand by these large employers and their consultants for self-funded arrangements such as administrative service only (ASO) plans and minimum premium plans. The employers often purchased stop-loss insurance to provide protection for catastrophic claims (specific stop-loss) or for the risk of high total expenses (aggregate stop-loss). As healthcare cost and inflation trends increased during the 1980s, these large employers looked to managed care as a means of keeping healthcare costs under control. This usually implied passing the risk back to the managed care organizations.

In recent years, particularly for the individual and small group markets, many states have passed reform legislation that prevents carriers from engaging in many of the practices used in the past to select the best risks. Some states do not allow the use of medical underwriting and do not allow carriers to decline groups or individuals. Several states limit the rating variables that carriers can use or place limits on the variation in rates from the highest rate charged to a group to the lowest rate charged to a group. In some states where small-group reform has been enacted, rating variables might be limited for small groups to age and sex characteristics, geography, and plan design. In addition, some states impose limits, such as a 2:1 variation on rates charged to small groups due to age and sex differentials even though from an actuarial perspective the rate variation should be closer to a 5:1 variation.

In connection with such insurance reforms, states have experimented with reinsurance pools and risk adjustment. Reinsurance pools have been used to fund high-risk cases that carriers' previous underwriting policies would have declined. Risk adjustment has been used as a means of transferring monetary payments between carriers so that carriers with a disproportionate share of high-risk enrollees are not forced to charge the highest community rates.

A recent Government Accounting Office (GAO) report concluded that, "Unless payments received by insurers are risk adjusted, the goal of community rating—to have affordable, comprehensive health insurance available to those who need it most—may be compromised. Community rating creates strong incentives for insurers to avoid the less healthy, which conflicts with the concept that community rating would expand access to those same beneficiaries."[1]

With managed care has come the movement to pass the risk on to providers through capitated arrangements. In its simplest sense, capitation is like a community-rated premium, ignoring for the moment any type of risk adjustment. Thus, both capitation and premium are paid upfront for each member of an insured population. The risk-taking organization assumes the risk of all medical services for the insured population in exchange for this upfront payment.

Providers are looking to capitation to increase their revenue, which is declining as a result of managed care. The above historical perspective raises important questions for the provider community, such as

- Why did carriers underwrite to exclude high-risk individuals?

- Why did carriers vary their premiums by age, sex, industry, experience, and health status?

- What are the implications for providers that are currently accepting capitation without any adjustment for the types of risks?

- What does the lack of risk adjustment imply for the quality of care and the providers' ability to serve the high-risk population?

Risk adjustment

Several managed care organizations that are reimbursing providers using capitated arrangements include some form of risk adjustment.

Most capitated arrangements include a form of reinsurance, where the managed care organization may assume the risk of claims of more than a specific dollar amount, measured on a fee-for-service (FFS) equivalent basis. For example, for hospitals, claims of more than $50,000, $75,000, or $100,000 may be subject to the reinsurance. Primary care physicians (PCPs) claims of more than $10,000 or $15,000 may be subject to the reinsurance. Another simple risk-adjustment mechanism uses age/sex adjustments.

Other managed care organizations are offering providers a percent of premium. To the extent that premium may be age/sex or experience adjusted, this becomes a method of risk adjusting the capitated payments. In other words, to the extent that the premium has been developed in accordance with actuarially sound methodology, the premium development has probably accounted for the need to match expected claims experience for the population to be insured with the premium. However, there are two dangers. One is that whereas the premium in total is correct, the premium is not correct for a particular provider, since that provider's patients do not reflect the average expected claims costs. The other danger is that the carrier may underprice its products during periods of competitive price wars.

The more sophisticated forms of risk adjustment are currently more art than science and involve some analysis of prior claims or diagnosis history. Thus, they are very data intensive.

Examples include ACGs—Ambulatory Care Groups, which classify individuals according to a combination of age/sex characteristics and prior ambulatory care diagnoses—and DCGs—Diagnostic Care Groups, which use both inpatient hospital care diagnoses and ambulatory diagnoses for classification into risk groupings.[2]

Any of these risk-adjustment methods could be used to adjust capitation payments to reflect the risk characteristics of the enrolled population. For example, age/sex factors are often used to adjust capitation payments for the expected claims costs of specified age/sex cohorts.

Assuming that an average capitation payment unadjusted for age/sex differentials is $100, then some sample capitation payments would be calculated as shown in Table 1, using illustrative factors and age/sex groupings.

It is important to note that the age/sex factors in Table 1 were derived from claim payment data truncated at $25,000. The factors should be calculated using the experience of the particular population to be covered and should account for the amount at-risk (i.e., whether any stop-loss is also involved) as well as plan design features.

TABLE 1
Age/sex risk-adjusted capitation example

Sample age group	Sex	Illustrative age/sex factor	Illustrative adjusted capitation
0	M/F	.70	$70.00
1–9	F	.35	$35.00
10–19	F	.70	$70.00
20–29	F	1.35	$135.00
30–39	F	1.35	$135.00
40–49	F	1.40	$140.00
50–59	F	1.80	$180.00
60–64	F	2.25	$225.00
1–9	M	.45	$45.00
10–19	M	.60	$60.00
20–29	M	.50	$50.00
30–39	M	.70	$70.00
40–49	M	1.00	$100.00
50–59	M	1.70	$170.00
60–64	M	2.50	$250.00

Using sample factors developed as described in Table 1, the capitation payments using illustrative ACG factors and groupings are shown in Table 2.

In Table 2, ADGs refer to Ambulatory Diagnostic Groups, which is a 34-group classification system for ICD-9-CM codes denoting primary diagnoses or subsidiary diagnoses.

Note that the previous age/sex and ACG factors are purely illustrative and are not appropriate for general use due to the truncation at $25,000 of the claims experience base used to develop these factors and the particular plan designs, population, and geographic areas represented by the claims experience.

Distribution of claims

In a typical insured plan, 4 percent of the claimants generate approximately 50 percent of the claim costs. These types of statistics led the insurance carriers to attempt to predict the individuals who would be likely to incur these high-amount claims. Such individuals were either excluded from coverage or charged higher-than-average rates. For example, some carriers engaged in "cherry-picking practices," such as medical underwriting to exclude such individuals, nonrenewal of particular employer groups, or renewals with 300 percent rate increases for employer groups with unfavorable past experience.

The financial implications of these high-risk individuals are now being passed from the carriers to the providers—a result of healthcare reform that prevents insurance carriers from either excluding these

TABLE 2
ACG risk-adjusted capitation example

Sample ACG group	Description	Illustrative ACG factor	Illustrative adjusted capitation
1	Acute minor, age <1	.30	$30.00
4	Acute major	.70	$70.00
12	Chronic specialty, unstable	1.00	$100.00
18	Acute minor and acute major	1.00	$100.00
28	Acute major and likely to recur discrete	1.00	$100.00
43	4–5 Other ADG combinations, age 17–44	2.10	$210.00
50	10+ Other ADG combinations	5.55	$555.00

high-risk individuals or charging higher rates to such individuals and carriers from offering capitated contracts to providers.

If providers react to these implications the same way that the insurance carriers reacted in the past, providers would avoid high-risk categories of patients or give inferior service to such patients in an attempt to cause them to switch to other providers.

Risk adjustment would reimburse providers more for the high-risk patients, and thus align the financial incentives with the public policy direction of guaranteed issue and portability of coverage.

Adverse selection

In simple terms, adverse selection can be described as a situation that causes a nonrandom selection of individuals for a particular carrier or provider.

For example, many employers currently offer their employees a choice of health insurance plans that may include indemnity plans, preferred provider organization (PPO) plans, and HMOs. Many of these employers can document that the higher-risk individuals tend to select the plans with the widest choice of providers and the richest benefits, causing a situation known as adverse selection. For example, when an indemnity plan is offered in addition to an HMO, the plan design and managed care features can be modeled actuarially to develop equivalent premiums for the two plans. However, adverse selection could result in premium differentials of as much as 100 percent.

If all risk selection were random, risk adjustment would not be necessary. However, just as certain carriers attract the high-risk population due to their broad networks or rich benefit designs, certain providers such as cancer or heart-disease specialists also attract the high-risk population. These providers should be extremely careful in the design of capitated arrangements.

Adverse selection in the Medicare population has been widely studied. A Mathematica report concluded that Medicare risk plans are experiencing favorable selection. The study found that "enrollees in Medicare risk plans were less likely to report poor health, to report functional impairments, to have a history of serious illness (cancer, heart disease, or stroke), and less likely to die in the nine-month period after the survey interview."[3]

The study also found that "the actuarial risk factors used to determine AAPCC [adjusted average per capita cost] rates failed to account for the better health status and, hence, lower costs of enrollees . . ." Finally, the implication of the study is, "The results indicate that it may be necessary to incorporate some type of health status adjuster in the payment methodology."

The Government Accounting Office (GAO) has recognized the implications of adverse selection in Medicare risk program. Currently, payments to managed care organizations participating in Medicare risk programs are risk adjusted for age, sex, Medicaid eligibility, disability, institutionalized status, and working age-status.

A GAO report mentions several other forms of risk adjustment that were considered, which include

1. Clinical indicators combined with demographic variables. The clinical indicators are simple indicators of a history of a specific health problem termed a tracer condition (e.g. heart disease, cancer, and stroke)

2. Mortality adjustment (based on last year's mortality rates)

3. Ambulatory Care Groups (ACG)—categorizes patients into 51 cost groups based on clinical diagnosis codes and the individual's age and sex

4. Clinical complexity index—panels of participating physicians assign severity codes to medical diagnoses, according to the resources needed to treat the case

5. Prior utilization—base HMO capitation payments on services used by the beneficiary in a previous period

6. Diagnostic Cost Group (DCG)—clinical and utilization measures for inpatient stays

7. Payment amount for capitated systems (PACS)—combines information on demographics, inpatient and outpatient utilization, clinical diagnoses, urban and rural indicator, and wage index

8. Lifestyle or socioeconomic factors—risk of lifestyle factors such as smoking, occupation, marital status, and education

9. Functional status—ability to perform activities of daily living such as grocery shopping, eating, dressing, housecleaning, and preparing food

10. Self-reported health status—based on a questionnaire such as the SF-36, which requests information from the patient on physical functioning, bodily pain, limitations due to physical, personal, or emotional problems, general mental health, social functioning, energy and fatigue levels, general health perceptions, and the patient's perception of change in health status

The report concluded that only four of the above 10 alternatives were the most promising for improving the current system, including self-reported health status; clinical indicators, such as indicators of heart disease, cancer, and stroke; the ACG method; and DCG method.

The report also stated that "under HCFA's current rate-setting method, HMOs have a strong financial incentive to attract the healthiest possible Medicare client. When a relatively healthy Medicare patient joins an HMO, the HMO will provide less treatment than for the average patient, but HCFA's capitated payment for that person will not fully reflect the lower expected costs."

Other criteria mentioned in the report for a risk adjuster include inexpensive administration, reducing favorable selection, creating incentives for HMOs to provide appropriate care, and excluding manipulation by participating HMOs.[4]

Medical management

While medical management cannot change the fact that the sickest 4 percent of the population consumes 50 percent of the healthcare dollar, medical management interventions can have a significant impact on the total dollars expended in capitation. These interventions include maintaining the health of a population, providing primary care, and reducing variation in clinical practice.

HEALTH MAINTENANCE

In a FFS setting, there are few incentives to implement measures that reduce utilization. In contrast, the logic is reversed in capitation.

Managed care organizations and providers are in part rewarded for maximizing health (i.e., helping the patient prolong the length of time between visits to healthcare professionals). The strategy has been centered around cost-effective screening and preventive strategies such as childhood immunizations, adult flu and pneumococcal vaccinations, screening for cervical and breast cancer, screening for hypertension, counseling for smoking cessation, and seatbelt use.[5]

More recently, there has been increased interest in patient education for self-care—for so-called demand management programs.[6] Early interventions by several managed care organizations consisted of providing members with self-help books, such as *Take Care of Yourself,* a self-help book on when to call a provider, or *What to Expect When You're Expecting* for pregnant women. There have been several studies that have demonstrated lower rates of utilization by patients when they have been provided with objective information about appropriate self-treatment and information about when to seek professional help.[7]

These programs have been expanded recently to include 24-hour, phone-based patient help lines designed to provide decision support to patients at the time they contemplate seeking care. These services are usually staffed by trained nurses using peer-reviewed medical literature or practice protocols. Ideally, this clinical information is reviewed by the local medical management or medical advisory committee of the managed care organization providing the service. These services are typically nondirective and provide options rather than prescribe treatment to avoid the attendant liability issues. These enhanced patient education programs are still too new to have had rigorous evaluation of whether or not they have a significant additional impact on reducing demand for services from patients.

PRIMARY CARE

In FFS, the controls over utilization have been precertification and prior authorization because of the incentives to do more. With the advent of managed care, capitation, and alignment of economic incentives, the primary care gatekeeper model to control utilization has been adopted by 90 percent of HMOs.[8]

These primary care gatekeepers include family practitioners, internists, pediatricians, and, in some settings, obstetrician-gynecologists. The

Institute of Medicine Consensus Conference defined five key attributes of primary care: accessibility, accountability, comprehensiveness, continuity, and coordination.[9]

One aspect of the Rand Health Insurance Experiment, a randomized trial conducted by the Rand Institute in the early 1980s, examined the effect of primary care gatekeepers on utilization. They found that HMO patients assigned to gatekeepers were hospitalized 40 percent less often than those patients assigned to a FFS group without a gatekeeper.[10]

Further evidence of the cost-effectiveness of primary care came from the Medical Outcomes Study (MOS), which adjusted for variation and severity of illness among patients who had diabetes and cardiac diseases. It examined the differences in care provided these patients by internists, family practitioners, cardiologists, and endocrinologists. They found that the number of office visits, the percentage of patients tested per visit, and hospitalization rates were higher among the specialists than among the generalists.[11] However, not all gatekeepers are created equal. Some are more cost-effective than others without apparent differences in outcome.

PROVIDER PROFILING

When confronted with the economic rewards and penalties commonplace in managed care capitated systems, providers often believe they have a preponderance of patients who consume a disproportionate share of resources. They make an implicit assumption that when confronted with similar patients, physicians practice in a similar fashion.

However, multiple studies have shown that variations in populations cannot account for variations in physician practice patterns. A study by Wennberg and Gittelsohn found that the rates of the three most common surgical procedures (i.e., hysterectomy, prostatectomy, and tonsillectomy) varied dramatically among the 193 small areas studied in the six New England states. The highest rates observed were six times higher than the lowest. These differences cannot be explained by the demographics of the population. The total rate was correlated most strongly with the number of surgeons and hospital beds per capita.[12]

In the face of such variation, profiling the practice patterns and feeding information back to physicians could educate physicians, reduce variation, and improve quality—especially if the appropriate incentives were in place, as they potentially are in managed care.

A whole industry has developed to meet the demand for these profiles. These systems predominantly rely on claims data. They generally use proprietary algorithms to group data by physicians and patients into diagnostic categories, adjust for severity or comorbidity, and then aggregate the financial information and compare actual to expected rates. Given that the source of these profiles is claims databases, there are serious limitations on the accuracy of the data[13] and in the full range of information on medications, postoperative care, and lab utilization.[14]

Given the lack of alternatives, provider and managed care organizations must use the currently available practice profiling systems, but those who use them should thoroughly understand the limitations of the systems they have purchased before they disseminate the resulting profiles back to clinicians and potentially to employers. Some of the limitations of these systems include

- Lack of credible data for small numbers of enrolled patients

- Most of the algorithms require a full year of data and understate the expected morbidity where less than 12 months of data is available

- Due to small populations, there may be "swings" in the indices of a particular provider from one period to the next

- Since these algorithms are so data intensive and require 12 months of data, there are usually substantial time lags between the claims experience period and the date the reports are generated. Since timely feedback is important in changing behavior, these time delays could be a serious problem

Any of the risk assessment methods discussed previously can be used for provider profiling, including age and sex, ACG, and DCG.

A simple methodology for comparing providers would be to calculate "assessment indices" for each provider's enrolled population and a per member per month (PMPM) index for each provider. A "risk-adjusted PMPM index" can then be obtained as illustrated in Table 3.

In this example, the population assessment index reflects the weights obtained by analyzing the provider's enrolled population by means of an assessment tool like the ACGs. The PMPM index would be the PMPM cost for the time period for the particular provider divided by the average PMPM cost of all providers.

TABLE 3
ACG risk-adjusted provider profiling example

Provider	Population assessment index (using ACG)	PMPM index	Risk-adjusted PMPM index
	(A)	(B)	(B)÷(A)
A	1.00	.9	.9
B	.50	1.2	2.4
C	1.30	1.1	.8

Note that Provider A has an average population and a PMPM index indicating lower cost. Thus, the risk-adjusted PMPM index also indicates lower cost. Provider B has a very healthy population, with a risk assessment index of .50. However, the PMPM index is 20 percent worse than average. When this index is adjusted for the better morbidity of the population, a risk-adjusted PMPM index more than double the average is obtained. Provider C has a population with an assessment index 30 percent worse than average. Provider C's PMPM index is 10 percent worse than average. The risk-adjusted index for Provider C is therefore 20 percent better than average.

Thus, these types of provider profiling analyses can identify providers that are overutilizers and are the best method available today of comparing providers on an "apples-to-apples" basis.

DISEASE MANAGEMENT

Disease management is another approach to medical management. As the name implies the approach is to manage a particular disease through its natural cycle (i.e., from self-care to acute care, to post-acute care, and back to self-care). These programs typically focus on chronic diseases (e.g., ulcers, diabetes, coronary artery disease, arthritis, and asthma). They are designed to prolong disease-free or symptom-free intervals of healthiness and speed healing once the disease returns. These programs can include all of the components of medical management mentioned earlier which include

- Educating the patient in self-care

- The use of literature and 800 numbers

- Designing specific practice guidelines to reduce variation with primary care and specialty physicians

- Building an information management system to feed the results back to the patients and physicians

Disease management can provide scientific techniques to develop the "ultimate" risk assessment method. If disease states could be sufficiently categorized, and medical protocols developed for each, then risk assessment would be based on the quantification of the cost of performing the medical protocols associated with each disease state.

Conclusion

To ensure proper financial incentives in healthcare delivery, risk adjustment of capitated payments is necessary. Although current methods for performing risk assessment and adjustment—such as age/sex, ACGs, and DCGs—are not as precise as would be desired, these methods are still preferable to no adjustments and provide good directional adjustments. These techniques can also be used to assist providers to better manage care, since these methods can be used for provider profiling.

NOTES

1. United States General Accounting Office, Health, Education, and Human Services Division, *Health Care Reform: Considerations for Risk Adjustment Under Community Rating* (Washington, DC: U.S. General Accounting Office, 1994), 94–173.

2. The John Hopkins University, *John Hopkins University: A Clinician's Guide to the John Hopkins Case-Mix System,* version 2.0 (Baltimore: John Hopkins University Press, 1993); and R. P. Ellis and A. Ash, "Refinements to the Diagnostic Cost Group (DCG) Model," *Inquiry* (Winter 1995): 32–34.

3. J. Hill et al., *The Impact of the Medicare Risk Program on the Use of Services and Costs to Medicare* (Washington, DC: Mathematica Policy Research, Inc., 1992).

4. United States General Accounting Office, Health, Education, and Human Services Division, *Medicare—HMO Rate Setting Method Needs Change* (Washington, DC: U.S. General Accounting Office, 1994), 94–119.

5. *Preventive Services Task Force, Guide to Clinical Preventive Services: Report of the U.S. Preventive Services Task Force* (Baltimore: Williams and Wilkins, 1989).

6. J. Fries et al., "Reducing Health Care Costs by Reducing the Need and Demand for Medical Services," *New England Journal of Medicine* 329 (1993): 321–25.

7. D. M. Vickery et al., "Effect of a Self-Care Education Program on Medical Visits," *Journal of American Medical Association* 250 (1983): 2952–56; K. Lorig et al., "Workplace Health Education Program That Reduces Outpatient Visits,"

Medical Care 23 (1985): 1044–54; T. Golaszewski et al., "Benefit-to-Cost Analysis of a Work-Site Health Promotion Program," *Journal of Occupational Medicine* 34 (1992): 1164–72.

8. K. M. Langwell, "Structure and Performance of HMOs: A Review," *Health Care Finance Review* 12, no. 1 (1990): 71–79.

9. Institute of Medicine, "A Manpower Policy for Primary Health Care," *National Academy of Science* (Washington, DC: Institute of Medicine, 1978).

10. W. G. Manning et al., "A Controlled Trial of the Effect of a Prepaid Group Practice on Use of Services," *New England Journal of Medicine* 310 (1984): 1505–10.

11. S. Greenfield et al., "Variations in Resource Utilization Among Medical Specialties and Systems of Care—Results From the Medicaid Outcomes Study," *Journal of American Medical Association* 267 (Washington, DC: GPO, 1992): 1624–30.

12. J. Wennberg and A. Gittelsohn, "Variations in Medical Care Among Small Areas," *Scientific American* 4 (Washington, DC: GPO, 1982): 120–34.

13. D. A. Brand et al., "Data Needs of Profiling Systems," *Physicians Review Commission*, no. 92–2 (GPO, 1992 Washington, DC), 20–45.

14. B. McNeil, et al., "Current Issues in Profiles: Potentials and Limitations," *Physician Payment Review Commission*, no. 92-2 (Washington, DC: GPO, 1992), 46–70.

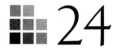

24

Minimizing employer liability in managed care arrangements

Sandra L. Berkowitz
Senior Vice President and Managed Care Practice Leader
Johnson & Higgins
Philadelphia, Pennsylvania

To CONTROL THE EVER-INCREASING COSTS of health-care benefits, many employers are turning to managed care organizations (MCOs) for assistance. One fear shared by many employers is that some emerging legal liabilities of their sponsored MCOs will be shifted to them. The good news for employers is that today, there have been no cases where employers have had to pay for injury to an employee arising out of use of the sponsored MCO. The bad news, however, is that employers are not shielded from risks or injuries sustained by an employee using a sponsored MCO on the basis of either vicarious liability or direct duty.

Under vicarious liability, the employee is judged to have received inadequate funds from the provider or the MCO to compensate for an injury and successfully demonstrates that the provider or MCO is an agent of the employer. Under direct duty, the employer is found to have breached a fiduciary duty to the employee by selecting the MCO in the first place. In either case, both employers and MCOs themselves can assess the extent of employer liability first by understanding the nature of an MCO's operations.

The nature of MCO risk

To understand MCO risk, view the organization as having a front and back end. Front-end operations include arranging for medical services in the following ways: creating a network of providers, credentialing providers, reviewing provider quality, and evaluating both the appropriateness and cost of care rendered. With a front-end problem, the result can be bodily injury to a member.

The back end, however, is an insurance operation. Regulated by state insurance departments, MCOs are required to maintain adequate surplus and financial reserves, develop adequate rate levels, market to and enroll members, determine benefit eligibility, pay claims, and buy reinsurance—typical insurance company functions. With back-end trouble, economic damages usually result (e.g., a wrongful determination of benefits). When an employer shares liability with an MCO, front-end operations (with their risk of bodily injury) are most likely to be involved.

How employers treat MCO risks

An employer's liability may arise vicariously or directly, but its methods to manage these liabilities are the same. The most effective risk treatment techniques are preventive, including

- Exercising due diligence

- Offering reasonable nonpanel options so employees cannot claim they were forced into a network

- Ensuring that providers and MCOs carry adequate liability limits so employees will not be tempted to seek recovery from employers seen as "deep pockets"

These risk prevention techniques, together with the risk transfer techniques discussed in this chapter, are employers' principal protection against managed care liability. Employers also benefit from ERISA (the Employee Retirement Income Security Act), federal legislation that restricts ERISA plan beneficiaries to recover only medical expenses from MCOs and, perhaps in the future, from the sponsoring employer that selected the MCO. However, not all employer groups are protected by ERISA (e.g., state and municipal governments and church groups). Federal employer plans are subject to similar protection by the Federal Employees Health Benefits Act (FEHBA).

Due diligence

Because steering employees to MCOs does limit employee choice, employers have some responsibility to ensure that the care provided (including the activities of network providers) does not harm employees. Employers typically seek assurances from MCOs that they have been accredited by voluntary not-for-profit organizations using defined, MCO-specific performance standards. The foremost accreditors are the National Committee for Quality Assurance (NCQA), the Utilization Review Accreditation Committee (URAC), and the Joint Commission on Accreditation of Healthcare Organizations (JCAHO). JCAHO's particular emphasis is on the delivery of care in an integrated delivery system, while NCQA focuses more on MCO administrative services that coordinate care.

Unfortunately, only a minority of MCOs are accredited. Without accreditation, employers must exercise due diligence, which involves close collaboration between the risk manager and the human resources manager. Together they review a full range of front- and back-end operations with special attention paid to provider credentialing and utilization review.

PROVIDER CREDENTIALING

Understanding an MCO's provider selection process is a high priority for employers, usually through a request to review its written policies and procedures. Employers will ask what selection criteria are used, whether on-site visits are performed, how frequently providers are recredentialed, and what minimum malpractice liability limits are required.

Employers cannot possibly verify malpractice histories and insurance program limits of all members of the MCO's independent contractor network. Therefore, it is important to employers that MCOs confirm that sufficient liability limits will be available in the event of a negligent network provider. It is also in the MCO's interest to verify that adequate limits are available since it may become a deep-pocket target in the event a negligent network provider is uninsured. MCOs should collect evidence of provider insurance limits yearly.

Finally, the employer wants to know whether the MCO relies on claims histories furnished by providers (secondary verification) or whether it works directly with malpractice carrier or databank (primary verification). With primary verification, the provider has no opportunity to alter or omit claims information. Accreditation standards require primary verification efforts, but do not yet require a next step if the claims history is poor.

UTILIZATION REVIEW

While the most frequent source of managed care liability claims allege vicarious liability for the acts of negligent providers, the most costly awards have been in the area of utilization review, especially those that lead to a wrongful denial of benefits. Employers need assurance that utilization reviewers, in their verbal and written communications, state that the treating physician is the final decision maker with respect to the appropriateness of medical care.

The employer will also review the policies and procedures of the MCO to determine if denials are decided only by a physician who specializes in the medical problem at hand.

Finally, employers will be interested in any financial incentive arrangements MCOs set up with network providers and their medical directors. Disclosure of such arrangements would be required under patient protection legislation proposed by the American Medical Association. While case law holds that financial incentive arrangements are not negligent per se, it does acknowledge that such arrangements can be negligently designed, increasing the likelihood of harm to the patient. The more the financial risks and rewards of medical services delivery shifts to the provider, the more employers (and regulators) want to know what controls are in place to prevent underutilization.

In the seminal 1993 case of *Fox v. Health Net of California,* the HMO's medical director—not an outside review panel of appropriately matched specialists—determined that the proposed autologous bone marrow transplant treatment for a member's breast cancer was experimental and, therefore, was not covered. The plaintiff presented evidence that the medical director's decision not to cover that treatment was partly based on the director's compensation and money he saved the HMO. The jury awarded the plaintiff $12.3 million in compensatory and $77 million in punitive damages before the case was settled for an undisclosed sum. More recently, financial incentive concerns produced a $45 million verdict against Kaiser in Georgia (*Adams v. Kaiser*) and two more verdicts exceeding $1 million each by the same plaintiff attorney that litigated Fox and Gaines (*Ching v. Gaines*).

Contractual guarantees

Through contractual language, an employer can obligate the MCO to establish, maintain, and monitor compliance with those stated policies and procedures the employer relied on in selecting the MCO.

INDEMNIFICATION

When contracting with MCOs, employers often seek a provision holding them harmless for liability from injury arising out of the negligent acts of the MCO. Today this is a legitimate request for employers to make and one that most MCOs accept.

However, the employer may also ask to be held harmless for liability arising from the acts of an MCO's network providers. This can be a problem, because the network often includes providers who are independent contractors. The MCO can control its own activities, but cannot be expected to exercise the same level of control over the conduct of independent contractors. MCOs should not agree to indemnification provisions for liability arising out of the acts of nonemployed network providers.

Where does this leave the employer, then, who must accept an MCO network, including its independent contractor providers? Can the employer rely on indemnification agreements executed by smaller managed care carve-out organizations, such as behavioral healthcare firms, that may have limited financial resources?

EVIDENCING OF INSURANCE

For independent contractors and smaller carve-out organizations, employers rely less on indemnification agreements than on evidence of insurance. For front-line protection against deep-pocket liability, employers will insist the MCO and the general contractor require their providers' subcontractors to show evidence of adequate insurance limits. What the MCO considers adequate and how frequently it verifies that is subject to review as part of the employer's due diligence efforts.

A limit of $1 million per incident/$3 million annual aggregate per physician is the benchmark used today, but many MCOs accept lesser amounts. In some jurisdictions, such as Texas and Florida, MCOs may be forced to accept providers who evidence no insurance limits. In that case, the employer will want assurance that the MCO's own limits are high enough to form a strong second-line defense behind the provider's limits.

Today, how much insurance should an MCO carry? The jurisdictions in which an MCO operates and the limits purchased by providers are one consideration. Another is whether the company's employees are ERISA-exempt. The ERISA exemption exposes MCOs (and the sponsoring employer that selected the MCO) to awards for pain and suffering and even bad faith. Generally, claims involving plans covered by ERISA are not presented to juries and are limited to the recovery of the cost of denied medical benefit only. There is no recovery for pain and suffering and no punitive damages. But claims against ERISA-exempt or FEHBA-exempt plans (including Medicare and Medicaid) are not limited in the same way.

In a 1993 Johnson & Higgins survey of managed care organizations, IPA-model HMOs were found to carry an average professional liability limit of $10 to $15 million. Staff models carried malpractice liability limits similar to those carried by a comparably sized medical group. By 1994, one out of four respondents' professional liability limits had increased by at least $5 million, moving steadily upward in the wake of the $89 million California jury award against Health Net and a $26 million award against Lincoln National in Idaho. While both cases were settled for significantly lesser amounts, they raise the specter of inadequate MCO limits. As a result, there has been an increased interest in punitive damage coverage in jurisdictions where punitive damages are insurable (both of these cases involved substantial punitive damage awards).

Insurance protection for the employer

One traditional request of the MCO is that it add the employer to its managed care liability policy as an additional insured. Some carriers and some MCOs have no difficulty with this request, while others resist it strenuously. If the financial strength of the MCO is satisfactory to the employer, indemnification should be adequate. But for some employers, especially those who sponsor multiple MCO plans, the patchwork risk treatment offered by indemnification agreements is inadequate. These employers have purchased insurance protection in case MCO liability should come to rest at their doorstep.

Employers looking for insurance protection should first scrutinize their traditional insurance policies for the relevant coverage. However, pension liability carriers exclude coverage for bodily injury. General liability and umbrella liability carriers provide incidental malpractice coverage, but the employer's vicarious liability for the MCO or MCO provider negligence is not an intended part of these coverages. Often the employer's insurance carriers will resist responding to this kind of allegation.

Thus, employers are left with one final option: a customized "purchaser of healthcare services" liability policy. This coverage, issued in the employer's name, protects the employer from direct and vicarious liability arising out of the MCO plans they sponsor. It does not, however, protect the employer from malpractice claims against providers who work directly for the employer (e.g., in a workplace clinic). These specialized policies offer uniform managed care liability protection, which employers may find impossible to secure through either MCO indemnification or evidencing of insurance limits. The same carriers that lead the market in managed care liability policies will write these policies for employers. The challenge is persuading the underwriters that the risk is minimal. Until case law develops holding the employer liable, these arguments should be relatively successful.

Insolvency versus liability limits

Another important issue is an employer's need to know that the MCO will remain financially solvent. Solvency issues are typically reviewed as part of the employer's due diligence. Each state requires MCOs to demonstrate financial responsibility in the form of stop-loss coverage, insolvency insurance, parental guarantees, bonds, or letters of credit. Conscientious employers will know what is required in each jurisdiction where they use an MCO and require their MCOs to prove they are in compliance with the law. This assures the employer that sufficient MCO funds will be available to pay providers and, in the process, gives the provider confidence that established employee-provider relationships will not be precipitously disrupted.

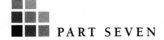

PART SEVEN

SPECIALTY AND ANCILLARY SERVICES CONTRACTING

25

Guidelines for subcontracting with specialty providers

Jonathan P. Solomons
Director, Ancillary Services
Independence Blue Cross and Keystone Health Plan East
Philadelphia, Pennsylvania

I N   A N   E R A   W H E R E   M A N A G E D   C A R E   companies are becoming increasingly popular among employers and other healthcare financiers, HMOs are becoming deluged with a variety of subcontractors bidding to deliver all or a portion of the HMO's covered services to its subscribers. These subcontractors range from full-service physician-hospital organizations (PHOs) to mental health and substance abuse, laboratory, dental, vision, and cancer therapy providers. Typically, these providers seek an exclusive arrangement with the HMO for a fixed capitation payment.

The frequent solicitation of HMOs by these subcontractors poses a set of challenges for a health plan. Essentially, the decision to subcontract is a make-or-buy decision. Does the subcontractor offer a certain expertise, quality, or cost-effective reputation that cannot be easily accomplished by the HMO directly? If so, is this expertise worth the expense of administration that must be funded by the HMO? Will the HMO's administrative costs for the newly subcontracted service decrease as expected?

This chapter reviews these questions as well as some of the reasons why HMOs choose to subcontract. It also explores why they may reject this option. Experience with an IPA-model HMO will also be cited to better understand the issues that must be addressed both in contract negotiations and implementation.

Advantages

Typically, HMOs are more receptive to subcontracting small portions of their business whose unique characteristics allow specialized providers to attain an expertise in network development and maintenance. Behavioral healthcare and dental services are probably the most commonly subcontracted services today.

Mental health and dental providers' demands on an HMO are distinct from medical providers and require individuals trained in these specialties to service them effectively. For example, dentists, who mostly provide preventive low-cost services, are quite concerned about copayments on specialty services and the scope of dental coverage since these areas significantly impact their total compensation. Mental health providers usually must work within the constraint of limited inpatient days and limited outpatient visit coverage. While HMO managers typically are well versed in medical provider issues, they are less sensitive to the unique aspects of the dental or mental health industries, and thus, the prospect of developing and maintaining networks for these nonmedical services is not attractive to them. However, the availability of a large number of mental health and dental providers with solid track records makes the decision to subcontract much easier.

A second reason to subcontract is the ability to shift financial risk to the subcontractor. Assuming that the capitated subcontractor is offering a large network that can effectively cover the HMO's service area, it makes little sense to contract with other providers. This would result in the HMO paying for the same member twice.

In return for exclusivity, the subcontractor is usually required to accept a fixed capitation payment for the HMO's members that does not vary with utilization. The HMO's cost of the subcontracted service is now predictable and can be accurately budgeted. The subcontractor, because of its expertise, is expected to manage utilization and control unit cost. This is accomplished by contracting with a network on a capitation, per case, or fee schedule basis and requiring the network to adhere to its utilization management policies.

A third advantage of subcontracting is the HMO's desire to create a barrier between itself and the servicing provider. In industries such as dental and mental health, where the payments are relatively low, the subcontractor is forced to address provider grievances. Any grumblings about managed care (e.g., infringing on a provider's practice or meddling) are directed at the subcontractor, not the HMO.

A fourth reason to subcontract is the HMO's expectation that its administrative costs of developing and maintaining its various networks will be reduced by passing them on to the subcontractor. In an extremely competitive market, the subcontractor must minimize its operating margin to bid for the HMO's business. In theory, the subcontractor's expertise and economies of scale (if it services several HMOs) should result in overall administrative cost savings.

A final reason to subcontract is that in the long run providers may be more effective at managing and policing themselves. Full-risk arrangements are being implemented with PHOs because HMOs are continually looking to develop low-cost products in response to employers' number one question—what is the premium? In theory, full-service PHO providers will be more sensitive to the cost of ordering tests or referring to specialists if they are at-risk for those costs. In addition, providers are more likely to change their behavior as a result of education by peers versus a "meddling" insurance company.

Disadvantages

There are many reasons HMOs reject the subcontracting option. The principal reason is that the HMO believes that it can manage the network better itself and that the subcontractor adds little value. For example, one large HMO planned to capitate physical therapy services. The organization looked at two options: recontracting with the existing freestanding network or exclusively contracting with one provider that owned several sites. Since this HMO already had a large network in place and was confident it could be maintained under capitation because of its market power, the decision to reject the subcontracting option was straightforward.

However, the HMO also decided to reject the prospective physical therapy contractor because the value added by the subcontractor (i.e., experience in managing physical therapists) was not worth the additional $.07 per member per month (PMPM) payout required to fund the subcontractor's administrative costs and profit margin. The HMO believed that it could hire and train an individual instead. Similarly, the HMO rejected a radiology management company's proposal to assume responsibility for a capitated radiology network because the HMO believed that it could exceed the $1.40 PMPM reduction in fee-for-service leakage proposed by the prospective subcontractor. The HMO subsequently hired a manager dedicated to its radiology network and was able to reduce leakage by more than $2.00 PMPM.

The HMO's decision to manage its existing physical therapy network revealed a third disadvantage of using subcontractors (only applicable if a network for the subcontracted service is already in place). By replacing its existing network with an exclusive contract with one provider, the HMO would have alienated its existing physical therapy network and may have unsettled its other specialty networks.

There are additional disadvantages in subcontracting to a full-service PHO. Even if the PHO only covers a small portion of the HMO's members, a significant amount of middle-management time and management information system (MIS) resources are consumed in implementing such an arrangement. This is particularly true if the HMO pays claims on behalf of the PHO but allows the PHO to develop payment arrangements that differ from those of the HMO. One HMO invested approximately $200,000 to enhance its MIS so that a PHO contract could be implemented. It also used the three full-time equivalents (FTEs) over a 12-month period to develop policies and coordinate operations with the PHO staff. One FTE was then needed to work with the PHO staff.

A second concern in implementing full-risk PHO contracts is an HMO's fear of spawning a competitor. Once the PHO hires staff and purchases a sophisticated MIS, it is well positioned to use its experience and the HMO's small membership pool as springboards to obtain additional contracts or become a licensed competitor. The PHO also is more likely to pursue independence once it is less dependent on the HMO's expertise, particularly in marketing, claims payment, and information reporting.

A final disadvantage of subcontracting to a PHO is the HMO's perceived loss of control over the network in terms of quality and service. The subcontractor may be less responsive to provider concerns and more eager to slash reimbursement as a means of preserving its profit margin. If the subcontractor is purely profit oriented, it may credential any provider willing to accept low fees. The addition of an intermediary leaves the HMO dependent on the subcontractor to manage the network effectively. If the subcontractor performs poorly, resulting in member quality complaints or spiraling utilization, the HMO will ultimately have to step in and assume the subcontractor's function. The decision to subcontract does not get the HMO off the hook in obligations to its members.

Another disadvantage is the complications that subcontractors bring. Regulatory bodies are increasingly sensitive to the need to monitor use of subcontractors. Some states, such as Pennsylvania, have demanded that HMOs develop strict subcontractor oversight guidelines. These guidelines, which are consistent with NCQA guidelines, require the HMO to closely monitor the subcontractor and its fulfillment of contractual obligations. Essentially, the HMO must validate that the subcontractor is adhering to quality assurance and utilization management policies as applicable.

In order to ensure that providers are not left "holding the bag" by an insolvent unlicensed subcontractor, states have insisted that HMOs retain contracts with the subcontractor's network and pay claims directly. The subcontractor is allowed to determine the payment terms (e.g., fee schedule) and the network configuration (e.g., determining which providers to contract with). Since subcontractors are not licensed HMOs, they do not fall under the oversight of the state departments of health or insurance. As a result, the HMO's subcontractor arrangements are closely scrutinized to ensure that the HMO regularly monitors the subcontractor's financial condition and provider network. Unfortunately for the HMO, these regulatory requirements further increase the administrative resources needed to support subcontractor arrangements.

Feasibility

In light of all the potential pitfalls and advantages, the decision to subcontract should be evaluated thoroughly before reaching an agreement. The decision process should consist of several components: (1) evaluating the subcontractor's strengths and weaknesses and its fit with the HMO's objectives (e.g., is the subcontractor an appropriate strategic partner?), (2) conducting due diligence on the subcontractor (e.g., analysis of financials, operations, caliber of management staff, quality of network, reference checks, and validation of the subcontractor's quality assurance plan), and (3) evaluating the impact on the HMO's existing operations (e.g., additional MIS system enhancements needed, staff training, and availability of staff resources for implementation).

During contract negotiations, the HMO should begin involving its managers in implementation planning. A task force consisting of representatives from MIS, claims, utilization management, provider relations, quality assurance, marketing, finance, and operations should be created and begin meeting regularly until full implementation. A full-service PHO subcontract can take up to a year to implement, particularly if major MIS changes are required (such as developing fee schedules unique to a selected pool of members). It is imperative that the task force understand the objective of the subcontract and how it fits with the HMO's overall mission. Lack of cooperation by any of these departments can quickly damage the relationship between the HMO and the subcontractor. A work plan detailing tasks, persons responsible, and deadlines should be developed and agreed to by the task force.

The task force should be given the opportunity to critique the proposed subcontracting arrangement and suggest modifications prior to contract execution. Frequently, the contract negotiations have omitted a key operational detail or may have proposed an arrangement that is unworkable. For example, one HMO task force rejected a proposed subcontracting arrangement involving two different utilization management systems with responsibility for claims payment and member services being split between the HMO and the subcontractor. The task force's recommendation was then passed on to senior management, which agreed to drop the proposal.

By involving an operations-oriented task force during contract negotiation, HMOs can more effectively assess whether the benefits of the proposed arrangement offset the costs. The cost of system enhancements is relatively easy to calculate once MIS realizes the proposed division of responsibilities. The investment in staff is not so easy to compute because most of the individuals involved in the project also have many other responsibilities; it is helpful if staff can log the hours expended on the subcontracting project.

A proposed subcontracting arrangement should be subject to the same return-on-investment analysis required of any major capital purchase. Unfortunately, because the benefits and some of the costs are not tangible and easy to measure, HMO management often ignores this analysis and shifts directly from conception to contract negotiation and implementation. The HMO should attempt to quantify the benefits and costs of the proposed arrangement.

First, the capitated investment must be computed. The investment consists of the staff hours required to design and implement MIS changes, develop and document changes to medical policy, negotiate and execute the contract, attend task force and sub-task force meetings as applicable, and conduct appropriate validation of the subcontractor's quality assurance plan (QA). Validation of the QA plan depends on the scope of subcontracted QA services but typically includes review of the subcontractor's credentialing process, its medical record audit process, utilization management policies and procedures, and compilation of utilization measures such as immunization rates, and bed days per 1,000 compared with utilization for the HMO's nonsubcontracted members.

The annual revenue stream is then computed, which consists of the percentage of premium retained by the HMO multiplied by the additional member months enrolled in the new products affiliated with the subcontractor. If the HMO's medical costs are expected to decrease under the new arrangement, these reduced costs should be added to the revenue stream.

Annual costs of the subcontractor arrangement should then be computed. As shown in Table 1, these costs are staff hours expended by various HMO departments on an ongoing basis. Additional staff and increasing responsibilities of existing staff may be required, and task force meetings will be required periodically to monitor the arrangement and to design and implement additional MIS modifications. A dedicated HMO liaison will be needed to resolve operating issues and relay PHO concerns to senior management and department heads. Additional claims processing time will be needed to orient processors on any new payment arrangement and to process claims generated by additional members.

Additional marketing staff may be required to market the new products. Medical management staff will need to interact frequently with the subcontractor's utilization management staff, particularly in the first year of operation, to ensure that medical policies are applied consistently. Additional provider relations staff will also be needed in the first year to interface with the claims department and ensure a smooth transition of provider relations functions.

Finance staff will be needed to calculate capitation payments and reconcile amounts owed to the subcontractor after claims payment and incurred but not reported (IBNR) claims are deducted. QA staff

TABLE 1

A full-service PHO arrangement

Capital investment	=	System changes	(Hours required × hourly rate of MIS staff)
	+	Medical policy development	(Staff hours × average hourly salary)
	+	Contracting	(Staff hours × average hourly rate)
	+	Task force meetings	(Number of meetings × average length × average hourly salaries)
	+	Legal review	(Staff hours × average hourly rate)
	+	Quality assurance review	(Staff hours × average hourly rate)

Revenue stream	=	Number of new member months × HMO retention PMPM (years 1–5) for all applicable subcontracting arrangements. (If separate capital investments are required for each arrangement, only member months applicable to each should be included.)
	+	Medical cost PMPM decrease × member months

Less annual operating costs	=	Task force meetings after implementation	(Number of meetings × average length × average hourly salaries)
	+	Staff liaison with PHO	(Staff hours × average hourly rate)
	+	Additional claims processing	(Number of claims × processing/claim hours × average hourly rate)
	+	Additional marketing	(Marketing staff hours × average hourly rate)
	+	Additional medical management	(Medical management staff hours × average hourly rate)
	+	Additional provider relations	(Provider relations staff hours × average hourly rate)
	+	Additional finance	(Finance staff hours × average hourly rate)
	+	Additional quality assurance	(QA staff hours × average hourly rate)

are needed to comply with subcontractor oversight guidelines, which usually include quarterly site visits and data review.

Once the net annual return is computed, net present value can be calculated. Management can then add intangible factors, such as the value of a strategic partnership or the risks of the subcontractor contracting with another HMO, to fully evaluate the logic of proceeding with the proposed arrangement. A make-versus-buy analysis is applicable when evaluating a limited service subcontract such as dental, mental health or substance abuse.

The contract

Once the decision is made to proceed, a term sheet should be submitted to the subcontractor that summarizes the HMO's contractual requirements and the subcontractor's obligations (see Exhibit 1 for example). Several safeguards are essential if the HMO intends on minimizing the reasons not to subcontract discussed above.

First, the HMO should retain claims payment, MIS, and marketing functions. These are appropriate HMO functions and what HMOs do best. The subcontractor is less likely to develop into an HMO if there is no reason to develop full-service capability. It will be difficult for the subcontractor to develop relationships with employer groups if the HMO retains responsibility for marketing.

The HMO will minimize system changes and operations headaches if it insists that the subcontractor develop payment arrangements consistent with the HMO. For example, the subcontractor should not be permitted to pay fee for service to a specialty capitated by the HMO. Similarly, the scope of capitated services within a specialty should be identical.

If the subcontractor chooses to perform utilization management (UM), which it should if it is assuming financial risk, it should be required to use the HMO's MIS and to adopt its UM policies.

It is critical that the functions performed by the HMO and the subcontractor be explicitly laid out in the contract. Exhibit 2 is an example of the format used by one HMO that divides the responsibilities for each key functional area: UM, provider relations, operations, member services, QA, finance, MIS, marketing, claims, and enrollment. If the HMO is required to provide all MIS reports, these reports should be listed, including examples of each and the applicable production schedule. Responsibility for developing additional reports and for the costs of hardware and software installation should also be spelled out.

Trust is essential between the HMO and the subcontractor for the arrangement to be successful. For products applicable to the subcontractor, the HMO should establish a maximum rate differential between its open panel and closed panel products. This will minimize the HMO's temptation to lowball the premium for products where the subcontractor is assuming significant risk. The subcontractor should also be permitted to review the HMO's rate filings and have veto power over filed rates that exceed the differential threshold.

The HMO should negotiate a long-term contract, of at least five years, that includes a provision preventing the subcontractor from submitting an HMO application during the contract. Standard termination clauses should be in the contract, including an explicit statement that the pool of members covered by the subcontractor is the HMO's members and revert to the HMO upon termination.

Performance parameters are desirable, although the HMO will also have to commit to certain standards. Essential performance parameters required of the subcontractor include network configuration (e.g., number and ratio of primary care physicians to specialists or number of dental offices), lab-test turnaround time, compliance with defined UM and QA policies, number of member and provider grievances covered by the subcontractor, promptness of grievance resolution, and financial performance. The HMO may have to commit to membership targets, accuracy and promptness of information reporting, and accuracy and promptness of claims payment.

In addition, regulatory bodies will typically require that clauses covering hold harmless language, compliance with state department of health or insurance regulations and directives, financial reserves, and grievance procedures be included in the contract.

Once the contract is executed, copies should be distributed to the task force with a full explanation of any changes from that originally proposed. The work plan should be tracked and updated as necessary. Each department must be accountable to complete its required tasks and report its progress to the task force.

Conclusion

HMOs should proceed with caution when entering into a subcontracting arrangement. The potential benefits (i.e., increased market share from an expanded product line or reduced medical costs) are often outweighed by the disadvantages—the MIS and staffing investment and the annual staffing required to implement the arrangement. The HMO should carefully assess the feasibility of such an arrangement and modify it when necessary.

When subcontracting, the HMO should not lose sight of its overall mission, to provide a high-quality, cost-effective product that combines the insurance and health delivery functions. The HMO's image in the market begins to diminish as more of its core functions shift to subcontractors. In an extreme view, the HMO merely collects premium dollars and holds the operating license while the subcontractors perform the functions abdicated by the HMO. The HMO's members affiliate more closely with the subcontractors from whom they are receiving services.

HMOs should never abdicate their obligation of developing innovative products and methods of managing medical costs. Subcontractors should be used when they clearly add value to the HMO's products and operations because of economies of scale or demonstrated expertise.

EXHIBIT 1

Date

Mr./Ms. _____
President and Chief Executive Officer
ABC Health Plan

Dear _____:

This letter of intent sets forth the general terms upon which Health Plan ("HP") will negotiate and execute with Sub Health Plan ("SHP") an agreement (the "Agreement") whereby SHP will be responsible for the provision of covered medical services to HP Medicare members residing in specific geographic areas surrounding _____ and _____ Hospitals. Such geographical areas may be expanded from time to time upon mutual agreement of the parties. Such members shall be enrolled in a closed panel arrangement (the "Plan"), under which Plan members will be restricted to providers designated as SHP network providers (the "Panel"). SHP will be paid by HP an agreed upon capitation amount that is not less than _____ percent of the monthly premium applicable to each member subject to deductions for covered services provided by HP.

Responsibilities of SHP

1. SHP will be responsible for member services, marketing, and billing (if applicable) to individuals (within designated service area), provider recruitment and relations, precertification, concurrent review, case management, enrollment, and development of marketing materials.

2. SHP will provide any additional information required by the Departments of Insurance and Health. HP will review this information and prepare and submit the application for state approval. It is understood that State approval will not be obtained until the contract is approved by HCFA.

3. SHP will comply with all HCFA and State requirements pertaining to member/provider grievances and appeals. SHP will also provide HP, on a timely basis, any information required by KePRO.

4. SHP will recruit providers for the Plan and will have the right to add or remove providers from the Plan's panel only so long as such providers have been credentialed and participate in HP. Panel primary care physicians must also meet criteria to participate in the HP65 product. Providers will sign an addendum to their HP contract specifying the terms unique to the Plan.

5. SHP will comply with all State and HCFA requirements to operate the Plan.

6. SHP will comply with all subcontractor oversight procedures agreed between the State and HP.

7. SHP will require that its providers limit referrals to those participating in the closed panel network for all nonemergency services that can be performed in-panel. Specialty services (e.g., bone marrow transplants) that cannot be performed in the panel will be referred to a HP participating provider.

8. The ID card and color will be consistent with all other HP ID cards with the HP and _____ logo on the top and the product name just below the logo. The product name should be HP 65 with a tag line specific to the panel hospitals. The SHP logo will also appear on the card. SHP will be responsible for generating the card.

9. SHP will use its own skilled nursing facility (once credentialed by HP) to provide skilled nursing services to Plan members.

10. SHP will not market the Plan to employer groups. The Plan will initially have a $ 0 premium with prescription drug coverage. The Plan benefits will mirror those included in other HP Medicare closed panel products to be marketed outside of the designated geographic area.

11. SHP recognizes and agrees that all Plan members are HP members and that HP is solely responsible for all interaction with regulatory authorities. Upon termination of this contract for any reason, SHP agrees not to market to or in any way contact then-current Plan members for a period of two (2) years.

12. SHP's UM activities will be restricted to panel hospitals.

13. SHP will complete all financial reports required by the Department of Insurance on a timely basis including quarterly reports and insurance "blanks."

Responsibilities of HP

1. HP will interface with KePRO and credential panel providers, perform all QA activities as required by regulatory and external review bodies, transmit eligibility information from CompuServe to SHP, supply the applicable subscriber agreement, and interface with HCFA and State regulatory bodies.

2. HP will not market a similar closed panel Medicare product within a mutually agreed upon, exclusive, geographic area but may market its HP 65 product or a commercial closed panel product within the designated area. Upon termination of this contract by breach of HP, HP agrees not to market a similar closed panel Medicare product within the designated geographic area for a period of two (2) years. HP will market the Plan to employer groups.

3. HP participating providers will initially provide home care, DME, laboratory, radiology, mental health, and dialysis services. Services can be added or deleted as mutually agreed.

4. HP contracted rates with participating hospitals and physicians other than panel providers must be used for services rendered to SHP closed panel members by such nonpanel providers. HP will provide SHP with the applicable Medicare rate on out-of-area admissions based on the DRG grouper and pricer.

5. HP will submit all applications and information required by HCFA and the State regulatory bodies. HP will make best efforts to obtain regulatory approval by _____.

6. HP will remit to SHP a monthly capitation amount within 10 days of receiving such from HCFA less deductions for claims (including an IBNR reserve) or capitated services paid by HP on SHP's behalf. HP will also retain reserves to pay two months of expected claims.

7. HP will provide UM services for Plan members receiving services at nonpanel providers.

The final terms and conditions of any arrangement agreed to by the parties shall be reflected in a final definitive agreement subject to regulatory approval. HP and SHP agree to work diligently and in good faith toward executing such an agreement. Such agreement shall be executed no later than _____.

Please indicate your agreement with the foregoing by signing below.

Sincerely,

Approved:
ABC Health Plan

By: _____

Senior Vice President
Health Plan

Title: _____

Date: _____

EXHIBIT 2
HMO/PHO division of responsibilities

Activity	PHO	HMO
Utilization management		
Precertification—panel providers	■	
Precertification—out-of-panel providers		■
Concurrent review—panel provider	■	
Concurrent review—out-of-panel providers		■
Case management	■	
Provider relations		
Recruit panel providers	■	
Orient panel providers	■	■
Service panel providers	■	
Develop/update panel provider directory		■
Approve panel provider directory	■	
Handle initial phone inquiries—panel provider	■	■
Follow-up—panel provider phone inquiries	■	
Complete panel provider change sheet	■	
Input panel provider changes in MIS		■
Handle informal panel provider complaints	■	
Handle first-level panel provider complaints	■	
Handle subsequent level panel provider complaints		■
Determine capitation and fee schedule—panel provider	■	
Input capitation and fee schedule changes		■
Approve exception payments to panel provider	■	
Approve exception payments to nonpanel provider		■
Update fee schedule	■	
Maintain provider manuals		■
Approve provider manual references to PHO products	■	
Provide copies of all general provider mailings		■
Provide copies of medical policy updates		■
Operations		
Approve panel facility payments more than $50,000	■	
Approve nonpanel facility payments more than $50,000		■
Approve panel physician claims more than $1,000	■	
Approve nonpanel physician claims more than $1,000		■
Negotiate nonpar provider claims		■
Supply missing fees for suspended claims	■	
Process suspended claims for missing fees		■
Develop and revise suspense criteria		■
Maintain error codes, EOB, statement of remittance messages		■
Conduct periodic audit of claims		■
Review and approve ER payment (non-auto-pay)		■
Approve payment of medical record invoices		■
Coordinate claims adjustment due to retroactive UM decisions		■

EXHIBIT 2 (CONTINUED)

Activity	PHO	HMO
Operations (cont.)		
Handle inquiries regarding HMO employees who have selected panel PCP		■
Pursue COB and subrogation		■
Retain COB and subrogation collected	■	
Process panel member enrollment		■
Process panel member PCP changes		■
Process all provider claims		■
Generate ID cards		■
Generate capitation payments		■
Member services		
Handle panel member inquiries		■
Handle initial grievances		■
Handle grievance review		■
Approve exception payments to panel provider	■	
Approve exception payments to nonpanel provider		■
Update member handbooks and related materials		■
Quality assurance		
Credential and recredential panel providers		■
Develop and implement QA programs		■
Maintain subcontractor guidelines		■
Maintain member grievance log		■
Maintain provider grievance log		■
Conduct member satisfaction survey		■
Submit QA reports required by Department of Health		■
Sanction providers when applicable		■
Issue reports to HMO board of directors regarding services provided by PHO		■
Conduct focused reviews		■
Conduct studies on adverse outcomes		■
Evaluate sentinel conditions and target diagnoses for quality of care	■	
Review utilization and quality data on panel providers	■	
Finance		
Approve capitation and fee schedule changes		■
Load and update panel (system) profiles		■
Load and update hospital profiles		■
Reconcile claims estimate to actual		■
Maintain IBNR	■	■
File premium rates with Department of Insurance		■
Approve rate filing if meets differential criteria	■	
Provide copies of regulatory correspondence		■
Bill, collect, and reconcile group premiums		■
Obtain regulatory approvals		■

EXHIBIT 2 (CONTINUED)

Activity	PHO	HMO
Finance (cont.)		
Submit reports required by Departments of Health and Insurance		■
Assist in preparation of required DOH, DOI reports related to PHO products	■	
MIS		
Provide on-line access to panel member, panel provider data		■
Provide LAN and MIS system support		■
Provide training on use of data shells		■
Run data shells to support cost analysis	■	
Provide access to new data retrieval systems		■
Provide training on use of new data retrieval systems		■
Provide training on system menu-generated reports (e.g., daily hospital log)		■
Generate system reports	■	
Process system enhancement requests		■
Marketing		
Develop strategy and supporting materials		■
Approve strategy and supporting materials	■	
Approve underwriting guidelines if varying from standard	■	
Market PHO-affiliated product to groups and brokers		■
Conduct open enrollments		■
Health services		
Provide mental health and substance abuse services		■
Provide family planning services		■
Provide wellness services		■
Provide pharmacy, vision, and dental rider services		■

⬛ 26

Behavioral health capitation

Bruce Gorman
Vice President, Public Sector Programs
Merit Behavioral Care
South San Francisco, California

IN BEHAVIORAL HEALTHCARE delivery, many providers believe their growth, success, and ultimate survival depends on their ability to provide services under capitation. However, the percentage of providers in the behavioral healthcare industry who understand the risks associated with capitation, possess the systems to ensure success, and are prepared for capitation is relatively small.

This chapter describes the requirements of managing behavioral healthcare programs under capitation, when it is necessary and advantageous to enter into a capitated arrangement, the differences between capitation and subcapitation, the tools and systems that must be in place to enter into a capitation arrangement, and the unique features of capitation in behavioral healthcare.

Why consider capitation? Many behavioral healthcare providers and organizations consider capitation and subcapitation arrangements for inappropriate reasons. Some believe that without capitation, the provider will not survive in managed care markets. However, others believe capitation will enable the provider to

- Perform clinical services and operate its business as it sees fit

- Maximize its income and revenue

- Receive a cut of the large profits that managed care companies, insurance carriers, and HMOs receive

- Possess an inherent understanding of capitation because it already delivers services within a fixed budget (this is often cited by such non-profit providers as community mental health organizations)

- Have a distinct advantage over competitors in all markets

- Provide all the information and tools needed to capitate successfully

While elements of these conceptions about capitation or subcapitation may be correct, none of these assumptions are inherently valid. In fact, the opposite of each assumption may occur if capitation is poorly executed. Determining whether and where to enter into capitated arrangements requires careful analysis and forethought. This means analyzing purchasers' benefit designs (including out-of-pocket expenses required by the patient), risk profile of the population to be served, and expected utilization rates. It also means examining the nature of the provider network that will deliver services and the purchasers' objectives for access, cost, and utilization.

Some of the key factors to be addressed when considering capitation are whether

- Capitation creates a marketing advantage in terms of product differentiation

- Quality and appropriate care can be delivered under the proposed arrangement

- Actuarial experience and utilization information indicate the service can be performed within the negotiated capitation payment

- The necessary clinical, management, and financial systems are in place to manage the program

- Financial reserves or stop-loss coverage are sufficient to withstand unexpected or temporary losses or cash-flow problems

- Appropriate controls to identify and correct over- and underutilization are in place

- The population and delivery system are sufficiently understood to improve outcomes

Alternatives to consider

Organizations must assess the feasibility of providing services under capitation because such arrangements may demand considerable investment in clinical and management systems. The needs and desires of the market, the purchasers, and the covered members should also be considered. In addition to making this assessment, providers should recognize that other forms of reimbursement, including those that have elements of capitation but tend to limit risk, are also possible. Some of these include

- *Case rates.* These are arrangements whereby the provider or organization is reimbursed a flat amount for providing a specific level and amount of service for a patient (e.g., outpatient therapy) regardless of the number of sessions required

- *Retained providers.* These providers devote a specific amount of their professional time to providing services to a payer group or population. For example, a provider may deliver services exclusively for a managed care company's beneficiaries for a certain number of hours per month and be paid a flat amount for that time. In other words, such providers contract out blocks of time for a fixed fee, regardless of number of patients seen in that time. Sometimes providers are designated as key provider groups (e.g., anchor groups or regional service groups) in a similar arrangement

- *Risk and reward arrangements.* In these arrangements a percentage of the provider's reimbursement is based upon some financial and clinical performance objective. For example, if the cost of delivering services falls within an expected range, and the provider's patients achieve expected clinical outcomes, the provider is paid an additional payment over the previously negotiated fee. In contrast, if treatment objectives are not met, the provider will be paid less than the expected amount

- *Withhold.* This method is used extensively by medical individual practice associations (IPAs), whereby a percentage (e.g., 10 to 20 percent) of the negotiated fee-for-service payment is withheld and then issued if clinical outcome and financial performance objectives are met

By understanding available options, providers can consider an alternative to capitation, such as when adequate claims and utilization information are not available, when a provider is asked to assume risk for services that it does not deliver, or when the provider is unprepared to accept capitation.

In addition, recognizing the difference between capitation and subcapitation is important to determine whether to enter into a capitation arrangement and what resources will be required. Where capitation refers to financial and clinical responsibility for all covered health services for a given population, subcapitation refers to providing a limited type of service (e.g., outpatient services) or providing services in a geographically limited area within a community on a capitated or per member per month (PMPM) basis. In general, the risk and related management requirements are greater in a fully capitated program than in a subcapitated relationship because of the complex clinical and financial management requirements involved in full capitation.

Capitation readiness

A key difference between physical healthcare and behavioral healthcare is that behavioral healthcare practices are guided more by each provider's clinical philosophy, orientation, and training than in general medicine. Unlike medical-surgical conditions, the signs and symptoms of mental illness do not lend themselves to precise or direct measurement. Hallucinations, unlike fevers, lack diagnostic specificity and reliability due to their variable interpretations and the paucity of objective (as opposed to subjective) signs and symptoms. Further, the specificity of behavioral interventions is variable. For example, the clinical response of depression to medications or psychotherapy can be virtually equivalent. A chemical dependency program oriented to a particular treatment regimen will likely take an allotted number of days as compared to a program progressively based on a continuum of care.

The behavioral healthcare organization must have a flexible clinical philosophy that is consistent with both a capitated arrangement and the needs of the purchaser. For example, many HMOs only cover crisis-related services, and the provider must be prepared to render services accordingly.

Generally, in order to work successfully in a behavioral health capitated environment, it is essential to offer the following: a full continuum of care, treatment in the least restrictive and most appropriate treatment setting, ability to measure and demonstrate improved outcomes, and procedures and programs to return the patient to maximum functioning as soon as possible. Therefore, the capitated provider must ensure that inpatient, partial hospitalization, day treatment, intensive outpatient, and similar nontraditional services are available. It is important for the capitated caregiver either to deliver or to arrange for the delivery of these services. Reliance on a fixed and inflexible approach to treatment, such as providing services at a level of care that is inappropriate, is a prescription for failure under capitation.

Management information systems (MIS) that can track clinical, utilization, financial, and outcomes information are necessary for success in a capitated arrangement. However, many providers and organizations do not have the requisite MIS to evaluate their cost of delivering services, particularly in a capitation arrangement. Lack of this information can lead to financial or clinical failure of the program. For example, an inability to track utilization in inpatient and other higher-cost service settings can result in a squandering of resources. Under a full-risk arrangement, the capitated provider is responsible for covering all the costs of clinical services plus associated administrative expenses.

Cost overruns are also the provider's responsibility, who must make up the difference from other revenue sources or from purchased stop-loss coverage. To prevent this problem, the organization must have a system of authorizing, certifying, managing, monitoring, and evaluating its services. This requires a utilization management or review function, including the application of medical necessity or best practices guidelines. These support systems must also be able to meet payers' demands for data that demonstrate clinical, quality, and financial performance, such as patient satisfaction results, comparisons of cost required to achieve levels of patient functioning and analyses of recidivism (i.e., frequently returning to an intense level of care as a result of treatment failures at a lower level of care).

To be successful under capitation, the provider must ensure that a full continuum of care is available and consistent with the benefits available to the member. The organization or provider also must be aware of the range of available services, even those outside its own delivery system. Ensuring continuity (e.g., providing and coordinating care when, where, and to the extent necessary) and a full continuum of services (e.g., inpatient, residential, partial hospitalization, intensive outpatient, outpatient) is essential to providing high-quality, appropriate, and cost-effective services. Careful attention to discharge planning and active management of patient care are also crucial.

Developing and managing a wide-ranging network of providers requires much attention. Depending upon the services offered, the provider's responsibility can range from the actual development and management of the network of services to, at a minimum, understanding the level (e.g., inpatient, intensive outpatient) and quality of care provided by others. For example, even though the capitated provider may be responsible only for delivering outpatient services in a particular area, it must be intimately familiar with and prepared to determine which inpatient, intensive outpatient, and partial hospitalization services are delivered. This is especially true if the capitated provider is financially responsible for the levels of services that they don't provide.

Lastly, the provider must have the financial strength and stability or have sufficient stop-loss protection to implement a capitated arrangement. Even in the most effective, efficient, and well-underwritten arrangements there are likely to be months (and even more extended periods of time) in which financial losses are possible. This is particularly true when the capitated provider is fully at-risk for inpatient services or for an unusually high-utilizing population, such as Medicaid beneficiaries. Furthermore, there are always periods of time in which utilization, particularly expensive inpatient care, exceeds expectations. A carefully planned strategy to withstand these occurrences by spreading risk over a variety of programs or populations will increase the likelihood of success.

Clinical issues and system

The clinical elements of a successful capitated program include a comprehensive range of services and multiple levels of care integrated into the care delivery network. Most behavioral care capitated arrangements create benefit design flexibility to allow the provider or manager to use a wide range of settings and services. Known as flexing benefits or individual case management, these techniques allow the managed care company or capitated provider to arrange for services that are not specifically included in the benefits package, such as providing outpatient services in lieu of more costly, unnecessary inpatient services. This is key to the ability to improve quality, outcomes, and accessibility, while simultaneously creating cost efficiencies.

Another clinical element is a utilization management system. The capitated provider or organization needs to develop a method of determining reimbursement for services based on sound, documented medical necessity guidelines in combination with clinical judgment. In the absence of these guidelines and ongoing monitoring and correction, care may be delivered in ways that are not consistent with patients' needs or are not an effective use of benefit dollars. Management of these factors by clinicians focused on this activity are necessary to ensure both quality and cost effectiveness.

ORIENTATION TO CARE DELIVERY

Providers and organizations participating in capitated arrangements must have an orientation or clinical philosophy recognizing the need to deliver services consistent with the members' benefits plans in a cost-effective manner. Therefore, such concepts as medical necessity, clinical appropriateness, the least restrictive level of care, individual treatment planning, patient responsibility, and clinical efficacy must be embraced. Often this requires considerable provider education as well as adjustments in professional orientation and practice patterns. These activities can be accomplished through case conferences, managed care seminars, and consultation with managed care consultants.

APPROPRIATE MIX OF UTILIZATION AND COST OF CARE

When determining the proper level of capitation—or determining if an effective, high-quality program can be delivered within a certain capitation rate—it is necessary to forecast the appropriate mix of services to be delivered and the likely amount of services needed by the covered members. Therefore, precise forecasting of inpatient day utilization, intermediate care utilization (e.g., partial hospitalization, day treatment, intensive outpatient), and outpatient and community support services (particularly for Medicaid populations) is essential. Such forecasting depends on proper analysis of previous utilization data, estimates of the impact that careful management of care will have on utilization results, determination of the types and levels of care available, and study of the impact of changes in benefit design.

Table 1 represents an illustration of forecasting the impact of managed care for a managed behavioral care program and indicates the logic for developing a capitation rate.

Some of the key items to note include

1. The before-and-after effect of "managed activities"

2. The component costs of the delivery of care (e.g., days per 1,000, average length of stay [ALOS], and admits per 1,000) and changes in the cost of care (e.g., $750 per day negotiated to $625 for an inpatient day)

3. Benefit design changes are factored into the calculation (i.e., changes in coinsurance from 80 percent to 100 percent coverage)

4. The use of intermediate care (e.g., partial hospitalization, day treatment, intensive outpatient services) went from no utilization to substantial utilization under the managed care activities

5. The total cost of claims (delivery of services) in this scenario has been reduced by 36 percent, while the number of eligible members receiving outpatient care (this is sometimes known as penetration) increased by more than 20 percent. This is accomplished by decreasing unnecessary inpatient utilization, using intermediate care services, decreasing the average number of outpatient visits, and negotiating lower reimbursement for units of care

6. An increase in administrative cost (including profits) of 185 percent (this represents costs to manage an effective program). However, even with this increase, the overall aggregate cost of the program (i.e., claims and administration) has decreased by more than 30 percent from $11.74 to $8.16 PMPM

In many programs, the use of inpatient services is higher than necessary because of a lack of available alternatives, the failure to use inpatient services only when medically necessary, or benefit designs that create incentives to use inpatient care inappropriately. In some cases, inpatient days can be reduced 30 percent and more, using less costly settings. Forecasting requires the experience and the involvement of actuarial

TABLE 1
XYZ Corporation

	Unmanaged activities	Managed activities
Employees	1,000	1,000
Number of members	3,000	3,000
	Base	**Forecast**
Inpatient MH/CD		
Admits per 1,000	7.00	5.00
ALOS	12.00	10.00
Days per 1,000	84.00	50.00
Per diem with professional fee	$750.00	$625.00
Coinsurance	80%	100%
PMPM	$4.20	$2.60
Intermediate care		
Admits per 1,000		2.00
ALOS		15.00
Days per 1,000		30.00
Per diem with professional fee		$200.00
Coinsurance		100%
PMPM		$ .50
Outpatient MH/CD		
Percent of lives using care	6.2%	7.5%
Average number of visits	16.00	10.00
Visits per 1,000	992.00	750.00
Cost per visit	$87.00	$65.00
PMPM	$7.19	$4.06
Total claims cost	*$11.39*	*$7.16*
Administrative fee plus profit	$ .35	$1.00
Total cost	*$11.74*	*$8.16*

and financial analysts, clinical managers (particularly those familiar with the community, the types and levels of care available, and referral and treatment patterns), and operations personnel.

Another element of successful capitated programs is interaction with physical healthcare delivery systems. Behavioral healthcare providers and organizations must communicate with general medical providers and healthcare delivery systems to integrate care as fully as possible. A significant amount of interdependency between general health and behavioral health is best maximized when there is coordination of services. Several medical offset studies illustrate a significant positive relationship between the delivery of focused behavioral health services and the cost of medical care.[1] A significant portion of the illnesses for which patients seek primary care physicians (PCPs) include behavioral components. Additionally, PCPs often perform behavioral health services—most notably, administering psychiatric medication—although coding their services as regular office visits. It is imperative for capitated health providers to determine, in advance, if they are responsible for these services and how to accomplish the often difficult task of managing these relationships. Some ways to manage these relationships include in-service orientations with PCPs, developing protocols for sharing clinical information when a patient gives informed consent, and offering consults to PCPs.

Financial issues

There are several financial issues to be addressed.

RESERVE AND REINSURANCE REQUIREMENTS

A behavioral healthcare provider should have sufficient reserves or a stop-loss (reinsurance) policy to protect against unanticipated losses. For example, a reinsurance plan, which protects an at-risk provider against claim loss, may pay the cost of an individual or a group of claims (called aggregate stop-loss) 120 percent of anticipated costs. Adequate reserves or stop-loss coverage are particularly important if the organization is responsible for inpatient costs or the cost of the delivery of services that they do not provide or manage themselves. Even in a situation in which the capitated provider or organization has complete, reliable utilization data combined with a fully functioning management system, a significant probability persists that unanticipated losses or overutilization will occur at some point. A successful program must have financial contingencies (i.e., stop-loss insurance or reserves) to withstand these eventualities.

PROGRAM AND CONTRACTUAL SERVICE REQUIREMENTS

Managing the terms of the capitation agreement is crucial to a successful program. Understanding what benefits are to be covered, the extent to which benefits may be "flexed" to accommodate appropriate levels of care, coverage limitations and exclusions, eligibility requirements, and the ability of the capitated provider to determine which services are covered based upon medical necessity are of particular importance.

Behavioral healthcare benefits can range from coverage limited by dollar amounts (e.g., outpatient benefits up to $1,000 per year), crisis services only, a specific number of outpatient sessions and inpatient day limitations (e.g., 20 outpatient sessions per year and 30 inpatient days), and, in some cases, unlimited coverage.

Even when behavioral health treatment benefits are covered and reimbursed, they often must be certified as meeting medical necessity criteria. How medical necessity for reimbursement purposes is determined is often based on who holds the capitation risk in the relationship. Medical necessity for reimbursement determination by this definition should not be confused with the treatment provider's own clinical judgment.

COST OF SERVICE DELIVERY AND CLAIMS COSTS

This issue has significant impact on clinical requirements and financial success. Actuarial, financial, clinical, and operational analysis and projections must be performed to create a plan or operational assumptions consistent with the program benefits, delivery of quality, appropriate care, and client objectives. Developing these assumptions should be based upon cost projections, which, in turn, depend on utilization rates and unit cost of services. These assumptions can be expressed in a variety of ways (e.g., estimating inpatient use per 1,000 beneficiaries, determining the average number of outpatient sessions, and the utilization of other levels of care). In addition, direct administrative costs, overhead, and margins must be calculated. Clinicians who may be unfamiliar with these requirements or whose clinical patterns may not have the flexibility for responding to managed care techniques can fall short of meeting their financial objectives.

FINANCIAL GOALS AND OBJECTIVES OF PURCHASER

The capitated provider must recognize the unique financial and service objectives of the purchaser. For example, many HMOs try to keep behavioral health costs to a fixed percentage of overall healthcare costs. Large employers are more likely to be interested in a predictable cost trend while emphasizing access to services. Public sector purchasers are often concerned about overall aggregate costs of entitlement benefits and keeping these costs constant or below insurance trend inflation. Programs must be conceived with the purchaser's objectives in mind.

AVAILABILITY OF PREVIOUS UTILIZATION AND CLAIMS INFORMATION

The provider organization accepting capitation must persist in searching for and evaluating available data on previous utilization of its population. When the data are unreliable or incomplete, the capitated organization should look to its own experience with similar groups, consult with an actuarial or consulting firm, and search for public sources with usable information (e.g., public sector program reports and industry presentations). These data can be used as a baseline by which to build utilization and cost assumptions for capitated programs.

BEHAVIORAL HEALTHCARE COSTS IMBEDDED IN PHYSICAL HEALTHCARE EXPERIENCE

As a result of the difficulty and unevenness in coding behavioral health encounters, a large portion of these costs is not usually distinguishable from the overall health experience. For example, several health providers simply indicate that behavioral healthcare services were provided as an office visit without differentiating the service as a behavioral health or psychiatric visit. The capitated provider must be aware of this and ensure that a level playing field is created so that it receives the appropriate capitation for which it will be financially responsible.

Operational issues

There are numerous key operational issues to consider.

MIS EXPERIENCE AND REPORTING CAPABILITIES

To manage the clinical and financial risks associated with capitation, as well as learn about and report on clinical outcomes as necessary, the capitated provider must invest in the creation or purchase of a management information system (MIS). The MIS should provide real-time information on utilization, quality, and performance against forecasts or plan estimates;

identify clinical outliers; and track patients who move through the system. It is important to recognize, however, that the presence of an MIS is not adequate without the commensurate management system to address and resolve issues reported by the MIS, such as overutilization.

No single behavioral care MIS or set of reports has yet set the industry standard. A wide variety of internal and external reports address such diverse issues as utilization, clinical outcomes, phone response time, adequacy of provider networks, tracking of grievances and their resolution, penetration (i.e., the percentage of beneficiaries who utilize behavioral health services), and provider and beneficiary satisfaction. MIS needs and resources must be addressed on a case-by-case basis for each organization, consistent with purchaser needs.

INTERNAL AND EXTERNAL REPORTING REQUIREMENTS

The ability to report on performance, utilization, penetration, and outcomes is essential as well as being a strong indicator of quality and capitation readiness. While some smaller capitated and subcapitated arrangements may not require the provider to submit reports, an internal report generation capability must be developed for self-monitoring and evaluation purposes. Increasingly, however, purchasers are demanding sophisticated reports to assist them to evaluate the effectiveness and value of their healthcare services. It is now common for payers to also require specific reports.

Employers are concerned with clinical and financial performance for their own employees and dependents. The Health Plan Employer Data and Information Sets (HEDIS) now required of behavioral health providers for several HMOs exemplify employer concern.

MANAGEMENT INFRASTRUCTURE FOR CLINICAL SYSTEMS, UTILIZATION, AND QUALITY

The operational component of managing a capitated arrangement must be carefully aligned with the clinical management system to ensure appropriate services are delivered, monitored, and evaluated in a timely fashion. Checks and balances must be present to ensure that all actions and outcomes are carefully monitored to achieve the desired outcome. Meeting their clinical objectives requires clinical monitoring, case conferences, consults, and similar activities.

CLAIMS PAYMENT

Unless a single provider organization will be delivering services, claims will need to be paid to other providers and provider organizations. Capitated provider must decide if they wish to purchase claims services or perform these services themselves. However, even if the capitated provider is not responsible for claims payment, it must have a knowledge of claims systems and their proper management. For many behavioral healthcare organizations, inadequate claims systems are significant barriers to the successful operation of capitated arrangements.

When providers are not paid in a timely or correct fashion, significant customer service failures result that compromise the provider organization's ability to provide overall effective clinical services. In addition, when claims' payments are not tied appropriately to the delivery of services that have been certified as medically necessary, the capitated provider may pay for services for which it should not be responsible.

QUALITY MANAGEMENT AND PERFORMANCE OBJECTIVES

Many capitated providers are required to include administrative performance objectives in their contracts. These include such items as telephone response time, time spent between appointments and the scheduling of other visits (e.g., 5 days for routine appointments), turnaround time on claims payment (e.g., 30 days), responsiveness to beneficiary complaints (e.g., within 24 to 48 hours), and proper handling of member communications. Also, operating the organization consistent with total quality management or continuous quality improvement principles is a barometer for clinical and program performance.

Conclusions

The challenge of managing a capitated arrangement for behavioral healthcare services is complicated by the subjectivity inherent in behavioral healthcare delivery, the lack of agreement on what appropriate outcomes should be, and the debate regarding where to allocate scarce benefit resources among competing services. Behavioral healthcare providers and organizations are vulnerable to allocation decisions being made by those who may have limited knowledge about the efficacy of behavioral healthcare.

The ability to manage a capitation-based program to deliver these services provides the behavioral healthcare industry an opportunity to illustrate the value of its services while creating a range of treatment options that meet the needs of each individual member.

To make capitation a successful experience for everyone involved—for providers, for purchasers, and, most importantly, for patients—the capitated provider or organization must be prepared to accept responsibility for care and the accompanying risk by fully addressing all the complexities of these arrangements.

NOTES

1. See, for example, N. A. Cummings, PhD, "The Successful Application of Medical Offset in Program Planning and in Clinical Delivery," *Managed Care Quarterly* 2, no. 2 (1994): 1–6.

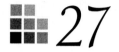

27

Ancillary medical service strategies

Robert M. Kisabeth, MD
Medical Director, Mayo Medical Laboratories
Mayo Clinic
Rochester, Minnesota

THE PURPOSE OF THIS CHAPTER is to review alternative strategies for the purchase, utilization, and provision of ancillary medical services. Services that have been considered "ancillary" include radiology, electrocardiography, electroencephalography, physical therapy and other rehabilitation services, pulmonary therapy, and nuclear medicine and imaging. Each of these disciplines can illustrate the positive and negative ramifications of specific purchasing patterns.

Negative ramifications in quality and cost are most apparent when capitation is used to purchase ancillary services separately from the purchase of other medical services. Today there is much emphasis on how integrated payment can, when carefully designed and implemented, facilitate integrated practice and how disease management strategies can facilitate reduced cost and enhance quality of medical care. This chapter will highlight ways in which other capitation plans have the potential for increasing overall costs and negatively affecting quality of care.

To consider the possible advantages and disadvantages of alternative capitation scenarios, it is helpful to review the unintended consequences of fee-for-service (FFS) purchasing methods.

Prior to the explosive rate of technological progress of the last 30 years, purchasing medical services from physicians and other providers constituted a mutually satisfactory method of payment. Payments were made largely for services that the patient had experienced firsthand and from which the patient had derived some tangible benefit, albeit frequently limited to consolation, reassurance, or advice. As technological advances ensued, more and more of the bill received by the patient or third-party payer reflected services that had very little tangible or understandable benefit to them. For example, a patient might have received a bill for bone densitometry (i.e., modern radiologic technique for evaluating bone loss), or tonometry (i.e., simple measurement for intraocular pressure), HPLC-Drug Level (i.e., not for drug abuse, but for a therapeutic drug a patient was receiving), or PCR-*Borrelia burgdorfii* (i.e., Lyme disease test). In general, the patients could not identify the benefit to such procedures and in most cases did not know if or why such tests might have been done. This gap between providers' and patients' levels of understanding vis à vis the value of increasingly complex procedures, tests, analyses, and calculations—and their respective interpretations and correlations—has continued to grow.

As a consequence of this growing knowledge gap between patients or payer and provider, the healthcare industry embarked upon the task of developing relative value scales to be used in conjunction with a consistent conversion factor to calculate payment for a particular service. The common procedural terminology (CPT) system, developed and maintained in cooperation with the American Medical Association, was used to facilitate billing for the myriad of procedures and services that might be used during an episode of care. Such CPT codes tend to enumerate the tangible products associated with a service, often excluding the more deliberative or contemplative services.

Although technological procedures such as serum protein electrophoresis and endoscopy were assigned CPT codes, there were in many cases no analogous codes for the integration of these test results with other tests, the patient's history, and other clinician findings.

At the same time, the resource-based relative value scale (RBRVS) was developed. The term "value" is an unfortunate choice—units assigned to medical services are more correlated with cost than with value. The patient history and physical examination, for example, received relatively paltry remuneration in the RBRVS even though the services were very highly valued by patients and widely accepted as being the most important and cost-effective processes in providing quality care.

The subliminal message inherent in the RBRVS, particularly in conjunction with a procedure-focused CPT coding system, was that patients and payers placed high value on procedures and low value on such activities as spending time with patients or performing thorough physical examinations. There was, for example, no CPT code assigned to "searching index medicus for articles relevant to dealing with a patient's unusual mix of disease processes," or to "prolonged discussion necessary to help patient decide between two therapeutic approaches, each having very complex ramifications," or "discussing with a family a disease process such as connective tissue disease, which in many cases requires aggressive pharmacologic therapy but has no specific name."

A principal consequence of this method to determine reimbursement to providers was that physicians engaged in the procedure-intensive specialties received higher total reimbursement per patient than those in less procedure-intensive specialties; and those healthcare institutions providing support for the more procedure-intensive specialties received higher total reimbursement per patient.

As a result, a variety of changes in physician and hospital practice patterns evolved. Medical school graduates increasingly pursued the more highly "valued," more procedure-intense specialties. This trend was exacerbated by a decision by the U.S. government to encourage (through grants) the training of more medical students in an attempt to saturate the provider market and drive down the costs of medical care.

Physicians generally committed less time to history, physical exam, and patient-counseling activities and began to focus their efforts on the more highly valued activities within their specialty fields. For example, many pathologists previously had been involved in the clinical laboratory and had made valuable contributions toward test development, implementation, selection, and interpretation—the cognitive practice of laboratory medicine. This facet of pathology practice was designated "clinical pathology," a discipline requiring formally approved residency training to qualify for certification by the American Board of Pathology. As the RBRVS and CPT code systems failed to acknowledge the value of such cognitive skills, many pathologists who previously had focused their efforts on the clinical pathology disciplines began to shift their efforts toward surgical pathology and cytology—activities that, although highly cognitive and deliberative, were easily quantifiable in the minds of those assigning value.

Procedure-intensive specialists began to move their practices to locations away from the traditional medical center to "boutique" practices (e.g., surgicenters, hernia repair centers, and cataract institutes). These stand-alone centers, which were unburdened from the high operating costs of a full-service community medical center, became very profitable, leaving the medical community with most of its preexistent fixed costs but with significantly reduced means for being reimbursed.

First-generation health maintenance organizations (HMOs) arose in an effort to introduce purchasing power into the marketplace and control costs by negotiating lower prices for a largely disintegrated assortment of medical services.

These activities characterize the "commoditization" of healthcare, a phenomenon that has proven to benefit neither patients nor healthcare purchasers. This commoditization, which fostered a financial windfall for procedure-intense medical specialists, resulted in a disintegration of delivery systems and a reduction of focus on activities that were most valued by patients. Healthcare providers are therefore increasingly perceived by patients as insensitive to their interests, needs, and desires.

Nowhere in medicine has this commoditization proceeded with such alacrity as in the fields of laboratory medicine and other ancillary specialties. The extraordinarily large and ever-growing number of CPT codes assigned to its even greater number of tests and procedures has encouraged the commoditization of laboratory medicine.

Because such large numbers of laboratory tests are performed and can be sent long distances, large national commercial laboratories have emerged. Their rapid growth was further facilitated by the following factors:

- Automation of high-volume tests tended to accentuate the "economies of scale" (regarding testing) that characterized large central laboratories remote from the patient care site

- The providers' ability to purchase laboratory tests at low prices from such facilities and in turn sell them at substantially higher prices to their patients (serving therefore as a source of significant net revenue to the provider) encouraged outsourcing

- The rapid proliferation of new tests in the absence of well-defined community standards for their use or well-designed clinical studies establishing their clinical utility resulted in overutilization of tests of questionable clinical value (e.g., serum CA 15-3, serum cathepsin D, and RAST testing in absence of clinical history)

- A widespread failure to recognize the unintended or "downstream" costs that result from the disintegrated use of diagnostic services

These problems have been exacerbated by large multitest panels popularized by the large commercial laboratories: the greater the number of tests in a panel, the greater the probability of an erroneous finding. Although similar problems are encountered with local community-based laboratory performance of tests, the potential costs can be significantly reduced by active consultation between community laboratorians and their clinicians regarding unanticipated test results. Downstream costs, which result from outsourcing, also include prolonged hospitalization resulting from delay in test reporting. With the cost of a hospital day readily exceeding $700, substantial savings can result if even a small number of patient days are avoided by the provision of timely laboratory tests.

The vertical integration of clinical laboratory and other support services results in cost savings and quality enhancement, with a relatively minor cost reduction from reduction in duplication of tests. There is, however, a far greater potential for savings that results from a reduction in office visits, improved turnaround times, and a reduction of unindicated work up of spurious or erroneous test abnormalities. A parallel benefit accrues vertically in an integrated community-based laboratory—its fixed costs of operation can be spread across a much larger pool of tests, resulting in substantial reductions in cost per unit of service.

Capitation

It is within this context of highly commoditized and disintegrated healthcare that managed care plans have begun to experiment with capitation of ancillary medical services. These attempts have been largely confined to the procurement by carve outs of outpatient laboratory services in an attempt to increase savings by placing the provider at-risk. It is important to realize providers of laboratory services are, in this setting, at-risk only for testing costs that are relevant to the contract in question. They are not exposed to the downstream or unintended additions to the

TABLE 1
Test turnaround time: Financial impact

Community laboratory

Capitated daily census	65%	75%	85%
Available beds	1,320	1,320	1,320
Average daily occupancy (65%)	858	858	858
Capitated daily census	558	644	729
Average cost per day estimate	$738*	$738*	$738*

If enhanced lab service (i.e., decreased turnaround time) decreases capitated patients' length of stay by one day:

	1 percent		
Daily costs	$4,118	$4,753	$5,380
Annualized costs	$1,503,070	$1,734,845	$1,963,700
	5 percent		
Daily costs	$20,590	$23,764	$26,900
Annualized costs	$7,515,423	$8,673,714	$9,818,500
	10 percent		
Daily costs	$41,180	$47,527	$53,800
Annualized costs	$15,030,846	$17,347,355	$19,637,000

Source: AHA Monitrend II: Hospitals, October 5, 1992.

aggregate cost of care that their tests or their patterns of service might produce. In this setting, where laboratory testing represents a small fraction of the total costs and therefore aggregate risks to which a managed care system is exposed, such an approach to the purchase of laboratory services is ill advised.

To obtain the full potential benefit of capitation methods as they apply to purchasing ancillary medical services (particularly those services with potential for affecting total medical costs in ways other than their direct costs), ancillary services should be purchased under the overall capitation of the provider. Such an approach places the testing facility, either as part of a fully integrated health delivery system or as a contractor to the provider, at full risk for the aggregate cost of medical care provided.

Including outpatient and inpatient ancillary services as part of the overall provider agreement achieves the following operational, quality, and cost-control objectives:

1. The ancillary medical service becomes responsible for controlling the unit cost of its service within the context of achieving the overall goals

of the vertically integrating healthcare provider. Cost control is exercised within the context of patient-care goals established collectively by the community. Balance can then be achieved between the costs that can be afforded by a community and the quality of care it receives. Decisions can be made prospectively about allocating financial resources, not for procedures but for specific illnesses or patient presentations. Integrated payment frees ancillary services of conflicts of interest in developing "disease management strategies" and facilitates integrated practice

2. It is difficult to design cost objectives for outpatient care until the specific roles of support services, such as laboratory, imaging, EKG, EMG, and EEG, are outlined in disease management strategies. The reduction in access to outpatient lab services that results from capitation rates for carved-out outpatient laboratory services might result in substantial increase in other medical costs

3. Vertical integration and attendant cost savings are accelerated. Healthcare providers try to find new ways to prove their value, not only by demonstrating the ability to control their direct costs but by more effective coordination of their services with those of others

Attempts by the community-based clinical laboratory to facilitate reduction in downstream costs can take many forms:

Example 1:
The community-based laboratory should develop a "formulary" of laboratory procedures and tests representing a consensus of that medical community as to what comprises truly useful tests within the context of their practice. This list might also articulate what tests are considered of no value and describe the process by which a physician must request a test not on the list. Such lists are virtually ubiquitous among medical center pharmacies. This ongoing review of the test formulary should be required of the laboratory medical director and must be accomplished in full cooperation with the medical staff, preferably through group discussions.

Example 2:
The clinical laboratory should carefully review the ordering patterns of its clinicians, searching for wide deviations in test ordering in a specific clinical setting. Such variations might suggest the need to develop

with the medical staff a carefully reasoned standard approach appropriate to that community's unique mix of medical resources as well as diagnostic and therapeutic resources. These community standards, or disease management strategies—analogous to the informal community standards of the past—are not intended to be followed rigidly. They serve as an essential resource to all ancillary medical services as they repackage and redesign their service delivery patterns to keep the overall service plan up to date.

Example 3:
The development of disease management strategies is of particular importance to quality and cost optimization when treating chronic diseases. Such diseases represent a major portion of healthcare expenditures and the manner in which they have been addressed has been largely by episodic intervention. There has been little in the way of long-term strategies to deal with long-term diseases. More recent advances toward understanding the pathophysiology of such diseases, particularly as they relate to long-term consequences of chronic disease, provide an opportunity to devise treatment plans that more effectively prevent long-term and costly complications. The consistent execution of chronic disease management strategies is the most successful way to effect such savings. The following case study of hypertension illustrates an example of how capitation could encourage a longer-term strategy.

CASE STUDY: HYPERTENSION
Among the 30 to 50 million hypertension patients in the United States who are treated with a drug, approximately 50 percent will stop taking their prescribed medication. It is probable that such patients, when "lost to follow-up," may comprise a significant portion of 3.8 percent of hypertensive patients who account for 40 percent of the total funds spent on hypertension.[1] These patients are those who are hospitalized with evidence of hypertension-associated end-organ failure, such as kidney failure or congestive heart failure. Disease management strategies directed at reducing these unfortunate and costly consequences can accomplish the following

1. Identify causes of hypertension that are not amenable to pharmacologic treatment

2. Identify causes of hypertension related to patient's current drug therapy, which are often most effectively and economically treated by
removing or changing the offending agent

3. Reveal surgically curable abnormalities

4. Detect and minimize noncompliance with therapy

5. Determine, prior to beginning therapy, baselines for those laboratory
tests essential to preventing hazardous and costly complications of
therapy

Hypertension provides a good opportunity to consider the potential
obstacles facing even integrated medical practices in attempting to assess
the relative cost effectiveness of each potential diagnostic and therapeutic component. Below is a list of procedures that typify the basic evaluation of patients found to be hypertensive:

- CBC

- Fasting glucose

- Potassium

- Uric acid

- Cholesterol (total, HDL)

- Triglycerides

- Calcium

- Creatinine

- Urinalysis

- EKG

Because such simple and relatively inexpensive tests are so essential to
the initial workup of patients with hypertension, this list of tests is commonly included in hypertension disease management strategies, even if
the cost of performing such tests is unknown to those determining such
a strategy. When clinicians ask about the cost of performing such tests,
they are frequently told the price, not the cost of such a profile. Prices
bear little relationship to cost.

The dramatic paradigm shift from FFS indemnity healthcare to fully capitated managed care requires special attention to terminology about price versus cost. The director of an ancillary medical service, such as the clinical laboratory, may know the current costs of a given profile; but what needs to be considered is the cost for that profile if a proposed disease management strategy is implemented. In the workup of most hypertensive patients, little cost difference should be anticipated between the old and the new payment structures. However, the cost versus benefit challenge is accentuated when they consider whether or not to make changes in a pattern of care that was previously fee for service and thought to be cost effective. Consider for example whether or not it is reasonable to include the following intermediate group of tests in the routine evaluation of patients presenting with hypertension:

- Basic lab assessment

- Echocardiogram

- 24-hour urine sodium

- Urine microalbumin

- Peripheral vein renin

If the working group inadvertently reviews the price of the above group of tests, they might be presented with an aggregate price greater than $250; and such a sum might quickly be regarded as unacceptably expensive for routine use. What will happen to the unit cost of performing a 24-hour urine sodium or urine microalbumin among the hypertensive population? Determine if the benefits obtained by the routine implementation of such tests might justify more routine application in the context of lower projected unit costs of testing. In the case of urine microalbumin, which should prove to be a reliable indicator of renal hyperperfusion phenomenon (i.e., a predictor of renal failure secondary to hypertension and/or diabetes mellitus), the working group might consider its routine application to patients with hypertension. It is likely that in hypertension, such findings would cause the clinician to change the patient's drug regimen to an agent that, although more expensive, tends to reduce hyperperfusion and avoids subsequent costly renal failure.

Cost savings in a managed care environment are clearly affected by reducing duplication and use of ancillary medical services that have little value. However, carefully derived disease management strategies may (particularly when addressing chronic disease) mandate additional testing. In the case of hypertension, such new strategies and their testing patterns may significantly reduce the need for hospitalization or dialysis with end-organ failure.

An additional question arises about the follow-up of patients with chronic diseases such as hypertension as to whether an ancillary medical service should consider expanding its support for such patients. Hypertension patients are seen routinely in the laboratory for follow-up of their drug therapy, during which visits such simple tests as potassium or liver function tests are performed. Such follow-up investigations are pursued primarily in an effort to assure the attending physicians that the therapy they have initiated is being complied with, is effective in reducing the patient's blood pressure to an acceptable level, and is causing the patient no harm.

In FFS arrangements, the clinical laboratory has limited its function to drawing blood or urine specimens and performing laboratory tests on those specimens (returning the potassium or liver function test results to the attending physician). This largely iterative activity (i.e., patient visiting laboratory, laboratory sending results to physician, patient visiting physician) results in unnecessary physician office visits with very little quality patient-physician interaction. It is appropriate that the clinical laboratory, in this circumstance, consider the addition of blood pressure measurements and patient interview in connection with the visit already necessary to acquire patient specimens: patients who lie outside acceptable ranges, as determined by clinicians, would be referred for a quality visit (i.e., greater amount of time and interaction) to their doctor. It is well known that a patient who does not show up for a scheduled laboratory appointment has a higher incidence of noncompliance with therapy, and the laboratory should call such patients, making every effort to reschedule appointments and to reinitiate compliance with the attending physician's prescription. It is this kind of systems redesign in the delivery of ancillary medical services that will effect downstream savings of great magnitude.

Laboratory "critical pathways" and "reflex testing algorithms" should be implemented in conjunction with disease management strategies. Such protocols substantially reduce the amount of time and number of patient visits necessary to establish diagnosis and begin therapy. The exhibits following this chapter show examples that are typical of critical pathways that can be arrived at by consensus within an integrated medical practice. Such pathways accomplish the patient's diagnosis in the most consistent, rapid, and cost-effective manner possible while fully respecting the individual physician's need to deviate from such patterns when necessary.

The greatest obstacle to realizing the full potential of disease management strategies and critical pathways within the context of a fully integrated medical practice lies in the failure to redesign systems that encourage compliance by physicians and other healthcare professionals with the diagnostic and therapeutic plan. Clinical laboratories and other ancillary medical services must repackage the delivery of their services and redesign the manner in which these services are requested in order to minimize wasteful misutilization and associated downstream costs.

The greatest barrier to achieving optimal healthcare at optimal cost has been the lack of systematic delivery (i.e., teamwork). Capitation can play a very positive role by bringing together—rather than segregating—otherwise integrated medical practices with ancillary medical services.

NOTES

1. V. L. Burt et al., "Prevalence of Hypertension in the U.S. Adult Population," results from the third National Health and Nutrition Examination Survey, 1988–1991 in *Hypertension* 25 (1995): 305–13; and V. L. Burt et al., "Trends in the Prevalence, Awareness, Treatment, and Control of Hypertension in the Adult U.S. Population," data from the Health Examination Surveys, 1960–1991 in *Hypertension* 26 (1995): 60–69.

Exhibit 1
Connective tissue cascade

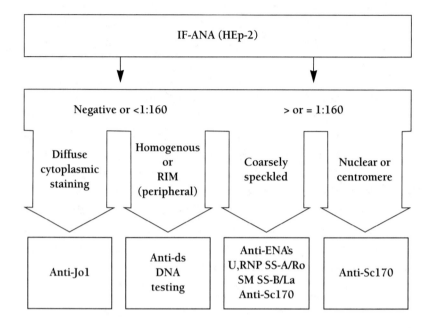

Reprinted, by permission, from H. A. Homberger, "Cascade Testing for Autoantibodies in Connective Tissue Diseases," *Mayo Clinic Procedings* 70 (1995): 183–184.

Exhibit 2
Proposed thyroid function cascade

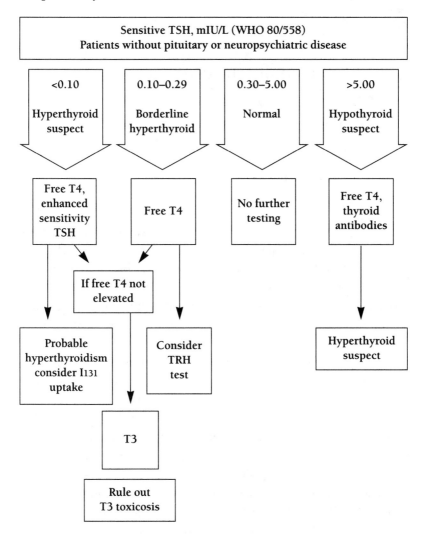

Reprinted, by permission, from George G. Klee et al., "Role of Thyrotropin Measurements in the Diagnosis and Management of Thyroid Disease," *Clinics in Laboratory Medicine* 13 (1993): 673–682.

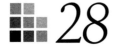

28

Capitated pharmaceutical pricing

Michael S. Miele
President
Capitated Disease Management Services, Inc.
Montclair, New Jersey

VIRTUALLY NO COMPONENT of healthcare has been protected from employer- or payer-driven reform. The past
year (1995) has been a particularly explosive year for capitated pricing
of healthcare services and supplies.

Payers have grown accustomed to flat or decreasing managed care
premiums and have been negotiating capitated contracts as a way to
continue to secure savings.

The pharmaceutical industry, not spared from this recent trend, has
been exploring capitated pharmaceutical pricing and "disease state management" to protect market share and to play a more active role in the
provision of managed care services. Under these arrangements, a manufacturer and a managed care organization (MCO) form a partnership
realizing the most efficient use of a product, aligning incentives, and
sharing gains and losses equally through risk-sharing contracts.

Capitation arrangements developed between MCOs and prescription
benefit managers (PBMs) are based on the total use of all prescriptions.
Those developed between MCOs and pharmaceutical manufacturers
are based on a therapeutic class of drugs (e.g., antibiotics or antidepres-
sants). These latter types of arrangements represent the first generation
of capitated disease state management (DSM) programs.

DSM represents a pharmaceutical industry initiative to extend beyond
the drug-related component of care (which represents 7 to 10 percent of

total healthcare expenditures) to the entire disease state. These types of arrangements require greater responsibility because they hold the disease manager responsible for patient outcomes as well as drug costs.

For example, if a therapeutic class of drugs is known to intervene and lower total medical costs associated with a certain medical condition, that therapeutic class could be capitated. Here, the pharmaceutical manufacturer accepts a fixed dollar amount (capitation) per member per month (PMPM) and accepts responsibility for the administration of the drugs by physicians and use of drugs by patients. If more products are used than anticipated, the pharmaceutical manufacturer will reimburse the MCO for the overage. If, on the other hand, fewer drugs are consumed than anticipated, the pharmaceutical manufacturer benefits financially. Although few of these arrangements have been made public, manufacturers are studying these types of arrangements and, in many cases, are engaging in pilot programs with interested MCOs.

Critical success factors

There are several critical success factors to develop a viable capitated rate structure between an MCO and a pharmaceutical manufacturer or disease manager. They are

- A well-conceived product concept that offers the customer reduced costs and enhanced quality of care

- An understanding of the capitation risks to the MCO and the manufacturer and strategies to manage these risks

- A method to collect available membership and claims experience to model financial results

- Effective contract language that can manage risk and still be attractive to the MCO and pharmaceutical manufacturer

- A practical method for implementing the program

This article describes the basic tenets to develop a capitated rate structure for a therapeutic class of drugs between an MCO and a pharmaceutical manufacturer.

PRODUCT DESIGN

By capitating the cost of a therapeutic class of drugs with an MCO, the pharmaceutical manufacturer agrees to provide an unlimited supply of products to treat a well-defined group of MCO enrollees for a multiple-year period. Products covered by the capitation arrangement could include competitor products.

This strategy represents a radical departure for most pharmaceutical manufacturers since these arrangements can yield higher profits even though pharmaceutical sales may have decreased (i.e., the pharmaceutical manufacturers receive the same capitated fee, regardless of the quantity of drugs sold) or by advocating the sale of competitor products if they achieve greater savings. Under these types of arrangements, the manufacturer partners with the MCO to manage utilization, monitor formulary compliance, educate physicians and patients, and emphasize wellness programs such as exercise, lifestyle, and diet. These arrangements are designed to offer the MCO immediate savings to keep its drug expenditures competitive.

Reaction

Today, many MCOs are not interested in buying insurance or shifting risk (i.e., capping costs at current levels plus some risk margin). The central issue is focused on shifting responsibility and seeking genuine productivity gains. Many MCOs are receptive to working with pharmaceutical manufacturers to lower drug and medical costs over time, as well as to ensure appropriate utilization and quality of care.

Product mechanics

Under these capitated arrangements, the manufacturer does not actually supply the pharmaceuticals to the MCO. Pharmaceuticals are acquired through their normal supply chain and claims are processed as they had been by the PBM, or the designated claims processor, with existing network pharmacy discount programs in place. The manufacturer will not offer rebates (cash returned by pharmaceutical manufacturers after utilization has been computed) as it had in the past to the PBM or directly to the MCO. Instead, these cost savings are incorporated into the capitation rate. Furthermore, the monthly capitated dollar amount is not actually paid to the manufacturer because the MCO continues to pay for the

TABLE 1
Calcium channel blocker example

Therapeutic class	Calcium channel blockers
Number of members	100,000
Total annual discounted ingredient cost for class	$1,895,000
Total annual current rebate for class	$95,000
Net cost for class	$1,800,000
Capitated cost PMPM	$1.50

After three months of the contract, the true-up would be computed as follows:

Actual member months for three months	300,000 (100,000 members covered for three months)
Capitation revenue	$450,000 (300,000 × $1.50)
Actual utilization cost (prerebate)	$475,000
Payment from manufacturer to MCO	$25,000 ($475,000 − $450,000)

products through the normal supply chain. Instead, the capitation revenue is theoretically calculated and compared to the actual utilization on a monthly or quarterly basis.

If the actual amount of drugs used exceeds the capitation, then the manufacturer will reimburse the MCO for the loss. These "true-ups," a method of settling gains and losses, can be calculated monthly, quarterly, or annually, although they are generally computed quarterly to remain consistent with certain Medicaid best-price calculations. Many of these arrangements incorporate risk sharing, in which gains and losses are shared equally by the partners. The example in Table 1 for calcium channel blockers (used to treat high blood pressure) illustrates an arrangement with no risk charges or administrative expenses.

This example demonstrates that the MCO is being indemnified by the contract because the net effective cost is $1.50 PMPM for the first three months of the arrangement. Alternatively, a risk-sharing formula could have been used where the $25,000 loss would be split between the MCO and pharmaceutical manufacturer.

RISKS OF CAPITATION TO THE MANUFACTURER

The pharmaceutical manufacturer is exposed to five principal types of risk that can be controlled through contract language to address roles, responsibilities, financial terms, aggressive management of the contract (i.e., profiling patients and physicians), and risk charges (i.e., additional revenues above expected costs that act as a buffer for fluctuations in

TABLE 2
Summary of risks

Type of risk	Description
Demographic	Age, sex, type of group (e.g., Medicare and Medicaid)
Customer performance	Adherence to the contract reporting requirements
Internal performance	Effective managed care interventions
Regulatory	State insurance law Medicaid best price
Insurance	Unexpected worst-case scenarios

expected versus actual costs). These issues are of utmost importance to MCOs when negotiating the details of the arrangement.

The five primary types of risk to the manufacturer are listed in Table 2.

Demographic risk

Demographic risks are the most basic considerations in any capitation arrangement. If the demographics are relatively unchanged for a given population over time, then the group's experience should also be stable. However, if these demographics change unexpectedly, costs could drastically be affected. For example, consider the information in Table 3 regarding the relative costs of calcium channel blockers by age.

These cost factors were developed for a specific 100,000-member group. The weighted average of 100 percent is an average risk. Members age 65 to 74 (e.g., a Medicare risk population) are 3.5 times or 350 percent more expensive than the average member.

To control for these demographic risks, the contract should contain a provision to allow for the capitation rate to be revised if the demographics change substantially over time. If the demographic mix changes during the terms of the contract (e.g., MCO expansion of a Medicare risk product that would attract older members), the contract should allow for a recalculation of the rate on some predetermined basis. More specifically, the contract could state that if the demographic index (a number initially set to 100 percent) changes due to changes in the demographic mix by more than a predetermined percentage, the capitation rate will be automatically recalculated using the following formula:

$$\text{New capitation rate} = \text{Old capitation rate} \times \frac{\text{New index}}{\text{Old index}}$$

TABLE 3
Relative calcium channel blocker costs by age

Age grouping	Relative cost factor (illustrative)
00–29	0%
30–44	75%
45–64	250%
65–74	350%
75+	275%

Customer performance risks

Reporting. Pharmaceutical manufacturers are generally willing to enter into these arrangements with groups that have a reasonable experience base (i.e., predictable, stable, and minimal variance) to review. However, this scenario can create problems for an MCO because script-level information (i.e., individual prescription claims data) by therapeutic class is generally not available through standard reports from the claims processor or PBM. If the MCO is using a PBM to process claims, obtaining this script-level information may require going back to the PBM for special reports. Even if the MCO processes its own prescription claims, compiling and deciphering this information generally requires special ad hoc programming.

MCO operational practices. Each MCO organization is unique in terms of enrollment, claims coding, pharmacy benefit management, rebate arrangements, and overall medical management. The manufacturer must understand the nuances associated with each of these capabilities in each of these areas to adequately form a baseline for the arrangement. For example, if during the arrangement claims-coding practices change, the manufacturer should retain the right to amend the contract and the capitation rate, if applicable.

Internal performance risks

Setting the capitation rate requires a firm understanding of how the pharmaceutical manufacturer plans to add value to the MCO. MCOs are generally not interested in buying insurance (i.e., setting a capitation rate at current trends and adding a risk margin) but want arrangements that provide upfront savings and guaranteed sustainable productivity gains over the life of the arrangement.

Because the pharmaceutical manufacturers have no hard data to assess if they can add value, they have had to make scientific estimates on the effectiveness of their interventions. Manufacturers are generally uncomfortable with this notion and have enlisted the help of qualified actuaries to build a financial argument to synthesize some of the clinical literature with historical experience. In many cases, the results of this analysis indicate that more drug therapy is required, often resulting in higher drug costs but lower overall medical costs. These projections can be difficult for the MCO to find credible and may result in the expansion of these types of arrangements to include other costs associated with a particular disease state.

For example, if clinical evidence supports more aggressive use of hypertensive and antilipidemic agents to lower the risk of heart disease, then perhaps the manufacturer can bear some degree of risk for the entire disease state as opposed to a calcium channel blocker capitation. Under this type of arrangement, the pharmaceutical manufacturer would encourage more use of pharmaceuticals and reap the financial benefit of lower mechanical costs associated with heart diseases.

Regulatory risk

Capitation is a form of insurance and is possibly subject to state insurance regulation. In some of the pilot arrangements, the MCO and the manufacturer operate under the assumption that the manufacturer is being subcapitated by the HMO, similar to other subcapitated vendors, not requiring the manufacturer to file as an insurer. The MCO and the manufacturer should seek legal counsel to assess if these types of arrangements are subject to insurance regulation.

The largest risk to the manufacturer is its exposure to Medicaid best-price rules. These rules require the manufacturer to supply Medicaid with pharmaceuticals at the lowest price available to the market. Some pharmaceutical manufacturers have taken a conservative view that capitating a class of drugs may potentially trigger a best-price scenario if the actual experience results in losses to the manufacturer. Table 4 illustrates this point using XYZ pharmaceutical manufacturer.

This example demonstrates a very large leveraging effect on the pharmaceutical manufacturer's best-price liability. A loss of $10 on a single MCO capitation contract could potentially trigger a $10 million loss.

There are two conclusions that can be drawn from this example: (1) because the manufacturer has to pay this tax only once, an argument

TABLE 4
Medicaid best-price liability

Negotiated capitation (includes a 5 percent rebate)	$100
Actual usage of XYZ product	$50
Actual usage of non-XYZ product	$60
Total actual cost	$110
"Loss" taken by the manufacturer	$10 ($110 – $100)
Possible interpretation by Medicaid	XYZ manufacturer supplied the MCO $50 worth of XYZ product for only $40 ($100 – $60)
Implied additional rebate	20% = 1 – ($40/$50)
Total effective rebate paid to MCO	25% = 5% (original rebate) + 20% (implied)
Current Medicaid best-price rebate	15%
Additional rebate payable	10% = 25% – 15%
Current sales of XYZ product to Medicaid	$100,000,000
Additional rebate to Medicaid	$10,000,000 = (10% × $100,000,000)

can be made for the manufacturer to either provide capitated products on a large scale or not at all, and (2) capitating the entire disease state could present less risk to the manufacturer by making the leveraging effect on best-price much smaller. In fact, by accepting responsibility for all costs associated with a particular disease state, best-price implications may not result because the product, at this level, appears to represent a "mini-HMO" rather than a pharmaceutical contract. These issues have to be reviewed by each pharmaceutical manufacturer's legal counsel.

Insurance risk

Capitated pharmaceutical products present risk to the manufacturer. Many of these risks can be limited through program design (e.g., benefit differentials for noncompliance), contractual provisions, and close monitoring of the contract. However, there is always the chance of experience fluctuation and unexpected worst-case scenarios.

These risks must be financed through a combination of risk charges and capital. Risk charges, depending on the type of risk, are imposed to cover small fluctuations in benefit cost. Capital or surplus (e.g., funds set aside from the normal course of business) is allocated to support the risk assumed for the worst-case scenario. These charges are developed based on the inherent risky nature of the arrangement and management's return on equity requirements and are dictated by state law where applicable. Since most MCOs are not interested in paying more than the current cost of the program (i.e., the add-on risk charge), the program can be difficult

TABLE 5
Capital requirement

Current cost of the program	$100
Negotiated capitation	$90
Expected actual ingredient cost	$80
Additional intervention cost	$5
Risk and profit charge	$5
Capital requirement to be set aside (as determined by the actuary or state law)	$10
Pretax return on equity	50%

to sell. To make these arrangements attractive and financially viable to the MCO and to cover risks, the manufacturer needs to retain some of these gross costs savings to cover these risks. Table 5 gives an example.

This analysis illustrates some of the tools needed to weigh the potential return on equity compared to other projects like developing a new innovator drug.

MANAGING AND MONITORING THE CONTRACT

After an arrangement is fully developed and the contract signed, the MCO has to provide timely utilization reports, work with the manufacturer to identify high-risk patients, cultivate support of the initiative with member physicians and patients, and, finally, relinquish some control to the manufacturer. Many MCOs have been reluctant to allow the manufacturer to literally manage patients. However, without the ability to intervene where appropriate, the manufacturer will not be able to add value required by the MCO. Ultimately, the MCO must render a business decision, weighing the benefits of pulling cost out of the system against the relinquishment of some control to the manufacturer. In theory, the more responsibility the MCO is willing to give the manufacturer, the better the capitation rate.

Conclusion

Capitation will undoubtedly make its way to the pharmaceutical industry. Based on the industry's interest in disease state management, combined with the potentially large risks of capitating only pharmaceuticals, manufacturers are realizing the need to take greater responsibility for the disease state than simply the drug component.

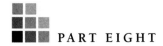

PART EIGHT

EPILOGUE

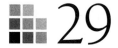

Ethical issues in risk-based contracting

Miriam Piven Cotler, PhD
Professor, Director of Bioethics Institute
Northridge Hospital Medical Center
Northridge, California

THIS CHAPTER DISCUSSES the challenges managed care poses to traditional medical ethics, including patients' rights to self-determination, the physician's obligation to act in the patient's best interest, provider autonomy, and social responsibility.

Ethics describes the community's common understandings of what is morally right for a given problem. It also provides a framework for resolving dilemmas that arise when there is more than one right option or no clearly good resolution—and action is needed. Healthcare ethics used to be associated with a professional code and physicians' responsibilities to each other, their patients, and society. In the last 30 years, the field has broadened to include moral dilemmas at the bedside, the community, and the society. We have more options now—and more constraints on medical decisions; those frequently require ethical choices.

Medicine has always been managed at the level of individual patient treatment decisions. However, management now includes financing and delivery of services. Some argue that these arrangements pose a prima facie threat to patients' best interests. It is not always clear whose interests are being served and whose autonomy compromised. There are also questions of social justice related to plans that see their primary obligation is to the company or the shareholders, rather than the community at large.

Thus, there are a number of internal contradictions and conflicts in the ethical management of healthcare that need to be made explicit, argued in a public discourse, and resolved or negotiated at the individual, institutional, and societal levels.

The following two cases are common and typical of the developing folklore:

Case 1:

Mrs. X is an HMO member, diagnosed with pancreatic cancer. The patient and her family want "everything done to help her live." However, her probable survival is six to eight months, and at the recommendation of the panel oncologist, she elects palliative radiation and comfort measures that will be provided in the hospital. The HMO hospital-based physicians who have assumed responsibility for her care strongly urge discharge home. They argue that she can be made comfortable there and allowed to die. The oncologist and nursing staff are extremely distressed at the refusal of care they believe indicated and appropriate to maximize the quality of her remaining life. They are also disturbed that this type of medical decision, based primarily on relative cost, has happened on several occasions, and one patient was recently discharged by the HMO physician over their objections.

Case 2:

Mrs. Y is a pregnant 35-year-old, insulin-dependent diabetic. Her last pregnancy was well managed by a high-risk specialist; it was uneventful until the 35th week when she became unstable and had to be delivered by a cesarean section. Under a new policy, her HMO will not refer her to a perinatologist or diabetologist, and she has spent 8 of her first 14 weeks of pregnancy in the hospital with wildly fluctuating hyper- and hypoglycemia. Her physician feels he can manage her care and rejects her requests for referral to a subspecialist and for a continuous infusion insulin pump. Finally, she sees her "old" specialist who recommends the pump. The HMO claims the pump is experimental and not a covered benefit. Mrs. Y's church raises the funds to purchase the pump. She does well, no further crises, and does not have to be hospitalized until the delivery of a healthy baby at 37 weeks gestation. After delivery, she hires an attorney who convinces the HMO to reimburse her for the pump and future associated costs.

These cases illustrate the ethical tensions among patients, healthcare plans, and physicians enrolled in either HMOs or fee for service (FFS). There is a perception that business and clinical priorities diverge, that goals are different among the groups, and that they are competing for relative autonomy and power. There is frequently doubt about whose interests are being served.

Healthcare has been perceived and treated as a basic social good, different from usual commerce. It has been dominated by medical professionals who have established codes of ethical obligations. The rights of patients and physicians have been negotiated based on professional norms and traditional relationships that emphasize patients' best interests. Perhaps the fundamental question is whether the integration of business efficiencies and cost containment with healthcare treatment decisions inherently compromise basic moral principles. The corollary is also important: are there also significant, common goals, risks, and benefits shared by clinical and business interests? The importance of these concerns has been underscored by legal and accreditation mandates, as well as patient and provider demands. Medical ethical questions often overlap with quality assurance and risk management; they are not abstract.

When healthcare management referred only to clinical practice and excluded organization or financing, ethics were centered around the individual patient, and the articulated principles were to avoid harms and promote the patient's best interests. Needs have been largely identified by physicians who have managed the clinical aspects of care, primarily through the private sector. Financial management of care has been at arm's length of clinical decisions. Although third-party payers have been part of the healthcare system, their relationship to patients, providers, and the community is largely based on contracts, and their ethical obligations to patients have been less clearly defined than those of providers. As long as third-party payers were a separate business, independent of the practice of medicine and with a relatively small market share, they were not perceived as a major threat to customary practices.

Management of care is no longer a locus of control or strictly clinically focused. The introduction of organizational efficiencies and rational planning clearly changes the equation by combining delivery and financing mechanisms into one organization. That integration challenges some basic ethical assumptions.

There are several managed care models currently used to lower costs, but they all combine responsibility for delivery with reimbursement and integrate payers and providers. These plans increase concerns about moral conflicts in caring for patients and with the business obligations associated with insurance. Medical codes of conduct and case law have supported the fundamental importance of independence between reimbursement questions and care of individual patients in both FFS and prepayment financing. However, discussion of ethical public policy becomes more complex and increasingly urgent as concerns with the ability of healthcare organizations and plans to survive, distribution of resources in the community, and reasonable costs to the payers challenge old principles.

The primary points developed in this chapter are

- Healthcare delivery has always been managed. Good management is desirable and necessary, and there are significant commonalties with other business demands for efficiency and effectiveness. Individual patient care practiced one to one at the bedside is a form of management, even though it is labeled clinical judgment, and it carries extensive financial implications. Decisions made at the bedside have largely ignored institutional or societal implications, because they have self-righteously claimed that individual patients' interests trumped all others

- There are challenges presented to *clinical* medical ethics by managed care delivery systems. Historically, patient care has been largely dictated by physicians who have acknowledged a fiduciary relationship to patients and a moral obligation to stewardship. However, the new healthcare systems are external to clinical settings. They thus challenge physician autonomy. They also encourage utilization of fewer services, not clearly in the patients' best interests.

- The moral, economic, and social risks and benefits of the new health plans must be addressed explicitly. Controversy exists at the levels of patient, institution, and community, at the expense of both moral and economic value. This will continue unless and until system goals are articulated and there is an agreed-upon process for setting healthcare priorities and for resolving disputes. Micromanagement of physicians and patients has discouraged both groups; it has also fostered gaming, continued unnecessary services, and added to moral confusion.

Background

Present market forces in healthcare have failed for several reasons.[1] Thus, there are at least two types of basic questions that need to be asked about how care should be managed regardless of setting. The first set of questions relates to scientific or medical values—effectiveness. Most bioethical dilemmas disappear when the medical facts are agreed upon by the caregivers and understood by the patient and the family. For example, given compassionate communication about prognosis, most patients and families accept the limitations of technologies and agree upon reasonably obtainable clinical goals. Often it is the physician who resists shifting from aggressive to palliative, comfort care.

The second set of questions challenges a consensus about moral or social obligations of the delivery system to individuals, the institution, and the community. The assumption has been that a patient's problem is evaluated in terms of differential diagnosis and need for care. It is also assumed that medical practices are based upon knowledge of effective clinical action as determined by objective measures. Until very recently, medical necessity was decided by the physician ostensibly based on scientific knowledge, community practice, experience, and judgment. Need, appropriateness, and quality presume to have answers that are grounded in science as demonstrated by: consistency in presentation, history, and diagnosis; objective measures; and outcomes directly related to the treatments. Ideally, medical appropriateness for a patient should be based on that individual's healthcare needs, independent of financing mechanism. Medical need has been the accepted criterion for service by the courts as well as insurance companies.

However, there are major problems with the assumption of independence between financial and clinical decisions. The FFS system reimburses after services have been provided. It thus contains financial incentives to overutilize, providers are paid for doing rather than not doing. When care is completely insured, more is requested, more is provided, and neither the doctor nor the patient appreciate the costs.

Also, there have been inadequate outcomes data to develop practice standards. Physicians place great emphasis on the uniqueness of each patient treatment decision that challenges consistent application of uniform guidelines. Without good standards, it is difficult to attack or defend the utilization differences as justified or unjustified; they simply are an act of physician clinical judgment.

The physician has little or no moral constraints concerning increased utilization when the obligation is to the patient who does not pay at the point of service. The increased costs of healthcare associated with these phenomena have been further justified by new technologies that seemed to promise more effective treatment and that more care is equated with better care.

Healthcare costs have increased significantly more than the Consumer Price Index annually for the last 25 years. Increasing numbers of people have been uninsured or inadequately covered and the nation's health status indicators do not show significant improvements. The inefficiency and perverse economic incentives have become a compelling problem for government and business, and both agree that system reform is urgent. They have turned to managed care delivery systems.

In its simplest form, managed care describes the planned allocation of health resources in a relationship between healthcare providers and third-party payers and through an administrative mechanism called "the plan." The formal, stated goals are a cost-effective system with targeted outcomes and appear consistent with clinical priorities. This efficiency seems to maximize quality of care using appropriateness standards and other practice guidelines. Certainly, those are admirable business goals and appear to be consistent with fairness and the public's best interests. Here, healthcare business and ethics appear quite compatible.

However, there is concern that the tools and incentives of the new management pose different threats to fundamental ethical principles and practices. While there are significant commonalties in goals between business efficiency and a just delivery system, there are also unique demands of healthcare to address basic human needs that conflict with administrative rationing and cost-control mechanisms.

Management by government, using diagnostic-related groups (DRGs) for Medicare or privately through health plans, appears to represent interests that are less pure and less concerned with the patients' good, because they are primarily cost driven rather than patient focused. Financial management and control of treatment decisions are outside the clinical arena, and they are seen by many physicians and some patients as hostile to basic ethical principles.

While managed healthcare systems are largely a response to cost inflation experienced by the employers and government who pay the bills, there has been a dramatic reversal of the dominant business philosophy regarding healthcare. In the last 10 years, hospitals have had to shift from "more and bigger" to "lean and mean" as the cost/benefit equation of a wide range of technologies is questioned. The pressures to reform the system have been further fueled from other sources by moral and economic concerns about the increased number of persons without health insurance or ability to pay for care.[2] As the direction to managed care is resisted by many healthcare providers and patients, is there an inherent moral conflict, or is it primarily a problem of power and control and a resistance to change from those who have been comfortable with the old ways? Is healthcare really different from other consumer goods, and if so, in what ways and to what extent?

Challenges

The traditional, dominant, ethical obligations of medicine have been to do no harm and to maintain confidentiality. They function to provide a professional framework that promotes trust, healing, and caring—the ultimate goals of medical care. With the technological explosion of the twentieth century, the increase in available treatment options, and rise of personal self-determination, the principle of patient autonomy has dominated healthcare ethics for 30 years. This much-misunderstood principle provides each person the right to be left alone, or to refuse recommended treatments or other interventions on their bodies and their psyches, which are presumed to be their private property. It does not acknowledge a right to demand inappropriate care as judged by the professional.

Cultural and religious differences among patients and caregivers have further fostered self-determination through patients' rights, informed consent, and advance directives. These rights have been accompanied by changes in who decides what constitutes a benefit, and a decreased belief that "doctor knows best." Physicians still decide medical appropriateness, and patients have legal and moral rights to accept or forgo the recommendations based on their values, perceived quality of life, and preferences.

With the successes in early detection, treatment, and cure or rehabilitation, patients' expectations have also changed. Thus, the successes of medicine, the relative freedom from price concerns allowed by third-party insurance, and the rise in consumerism have all encouraged patients to become more demanding of the healthcare system. Sometimes those demands are morally and practically problematic for the provider or the larger community. Often, they are primarily questions of control.

For example, how should need and appropriateness for formal rehabilitation, cardiac, or stress-reduction programs be determined when there are not good outcomes data? Patients as well as physicians demand technology of uncertain benefit. On the other hand, how responsible should patients be for their choice to continue smoking or for their failure to comply with treatment regimens?

Increased public and private third-party responsibility for paying the bills has also reduced professional autonomy. The assumption that physicians are motivated by the patient's best interest rather than their own self-interest is no longer blindly accepted. Physicians have to account for their interpretation of medical necessity and their responsibility to manage clinical care has been diluted as they are challenged by health plan administrators to defend treatment decisions. Thus, management controls such as utilization review and preauthorization appear to further compromise professional obligation to act in the patient's best interests.

Chronic illnesses are more varied than acute illness in onset, severity, and use of health services. As a result, costs increase and the number of remedies and prescriptions proliferate, without significant differences in outcomes. For the caregiver, there is increased uncertainty and legitimate variation in actual practice. Much of the variation in treatment modes and outcomes depends on patient characteristics, such as response to symptoms and adherence to treatment regimens. There is also variation associated with physician practice style or concerns about liability. Scientific and clinical uncertainty increase the legitimacy of questioning treatment and reimbursement policies.

In addition, with physicians determining "medical necessity" as the major reimbursement criterion, many physicians believe the patient's best interests gave the rationale to order and treat to the maximum benefit coverage, particularly given a lack of data and an acceptable range of treatment options. Thus there appeared to be an inherent moral tension between the payers and providers of care.

Because of this latitude in prescribing and treatment, managed care organizations justify limiting benefits provided and services authorized. As costs have escalated, the plans and payers increasingly challenge provider autonomy through techniques such as preauthorization and utilization review and also question the medical necessity, ostensibly without sacrificing patient health status. This era of discouraging utilization or substituting less costly providers of care and settings has been a major change.

Problem redefinition

There are several threats to the healthcare profession's obligation to serve the patient's best interest, sustain provider autonomy, and ensure the fair distribution of resources posed by managed care. As the financial opposite of FFS, rate setting calculates the loss associated with covered services, administrative overhead, and risk reserves. Risk-based capitation provides a variety of organizational tactics to lower the volume of service and costs and substitute lower-cost providers and services. Provider productivity standards may not promote patient or professional best interests.

The perception that risk-based capitation and other managed care arrangements encourage preventive services ignores the incentives to use fewer services. The managed care model has been inconsistent with early intervention or health promotion. On the one hand, financial risk seems to be a strong incentive to provide effective detection and preventive services that can save money in the long run. On the other hand, if the targeted disease or disability is not symptomatic for a number of years or if the case detection rate is significantly higher than the probability and cost of treatment, there may be disincentives to screen appropriately. When the financial costs are calculated within the cost/benefit equation, rather than separate from the medical risks and benefits, the relative value of screening underestimates the importance to patients and to the public health of the community. Also, insurance companies and many managed care plans have short time frames when calculating costs, which makes long-term prevention less attractive.

Among providers, there is the view that tools of managed care such as credentialing, case management, control of utilization, use of information systems, and total quality management have been used selectively with less caution and respect for confidentiality than FFS and have increased the administrative costs without advancing efficiency or effectiveness. Physicians and staff view these techniques as major hassle factors and do not appreciate diverting time and money away from patient care. Further, they argue that the doctor-patient relationship is undermined by demands that patients use only member physicians, that collegial communications are interrupted, and that treatment goals are defined too narrowly.[3]

Confusion accompanies this frustration. New authorization requirements, utilization and claims review, and reimbursement refusals make the scenario even more baffling. For example, many physicians do not yet understand Medicare DRGs and, as a result of hospital administration pressure to discharge, some believe they dictate a patient's length of stay. Patients, as well as providers, have responded by becoming even more demanding and litigious when coverage is postponed or denied.

The courts, however, continue to hold physicians liable for poor patient outcomes associated with failure to provide appropriate treatment. In the *Wickline* case (*Wickline v. State of California*), the court found the physician liable for damages to the patient but appeared to exempt Medicaid, the payer in this case. Although the physician had requested additional hospital days for Mrs. Wickline, the request had been denied, the physician discharged her home, and she developed an infection requiring an amputation of her leg. While the payer was not found liable in *Wickline*, in subsequent cases, courts have considered the possibility that the payer could potentially be held liable depending on the evidence. The number of lawyers who deal with these complaints and the lawsuits is increasing.

There is a seemingly inexhaustible supply of anecdotes from physicians about perverse incentives, undertreatment, and inconvenience in capitated arrangements. The extent and limits of physicians' liability are being tested along with their professional and moral duties. Should the gatekeeper's decision to consult a specialist be influenced by financial risk for referrals? How about the decision to hospitalize a patient, or to include nutrition and exercise counseling in the treatment protocol?

Physicians' evaluations of their competence to treat or refer a high-risk pregnancy, to advise radiation or chemotherapy, or to select a treatment plan should not be determined by finances. It is easier for the courts to be clear about that principle than for the individual plan or physician to internalize the moral mandate, especially when the bottom line is at stake and there are several treatment options.

The morally appropriate physician gatekeeper is parsimonious, orders only those tests and procedures that aid in diagnosis and treatment, and does not make clinical decisions for financial gain. Gatekeepers who deny appropriate care or who order excessively are both immoral.[4] But how are patients' needs measured and quantified? Particularly in chronic illness, indicators of need are inadequate and we measure how much healthcare is used rather than prevalence of illness. Need for long-term care has always been seen as less legitimate largely because of the subjectivity, variation, and unpredictability in the relationship between treatments and outcomes. The underlying pathology in chronic illness often makes it difficult for patients to function and seek care. Outcomes are further complicated by patients' social and financial needs, which are not well considered in the medical model or present payment system and have not been justified as moral obligations. Further, the community has not accepted responsibility to provide sufficient social services for long-term care.

There are serious concerns about healthcare management decisions that are based on statistics rather than on individual patient evaluation. Those based on statistics may ignore or not sufficiently appreciate important attributes such as need for a few additional days of rehabilitation to regain strength or palliative care that is implicitly factored into clinical judgment. Interpretation may be viewed as a professional skill or as an individual idiosyncrasy depending on what is portrayed. Much of the interpretation and decision to deny or authorize care depends on language and labels.

There are additional characteristics of treating chronic illness in managed care that make determination of benefits very complex. Insurance companies and HMO plans usually plan to meet expenses within a year or two, and that is a short time frame for long-term outcomes. The benefits of prevention, social services, and much of healthcare in general are achieved over a longer period of time. This poses a very significant difference in perceived obligations for the business as opposed to the clinical side. The obligation to provide social and other services, such as personal care for the patient or respite for the family, is even less clear, while moral hazard appears to be greater.

The abstract, subjective, self-reporting characteristics of long-term illness are used to justify increased administrative control and less respect for professional clinical judgment. However, because of its very subjectivity and variability, there is a more complex moral obligation to identify and separate specific interests and goals, financial or personal costs, and benefits in making treatment decisions. The variation in outcomes suggests to some administrators that such differences are random and therefore it does not violate a patient's best interest to impose external controls and substitute lower-cost services or providers. On the contrary, this increased variation is a compelling argument for morally responsible, professional clinical judgment. Benefit package limitations may not enhance clinical judgment or promote patients' interests, particularly when there is a range of acceptable treatments and dollars become the determinant of utilization.

There is no solid evidence that long-run costs are being contained or quality protected when adjusted for patient severity. Nor have plans decided whether to factor in, or how to weight, patients' values or the time the physician needs to tease out subtle but crucial patients' problems. Complex clinical judgment is especially important to provide an accurate differential diagnosis when there is concern about organic or physiologic components of illness, to make referrals, and to work as part of a team that develops appropriate treatment plans. The subjectivity of chronic illness demands increased, not decreased, clinical judgment. It also provides a strong moral argument for professional accountability.

These contentions do not advocate a return to FFS medicine with the obvious incentives to overutilize, but rather for professional accountability and a financing mechanism that reduces the relationship between treatment decisions and financial interests—in either direction. If decisions about what benefits to cover and how much care to authorize are determined by under- or overutilization of care, the system is both inefficient and immoral.

For acute as well as chronic illness, decisions to hospitalize, length of stay, readmission, and limitations on outpatient treatments are all profoundly influenced by financing. Care is complicated by substitutable diagnoses and treatments that encourage providers to label and treat according to defined benefits and to extend treatment time to the duration of coverage. In acting as the patient's agent, it may be morally appropriate for a physician to maximize insurance reimbursement as a way to provide access to a patient in need of care.

Case management and utilization review further challenge obligation to act primarily in the patient's interest. For whom do the reviewers work? Do they broker services? Are they reimbursed at a higher rate for individuals who are identified as more severely ill and less high functioning? If so, do they have an incentive to report and, thus, be paid accordingly? Case managers often do not even see patients, but employ computer algorithms to identify appropriateness of care. Data are submitted by practitioners who may be primary care physicians (PCPs) or supplied from questionnaires completed by the patients. Is this adequate clinical evaluation? The line between moral obligation and quality disappears. The General Accounting Office reports that utilization review is experienced by caregivers as providing the greatest intrusion into professional autonomy, and there is evidence that utilization review may provide a one-time-only cost savings. Physicians may be socialized to change behaviors over the long term, as long as they perceive no harm to patients or compromise to their basic professional duty. Established managed care systems such as Kaiser Permanente Health Plan have recognized professional integrity and have maintained arm's length relationships with the medical group.

There are also ethical concerns associated with the extensive use of innovative information systems in managed care. They may reduce costs, increase communication, and promote quality through patient information, but there is a real threat to patient confidentiality. There is obviously a basic moral obligation to protect patient privacy, and the courts are very strict about enforcing those rights, but with integration it is often difficult to establish or enforce a need-to-know only policy.

Another moral concern stems from the employer-provided insurance system.[5] Normally, purchases in the marketplace reflect consumer preferences. In the case of health insurance, the buyer is the employer, not the consumer. Patients, largely excluded from choice of benefits, lack the knowledge and discretionary choice that usually accompany decisions to buy. These qualities also discourage patients to shop.

There are additional institutional and societal ethical problems related to justice. There is good evidence that people with the greatest degree of physical and mental impairment are not enrolled in private managed systems because they do not work or do not have access, and mechanisms to lower costs may be incompatible with their healthcare needs.

Clearly, managed care organizations have to remain financially viable but also must consider the extent of their societal responsibility. Managed care traditionally enrolls a disproportionate share of the working well. Plans have a low proportion of poor, unemployed, chronically, and severely ill who are generally without any private coverage, and who need long-term care that is less discretionary and substitutable. Assumptions that people have access and transportation, are in the system, know how to use it, and will do so appropriately are less likely in closed private systems that are primarily financed through the workplace. Should the supervision of insurance companies, HMOs, and other managed plans be limited to monitoring fair business practices and reserves, or does the community have a right to demand that these plans accept a social obligation to cover risks that are not sound from an actuarial standpoint?

It has been argued that insurers must show why their interests are worth protecting in the face of complaints about injustice.[6] Insurers might ask the opposing questions: "Is there a compelling public right to demand that we jeopardize our solvency? Is it not our primary obligation to stay in business, particularly in the face of increased competition within the industry and with federal subsidy of self-insurance through ERISA, which limits further our market?" Like hospitals, all health plans deal with a product that is frequently nondiscretionary, where the consumer does not have sufficient knowledge to make an informed choice given the complexity of the system and the urgency or necessity of the problem and the solution.

Thus, the health economy fails to meet free-market criteria in an industry that is highly subsidized and yet resists accountability other than for banking reserves. Government subsidizes the private markets through significant subsidies by Medicare and Medicaid as well as tax exemptions, even while they complain about cost shifting. Medicare and Medicaid assume some high-risk patients, fill beds to cover fixed costs, and provide the safety net that allows the private sector to feel relieved of the burden to provide care to the uninsured poor.

But the public has not explicitly agreed to assume this responsibility. It has been piecemeal, subject to budget cuts, and criticized politically and socially from both liberals and conservatives. In an ethical, democratic system, the tradeoff to the public sector should be explicit. There needs to be agreement on what belongs in the public sector and what is to be handled in the private domain. To date, the process has not been deliberate, explicit, or coordinated. Gaps and fragmented coverage have left many people without good access to healthcare, and the split between the rich and poor, which is often the same as the split between the well functioning and the severely ill, has widened.

Are health plans responsible only to those subscribers privately enrolled in their system? Is there even an obligation to inform members about noncovered benefits? What about when enrollees' benefits are exhausted? How long does this obligation last? A priority-setting process should include discussion of responsibility for benefits, types of services, and groups of patients. It is very difficult even when the constituency includes the entire community. Medicare beneficiaries often have not been told, or do not understand, what they trade off in dollars, benefits, and choice when they enroll in HMOs. Nor do they appreciate that Medicare does not cover extensive rehabilitation or long-term care.

How should managed care companies contribute to the conversation about rationing and setting priorities to identify what services are most essential to cover? Managed care plans should not be expected to price themselves out of business. They do have an obligation to their board, stockholders, and employees, but those essential services that are rightfully financed in the private sector need to be identified. There must be a public dialogue and accountability, and all population subgroups need to be protected in one sector or the other.

Potential solutions

As a system, managed care contains many opportunities to enhance patient welfare through a more responsible, integrated clinical enterprise.[7] Managed care's primary ethical responsibilities include duties to provide competent physicians and staff, access to care, continuity, and confidentiality.[8] As with any healthcare system, managed care also has a compelling obligation to assure quality, which includes more than process and patient satisfaction, and to measure treatment effectiveness. The managed care organizations should take advantage of integrated systems to advance seamless, continuous care that promotes quality.

As an industry, managed care has the potential to advance professional skills and knowledge through interdisciplinary conferences and peer interaction. The HMO has a special opportunity to improve practice-based research through the study of subscribers who are users and nonusers of care and to analyze the implications of different structure and practice patterns on patient outcomes and costs.

Managed care provides a special opportunity to participate in an interdisciplinary effort toward developing data-based protocols that maximize patient welfare and professional satisfaction. Practice standards and guidelines not supported by sufficient data are indeed rules without reason, and there is little more than a random chance they are correct. Interdisciplinary dialogues could promote consensus on professional obligations and responsibilities under managed care. There is inadequate understanding of common clinical paths associated with better outcomes such as improved patient function, reduced family stress, or return to work. There should be discussion of long- and short-term noneconomic costs and benefits to patients associated with alternative treatments. For example, is it ultimately more or less costly financially, and clinically, to provide care in the home, rehabilitation unit, or nursing home for a particular chronic condition? Which subsets of patients are better managed where?

Managed care provides great potential to develop optimal patient care plans, target appropriate treatment goals, and monitor process as well as outcome. Costs can also be more explicit, and managed care is potentially well suited to the prioritizing consistent with professional and social values. Within the capitation model, clinical and business interests alike would be best served by intervention strategies consistent with patients' wishes and sensitive to social networks of the patients.[9]

Having respect for people means making their preferences explicit. Whenever possible, patients should participate in their own healthcare decisions, particularly if there are major differences in short- and long-term outcomes, likelihood of complications, or other risks and benefits from specific treatment decisions.

Patient privacy needs to be protected as well as public safety. Records should not be shared with the employer or anyone not directly involved with the care, including the family, unless the patient has given permission. Confidentiality promotes trust and, thus, healing.

In summary, the great advantage of managed care is ultimately its potential to develop comprehensive, coordinated systems of healthcare. Some other desirable characteristics of a good healthcare system, such as peer review and practice-based research, are facilitated through managed care. Similarly, there is a greater opportunity to assess and meet the healthcare needs of a population through integrated delivery systems. Physicians and other caregivers have additional moral and legal responsibilities under managed care. Some of these are to inform patients about reimbursement rules, to develop appropriate care plans and target treatment goals, to collaborate with colleagues to establish appropriate professional norms, to enforce professional standards, and to appeal reimbursement refusals for appropriate, indicated patients' services. Providers must learn the rules of the appeals process and how that process along with peer review of managed care can serve to advantage the caregiver and the patient.

Outreach to other professionals and communities is also important in managed care. It is essential that professionals within the system communicate with one another about patients and educate other providers. Managed care also provides an excellent opportunity to educate patients about the limits of healthcare. Patients need to accept individual and collective obligations to be more responsible for their own health and health status.

Finally, there must be acknowledgment that medicine is both an art and a science. Medicine is based on probabilities and professional status will not be diminished when uncertainty is admitted. That is an important step in making everyone's expectations more explicit, realistic, and achievable. An integrated healthcare system must include clinicians as well as administrators and must articulate and abide by clinical as well as business values. It is neither good management nor good medicine to function at the expense of important guiding principles that promote healing and trust.

NOTES

1. The failure is observed by inflation that is significantly higher than the rest of the economy, payer rebellion, and only slight marginal improvements in health outcomes as a result of increased services and costs. Failure has been acknowledged throughout the system and in reform attempts.

2. This unlikely partnership between public interest and social welfare groups, business, and government was also seen in the early 1970s with the passage of the original HMO legislation.

3. M. S. Jellinek and B. Nurcombe, "Two Wrongs Don't Make A Right: Managed Care, Mental Health, and the Marketplace," *JAMA* 270, no. 14 (Oct. 13, 1993): 1737–39.

4. E. Pellegrino, "Rationing Healthcare: The Ethics of Medical Gatekeeping," *Journal of Contemporary Health Law and Policy* 2 (1986): 23–45.

5. M. P. Cotler and B. Gould, "Setting Mental Health Priorities in the Private Sector," accepted for publication, *Hastings Center Report* 1/94.

6. N. Daniels, "Insurability and the HIV Epidemic; Ethical Issues in Underwriting," *The Milbank Quarterly,* no. 4 (1990).

7. M. P. McGovern, J. Lyons, and H. Pompage, "Capitation Payment Systems and Public Mental Health Care: Implications for Psychotherapy with the Seriously Mentally Ill," *American Journal of Orthopsychiatry* 60, no. 2 (April 1990): 298–304.

8. G. Povar and J. Moreno, "Hippocrates and the Health Maintenance Organization: A Discussion of Ethical Issues," *Annals of Internal Medicine* (September 1988): 419–24.

9. McGovern, Lyons, and Pompage, "Capitation Payment."

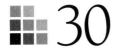 30

Economic incentives to do harm or good

John J. Mayerhofer
Principal
Mayerhofer and Associates
Oakland, California

THE NATION'S HEALTHCARE INDUSTRY is now swept up in a paradigm shift to capitation-based delivery reform. It is not predicated on population-based need and it may have little or no documentable outcomes for several generations. By surrendering healthcare reform to market forces, the healthcare industry will be subjected to a period of economic compression and dislocation. This compression may generate short-term profits for purchasers and payers, but, without a long-term view of the nation's aging population and corresponding population-based health needs, profits generated by capitation and converted into earnings per share will be just as oxymoronic as the "surplus" in the Social Security Trust Fund. The Social Security Trust Fund is currently building reserves, albeit at an insufficient rate. For-profit HMOs are required by the market to distribute profits rather than building reserves for the needs of an aging population.

Financial drivers

The financial driver for the growth from 5.2 percent of the gross domestic product in 1960 to 14 percent today was a system of payment that rewarded utilization.

Under fee-for-service (FFS) incentives, the first to enter a market with new services or technology sets the price. Competitors are forced to either offer service enhancements at no additional cost or the same service at lower costs. However, this "market pricing" is not without its hidden cost to the population. Unnecessary duplication of technology may result in lower prices per unit, but the ability of the providers to churn the patients or to unbundle pricing ultimately results in an over-all higher cost to the population.

Thus, beginning in the 1950s, America began a medical arms race that rapidly turned a cottage industry into a multibillion-dollar enter-prise fueled by the FFS business. Simply stated, the rules for success in the FFS healthcare delivery system were: "Get the bodies in, get the bills out, get the cash in."

Healthcare is a cash flow business with an unlimited ability to con-sume resources. What appear to be interim profits are really premature distributions. Short-term cash flow surpluses are being generated because capitated costs are less than capitated premiums, which still reflect FFS utilization practices. Likewise, under FFS as long as the pop-ulation of full-fee-paying patients continued to grow, healthcare pro-duced short-term financial gains. Yet, unless there is an improvement of the health status of the populations served, there will be no real short-term profit—just premature distributions from an underfunded health-care system.

The historical relationship between volume and profit is flipped under capitation. After fixed costs were paid for under FFS, profit was a func-tion of the volume of services provided. Under capitation, the more ser-vices that are generated after the capitation payment has been exceeded, the greater the loss.

Impact of aging

In 1996, the baby boom generation will start turning 50, an age where chronic problems typically arise, often requiring a need for acute care admission. Given the recent reductions in traditional admission rates under capitation versus FFS, the number of baby boomers entering their "golden years" will result in a reversal of the expected decline in the uti-lization of acute care services. Although genetic reengineering holds great promise for future generations, it will come too late to change the disease life cycle for baby boomers, thereby altering the inevitable increase in acute care utilization as baby boomers age.

At any point in time, individuals are in one of five stages of health as shown in Figure 1. The purpose of a primary care population-based delivery system is to prevent as many enrollees as possible from moving from a healthy state to an at-risk state or to an acute or chronic level of illness. If a patient progresses through risks and symptoms to an acute state, the objective of the delivery system is to return the patient to a healthy state as quickly as possible and to prevent as much chronic impairment as possible. However, even under a population-based disease life cycle approach, chronic care may be the only option.

Population-based planning seeks to identify and eliminate the socioeconomic factors that contribute to individuals progressing from a healthy state to a state requiring acute or chronic care intervention. However, while prevention and early detection services will help delay the progression from a healthy to a chronic state, the disease life cycle is primarily a function of age; lacking the discovery of a "genetic fountain of youth," boomers are aging and will soon enter the acute and chronic phases of their lives.

The market's current preoccupation with capitation is understandable when viewed as a paradigm shift caused by the anticipated demand for acute care services by the baby boomer generation. The FFS system was successful at creating capacity, but ineffective at controlling cost. Unless a system is put in place to limit the population-based growth in demand from those 50 years old and over, healthcare costs as a percentage of the GDP will exceed 20 percent shortly after the turn of the century. Capitation is seen as a panacea for the dual problems of excess cost and capacity. What is not clear, however, is how well capitation will address the

FIGURE 1
Disease life cycle and incentives under FFS versus capitation

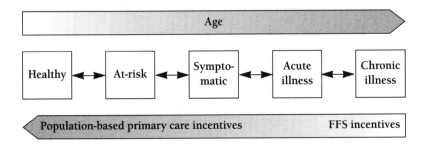

specific problems of an aging population and the challenges of managing a population-based disease life cycle.

New paradigm of reform

"A paradigm is: a set of rules, spoken or silent, that define the playing field, and the rules to win the game."[1] Paradigms define the boundaries within which the game will be played as well as the rules that must be followed in order to win the game (e.g., tennis is a simple paradigm, life is a forest of paradigms). The FFS payment system was the old paradigm, while capitation is the new paradigm. In a paradigm shift, there are some distinct stages that are typically followed in defining new and related rules. Thus, in the shift from FFS to capitation there are certain rules in the old game that must be abandoned and some other rules to be adopted.

For example, when the FFS delivery system was replaced by a market-driven capitated delivery system, it was anticipated that excess capacity would be squeezed out of both the physician and hospital delivery systems, premiums would be reduced for the employed population, but two fundamental systemic problems would remain. Because the capitated system failed to build reserves in anticipation of population-based needs, there may not be sufficient reserves to pay for services to the elderly, poor, or disenfranchised. Secondly, and more importantly, there has been no change in the overall health status of the population. Premiums have been cut, current expenditures are lower, but the population is no healthier than before.

The shift from FFS to capitation as both a delivery system and a payment methodology represents a paradigm shift equivalent to the shift from mainframe to microcomputer processing. Capitated systems such as the Kaiser Permanante Health Plan were viewed as aberrant when FFS dominated healthcare, but are now touted as the preferred delivery and payment systems. What makes the paradigm shift to capitation so powerful is the introduction of for-profit organizations, which have recognized that the financial incentives under capitation will greatly reduce utilization, thereby lowering the overall cost of the delivery system. Since capitated healthcare costs are expected to decline more rapidly than the premiums paid for healthcare, large profits will be earned that must be distributed to shareholders as dividends.

New paradigm under way

Capitation is both a philosophy of care (womb-to-tomb delivery reform) as well as a payment method (financing reform). As a payment method, capitation creates powerful economic incentives that can accomplish what FFS could not. Capitation removes the subsidization of excess capacity (e.g., hospital beds) and can forestall the acquisition of redundant delivery capacity (e.g., four MRI machines within a one-mile radius of each other). Capitation in more aggressive managed care plans has already caused the number of days of care (use rates) to plummet from 2,400 days per 1,000 members for the over-65 population to well below 900 days per 1,000. Even more dramatic reductions have been achieved with the under-65 population.

Economics of reform

The FFS mechanism produced a delivery system that exceeded the current expectations of consumers and purchasers. Healthcare has become too expensive, and the purchasers of care have chosen competitive market forces as a way to resolve the issues of excess cost and capacity. The silent partner in this rush to use market reform to lower cost is the federal government. Having created Medicare and Medicaid programs and having lost control of the regulatory process as a way to lower cost, the government has given control of the reform process to the market. It has also given control to the market without any accountability for adequate patient-focused healthcare or per member per month (PMPM) spending in the hopes that the market will deliver adequate and patient-focused healthcare.

The fact that healthcare has resisted market reform for such an extended time is a testament to the power of the FFS model and the political power of the provider community. However, no industry can ignore its consumers over the long term and expect to survive. Other industries such as railroads, banking, airlines, and trucking have gone through similar compression as they moved from monopoly to open markets and back to monopolies.

Healthcare passed through the regulation phase in the 1970s and the market innovation and product competition phases in the early 1980s. The introduction of selective contracting in the late 1980s, including

FIGURE 2
The regulatory cycle

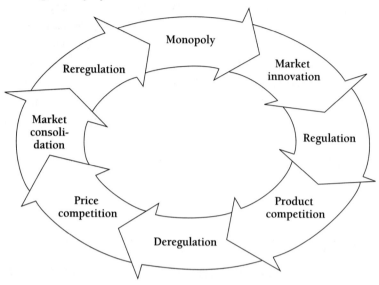

Medicare risk contracting, marked the deregulatory phase. Healthcare is now passing through the price competition phase of the regulatory cycle. The industry has shifted from regulatory compliance to market and price competition, which will lead to consolidation. The key question in this phase will be how to decide the winners of the competitive shake-out: how to value the quality and cost of the medical delivery system? The answer is price.

The industry has been unable to meet the purchaser's expectation for a defined change in health status with appropriate satisfaction at an acceptable price. As a result, purchasers, including the federal government, have chosen to let market forces do the sorting out of who will provide the greatest value where:

$$\text{Value} = \text{Change in health status} + \frac{\text{Consumer satisfaction}}{\text{Price}}$$

Since the healthcare community has not been able to adequately define quality and since it may take a lifetime to be able to document a true change in health status, the equation must be solved for price as follows:

$$\text{Value} = \frac{\text{Quality}}{\text{Price}}$$

Buy-sell relationship

In the new paradigm of market-driven reform, the personal trust of the physician-patient relationship has been replaced with the hard realities of the buy-sell relationship. In the FFS paradigm, management of care was entrusted to the physicians who in turn were responsible to the hospital's board of directors. The community service paradigm has been replaced by the buy-sell paradigm in Figure 3.

In this model, the purchaser only buys what it needs to meet the immediate needs of enrollees. Purchasers buy access and negotiation services from the premium collector (payers). Payers, in turn, buy only needed services from the providers. Providers, in turn, sell services to premium collectors and premium collectors sell access to the purchasers.

This system appears to be very crisp and works off the power of the market to manage through price. As currently structured, however, it is too narrow in scope and in focus. Healthcare must address the needs of the entire person. The human condition does not regulate itself in accordance with some payment PMPM schedule. Health status is a social good that will not be rationally allocated or improved by a capitation-based system, unless the incentives are applied equally to both the provider and healthcare consumer.

FIGURE 3
New buy-sell paradigm

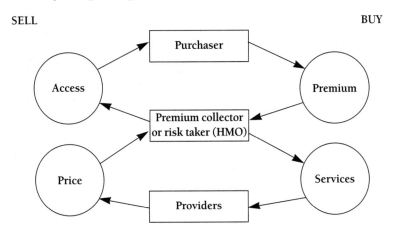

Given the difficulties of defining quality or measuring a change in health status, the process of valuing healthcare can be reduced to a single variable: price. Having chosen price as the key measure of value, the next objective is to prevent healthcare providers from unbundling services or artificially inflating volumes as a way to preserve cash flows. Capitation meets both needs: a fixed price for all services to a designated beneficiary.

Finance versus delivery

American medicine has become an entrepreneurial profession where financing and delivery are interwoven to such an extent that it is not possible to change delivery without changing finance. Thus, it is not reasonable to expect providers to change their behavior without the proper incentives to improve performance. While the market is effective at allocating limited capital resources at various levels of risk, it is not very adept at allocating social goods such as health status or wellness. There is a danger that a purely financial solution to the current surplus or maldistribution of provider capacity will yield a system that may cost less in the short term but has little long-term potential to finance healthcare for its community as it ages.

Assuming there is an appropriate number of primary care providers (PCPs) to care for the lives assigned to a delivery system, the incentives become very clear. A fixed amount of money is paid to each PCP for the care of the individuals assigned to them. The economic incentive is to avoid making referrals to specialists and hospitals. Subject to how the withhold agreements have been written, it may be possible for an aggressive PCP group to develop significant surpluses in the specialist, hospital, and hospital withhold pools, 50 percent of which would be given back to PCPs under a redistribution formula.

Capitation is intended to be a single payment for a full range of medical services. The provider community is given a single amount that is intended to cover the full cost of "womb to tomb" care. Capitation fixes the total amount of payment for healthcare services for a particular enrollee for a specific period of time, usually expressed as an amount PMPM. Controlling the cost of medical services delivered (i.e., the medical loss ratio) in the current period results in a surplus being generated between the capitation paid and the cost of care. What is not clear is whether the care rendered (or not rendered) is adequate for the disease life cycle realities of the population served.

Managing risk versus managing care

The three rules of success in capitation are very clear: enrollees, more enrollees, and still more enrollees. In order to prevent the risk of adverse selection, it is critical that the premium collector or risk taker be able to attract a sufficient number of enrollees to prevent any one segment of the population from adversely affecting the medical loss ratio (i.e., the percentage of the premium dollar actually spent on the provision of healthcare services). While various estimates of the number of enrollees needed for a sustainable HMO range from 50,000 to 400,000 members, it is easy to understand that $30 per month on 5,000 lives will not adequately cover the cost of providing intensive neonatal care for one premature infant (i.e., $150,000 to $200,000), let alone provide for the care of the remaining 4,999 enrollees.

Although there has been considerable compression in the HMO industry, with fewer HMOs having responsibility for more lives, the need to constantly manage adverse risk means that HMOs must constantly be marketing to new enrollees. With the exception of a few large and long-standing health plans such as the Kaiser Permanante Health Plan in California and Group Health Cooperative of Puget Sound, Seattle, other HMOs have not been in existence long enough to gather the longitudinal data to demonstrate that the capitation has effected the change in health status that a population-based health plan should be addressing. The Kaiser Health Plan in California has recently announced its intention to invest over one billion dollars in information systems to capture this data.

In response to the lack of data that differentiates the effectiveness of capitated care in changing the health status of a defined population, the HMO industry has developed "scorecards" to document a number of preventive measures being pursued by the HMO, such as pediatric inoculations, the number of breast cancer screenings, and the ratio of members to PCPs. Early scorecards indicated that capitated plans were having trouble tracking the members' PCP and vice versa. More importantly, because members will change plans for a premium differential as little as $10 PMPM and because more money can be generated by cutting payments to providers than investing in health status modification, plans may not have the incentives to invest time and money in getting a population healthy—only to have that population transferred to another plan with lower premiums.

Medicare risk plans

The ultimate perversion of the capitation paradigm is the current rush to Medicare Risk contracts. HMOs with Medicare risk capitation programs receive an amount equivalent to 95 percent of the average annual cost for all Medicare beneficiaries in a particular area. This average adjusted per capita cost (AAPCC) rate is a carryover from the FFS and cost reimbursement programs.

Under the Medicare Risk program or "no premium" Medicare, health plans are marketed directly to seniors as no-premium because the Medicare Risk plan pays the seniors' Part B coverage, deductibles, and coinsurance. The elderly well (just as the young working well did with HMOs in the 1980s) are choosing the no-premium Medicare plans. Conversely, the elderly frail are staying with traditional Medicare. The end result is that the AAPCC for Medicare beneficiaries still under the diagnostic related group-based FFS system rises, thus resulting in an immediate profit to the Medicare Risk HMO.

Purchasers are unwilling to pay for the constantly escalating cost of healthcare. The simple economics of the baby boom and the financial projections of the Medicare Trust Fund demand that expenditures be curtailed, or the trust will be bankrupt within 10 years.

A large segment of the American population is about to enter the "medical replacement" age, a time when one body system or another will fail. Since this population will have been too old to benefit from genetic reengineering, these baby boomers can be expected to progress down the path to chronic impairment with some predictability. Therefore any reduction to the medical loss ratio that is being generated today should be placed in trust for this future "incurred, but not yet manifested" liability.

Wall Street as the new regulator

In the nation's economy, where healthcare costs for auto industry employees exceeds the cost of steel used to manufacture the car, costs must be reduced.

Frequently, when there is no easy answer to a social conundrum, the market is called into force. No industry can ignore its consumer base. Therefore it is not inappropriate to use market-based price competition as a tool to eliminate excess capacity. What is called into question is the use of a pure price-driven model that may not make its allocation decisions on the basis of population-based need. Without a longer-term view of the disease life cycle and the population-based needs of enrolled members both today and in 20 years, the capitation paradigm may be short lived.

The American economic engine is fueled by capital, capital is fueled by Wall Street, and Wall Street is fueled by profits. Consequently, for-profit HMOs, which now dominate in many areas such as California, must prove to Wall Street that they can continue to generate a positive and increasing bottom line. To accomplish this they must do two things: gain more members to dilute the administrative cost of running the HMO and reduce the medical loss ratio (i.e., capitation payments to providers). The new rules of the game are quite straightforward: get the members in, keep the medical loss ratio low, and keep the profits high.

Health price negotiation organizations (HPNO)

HMOs are under pressure to reduce the medical loss ratio as a way to improve profitability. Purchasers demand that payers not only cut premiums, but also actually roll the premiums back. Given these pressures, the role of the payer is quite clear: to negotiate the lowest possible price with the provider community and to pass off as much risk as possible (in effect to retain no risk). It is not unreasonable then for the premium collector to view its business not as an HMO, but as an HPNO. With the rapidly consolidating buying power of the purchaser and payer amplified by the need for quarterly returns to stockholders, it is quite obvious what the results of the capitation experiment will be: decapitation to any but the most aggressive price negotiators.

Assuming value equals change in health status plus satisfaction over price, where risk is fully passed on to the provider community through capitation, the future becomes a series of rationing decisions. In essence, purchasers are paying Wall Street to discipline the industry to control its costs. However, instead of reinvesting the gains from cost reductions back into community-based health status improvement programs, profits will be redistributed to a broad range of investors. Since the New Age regulators (now called HMOs) will need to maintain a constantly increasing stream of earnings to meet the expectations of the Wall Street, and since purchasers will continue to demand that lower costs be translated into lower premiums, the end result can only be less money for healthcare delivery.

Capitation has the ability to transform the delivery system from a specialist-dominated, medical intervention system to a primary care, population-based health maintenance system.

As a negative reinforcer, however, capitation has the ability to cause the surviving providers to undertreat today to hold reserves for incurred but not yet manifested medical problems. More perniciously, services can be denied or unduly rationed so the surplus in the "withhold pool" can be distributed either to the providers, to the stockholders, or to purchasers.

As a type of financing reform, capitation has a limited future. At some point, the excess capacity will be eliminated and the sheer numbers of baby boomers will cause costs in the system to once again rise. Rather, even before the capitation paradigm fails to solve the cost of care problem through rationing, a new paradigm will appear that will most likely not be built around access to providers but on the effective use of information to bring about a change in health status. The key to success in delivery reform is not how much service is withheld in the name of economic savings, but how those savings will be reinvested today to assure the health status of the population tomorrow.

NOTES

1. J. Barker, *Future Edge* (New York: William Morrow, 1992).

Contributors

Editor

Peter Boland, PhD
President and Publisher
Boland Healthcare, Inc.
Berkeley, California

A consistently thought-provoking commentator and nationally recognized authority on managed care, Peter Boland forecasts industry trends and develops publications to improve healthcare management. He is the editor and publisher of *The Capitation Sourcebook* and *Redesigning Healthcare Delivery*, co-editor of *Physician Profiling and Risk Adjustment*, and was the principal author and editor of *Making Managed Healthcare Work* and *The New Healthcare Market*. He was also the founding editor of *Managed Care Quarterly*.

He received a PhD from the University of California, Los Angeles, a master's degree from the University of Michigan, and a postgraduate certificate from Harvard University's executive program in health policy and management. Often quoted in trade and news media, he frequently challenges the conventional wisdom and speaks regularly at industry conferences.

Authors

William Adamson
Chief Executive Officer
St. Joseph's Medical Resources
Stockton, California

William Adamson specializes in integrated delivery system formation, group practice operations, IPA development and implementation, and subcapitation models for evaluating provider efficiency. He is the chief executive officer of St. Joseph's Medical Resources, a physician group and IPA management company. Previously he was the administrator of an integrated group practice of primary care physicians in northern California and directed a 298-physician multispecialty IPA.

He has an MBA with an emphasis in accounting from California State University.

Lori Anderson
Assistant Vice President and Senior Consultant
Premier, Inc.
Westchester, Illinois

Lori Anderson directs consulting assignments for integrated delivery system design, managed care product development, reimbursement strategies, and contract negotiation. She is the acting chief operating officer of Atlantic Health, a large integrated delivery system in central Maryland.

She received a master's degree in hospital and healthcare administration from the University of Iowa. She is a frequent lecturer on capitation, managed care strategy, and integrated delivery system development.

Geoffrey B. Baker
Managing Director
Physician Management Alliance
Los Angeles, California

Geoffrey Baker focuses on MSO operations, physician network development, and capitation rate setting. He specializes in implementing managed care financial control and reporting systems. He worked for a staff model HMO, managed an IPA, and developed MSOs for AMI (Tenent), Massachusetts General Hospital, and Columbia/HCA.

He received an MBA from the Wharton School of Business at the University of Pennsylvania, has written numerous articles on integrated delivery systems, and presents on IPA and managed care financial topics.

Javon Bea
President and Chief Executive Officer
Mercy Health System
Janesville, Wisconsin

Javon Bea heads a rural 27-site health system in two states that includes more than 200 physicians, community clinics, and an HMO. He was executive vice president and chief operating officer at Providence Hospital and an administrator at Virginia Mason/Mason Clinic and the Mayo Medical Center.

He has a master's degree in hospital and healthcare administration from the University of Minnesota and is a fellow of the American College of Healthcare Executives.

Sandra L. Berkowitz
Senior Vice President and Managed Care Practice Leader
Johnson and Higgins
Philadelphia, Pennsylvania

Sandra Berkowitz directs development of the company's products and services to managed care customers. Her expertise includes manuscripting of specialty managed care coverages and creating alternative insurance vehicles to finance liability and reinsurance risks. Previously, she coordinated healthcare brokerage operations and practiced nursing as well as medical malpractice law.

She has a degree in nursing from the University of California, San Francisco, and a law degree from Temple University.

Dale Bradford
Vice President and General Manager, Cincinnati
ChoiceCare
Cincinnati, Ohio

Dale Bradford manages the health plan's operations for Cincinnati members and leads a team responsible for all strategy deployment. He was the vice president of finance at ChoiceCare and was responsible for negotiating the hospital network in addition to all financial activities, including actuarial, pricing and underwriting, financial reporting, provider reimbursements, budgeting, and financial analysis.

He received a master's degree in accounting from Brigham Young University, is a certified public accountant, and is a frequent speaker on capitation and managed care strategy.

Debra Carpenter
Director, Utilization Management
Blue Plus
Eagan, Minnesota

Debra Carpenter directs case management, referral management, and clinic-based utilization management activities for an HMO. She previously managed utilization and quality assurance activities at a teaching hospital.

She is an accredited record technician with a business degree from Augsburg College.

Francine Chapman
Director of Managed Care Programs
UCLA Medical Center
Los Angeles, CA

Francine Chapman directs managed care programs for the medical center and the medical group. She focuses on managed care strategies, payer relationships and contracting, and network development. She was vice president of Verti-Health where she developed systems and protocols for managing UniHealth's capitated hospital agreements.

She holds a master's degree from the University of California, Los Angeles.

David Chin, MD
Principal
Coopers & Lybrand LLP
Boston, Massachusetts

David Chin leads managed care and integrated delivery system engagements in the Northeast for the healthcare consulting group. He was president and medical director of the Harvard Community Health Plan's Health Centers Division in eastern Massachusetts and was president of Novalis Corporation, which developed HMOs and networks for insurers, hospital systems, and academic medical centers.

He is board certified in internal medicine, has an MBA from Stanford University, and has a medical degree from Harvard Medical School.

Miriam Piven Cotler, PhD
Professor, Director of Bioethics Institute
Northridge Hospital Medical Center
Northridge, California

Miriam Cotler teaches courses in healthcare ethics, organization, and policy. She is an ethics consultant to several healthcare institutions and is director of the Ethics Institute at Northridge Hospital Medical Center. She cochairs the Uni-Health Bioethics Institute and has been an advisor to the Hastings Center, the American Cancer Society, and Blue Cross. She serves on ethics committees of the Los Angeles County Bar Association, the Hospital Council, and the American College of Medical Quality.

She received a PhD in health services with an emphasis in policy from the department of health services at the University of California, Los Angeles.

Robert A. Dickinson
Director
BDC Advisors
San Francisco, California

Robert Dickinson leads implementation projects involving strategy, regional network and group practice development, physician compensation, and risk-sharing models for integrated delivery systems. He was formerly a consultant with APM and Andersen Consulting.

He received an MBA from the Harvard Business School. He has published in *Medical Network Strategy Report,* American Medical Association's *Legal Advisor,* and *Journal of the National Association of Medical Staff Services* and contributes regularly as an expert source to The Healthcare Advisory Board and *Medical Economics.*

Timothy J. Feeser
Consultant
Towers Perrin
Minneapolis, Minnesota

Timothy Feeser works with managed care companies on benefit plan design, pricing and claim liability estimation, and premium rate determination. He also assists PHOs in determining capitations and risk-sharing arrangements. He was formerly a benefits consultant at Touche Ross.

He is a fellow of the Society of Actuaries, a member of the American Academy of Actuaries, and a frequent speaker on developing actuarial cost models at industry seminars.

Susan J. Fox, PhD
President
Fox Systems, Inc.
Scottsdale, Arizona

Susan Fox specializes in defining data and information management requirements for state Medicaid agencies and capitated health plans. She is a frequent presenter at national Medicaid conferences on applying healthcare information technology.

She has a PhD from the University of California, Berkeley.

Henry E. Golembesky, MD
Principal
APM Incorporated
San Francisco, California

Henry Golembesky assists physician group practices transition from fee-for-service to risk-based reimbursement. He was the board chair and medical director of SHARP Rees-Stealy Medical Group in San Diego and president and chief executive officer of UniMed America in Los Angeles.

He has a medical degree from the University of New Mexico School of Medicine and is board certified in pediatrics and medical management. He is a fellow of the American Academy of Pediatrics and the American College of Physician Executives.

Bruce Gorman
Vice President, Public Sector Programs
Merit Behavioral Care
South San Francisco, California

Bruce Gorman is responsible for provider organization relations, public-private integration issues, and the development of contractual arrangements with network providers. He was formerly with Aetna Life Insurance Company, where he oversaw managed care operations on the West Coast.

He holds a master's degree in city and regional planning from Rutgers University, publishes in healthcare and behavioral healthcare journals, and presents on managed care and health economic issues.

James Wm. Hager
Director of National Business Development
Blue Shield of California
San Francisco, California

James Hager directs national business development activities and works jointly with providers, other health plans, and organizations to meet employer and member needs. He was formerly interregional contract management consultant with Kaiser Permanente, where he coordinated national contracting efforts and established a center of excellence network of transplant service providers.

He has a master's of public administration with a concentration in health policy from the University of Southern California and completed the executive program of the Stanford University School of Business.

James A. Hester, Jr., PhD
Vice President of Network Development
ChoiceCare
Cincinnati, Ohio

James Hester is responsible for developing and maintaining provider networks that support both commercial and Medicaid product lines. He oversees the implementation of provider capitation including specialty reimbursement and global incentive programs. He held senior management positions at Pilgrim Health Care, Harvard Community Health Plan, New England Medical Center, and Kaiser-Permanente.

He received a PhD in planning from the Massachusetts Institute of Technology and has published in *Medical Care, Millank Memorial Fund Quarterly*, and *Business and Health*.

James O. Hillman
Executive Director
Unified Medical Group Association
Seal Beach, California

James Hillman directs a national association of capitated medical groups and IPAs that offer educational programs and capitation expertise to members. He was formerly the administrator at Harriman Jones Medical Group and led its transition from exclusively fee-for-service to predominantly prepaid healthcare.

He is a certified public accountant, a frequent writer on capitation, and a founding member and president of the Medical Quality Commission, a nonprofit organization that promotes quality improvement in managed care.

Margaret Houy
Manager, Network Development
Harvard Pilgrim Health Care, Inc.
Quincy, Massachusetts

Margaret Houy develops and manages commercial and Medicare risk sharing arrangements with network physicians and hospitals and specializes in structuring budgeted capitation arrangements with participating providers. She previously practiced and taught health law.

She received a law degree from the University of Michigan and an MBA from Simmons College Graduate School of Management.

Cal James
Principal
APM Incorporated
San Francisco, California

Cal James specializes in medical group management—management services organization (MSO) design, implementation, and operation—and health system development. He was formerly president and chief executive officer of Alta Bates Medical Resources and executive director of the affiliated medical groups, implementing an MSO for regional managed care contracting and practice management operations.

He has an MBA from the University of San Diego, a master's degree in management science from the University of Southern California, and speaks widely on physician organization issues.

Michael K. Kaplan
Senior Associate
APM Incorporated
San Francisco, California

Michael Kaplan leads client engagements on integrated delivery networks, including physician network development, contract negotiation, and medical management techniques.

He has an MBA from the Stanford Graduate School of Business and speaks often at industry conferences, particularly on issues of physician incentives.

Kevin M. Kennedy
Manager
ECG Management Consultants
Seattle, Washington

Kevin Kennedy consults on strategic planning and organization design and development for healthcare clients. He has assisted medical groups, physician-hospital joint ventures, and health systems in creating compensation plans for physicians at all levels of capitation.

He has an MBA from the University of Chicago and is a frequent speaker at industry conferences on healthcare integration, managed care operations, and physician strategic issues.

Robert M. Kisabeth, MD
Medical Director, Mayo Medical Laboratories
Mayo Clinic
Rochester, Minnesota

Robert Kisabeth directs the clinic's laboratory outreach programs and assists community laboratories in executing fee-for-service plans and capitated agreements. He previously practiced general pathology in a large community hospital.

He has a medical degree from the University of Tennessee and speaks frequently on the role of community-based ancillary services in reducing costs while designing and executing disease management strategies.

Peter Kongstvedt, MD
Partner
Ernst & Young LLP
Washington, DC

Peter Kongstvedt leads consulting projects on HMO operations and integrated delivery systems. He was the chief operating officer of a Blue Cross Blue Shield health plan and chief executive officer of an HMO. He has served on a number of state and national healthcare policy and strategy committees.

He received a medical degree from the University of Wisconsin, is a board certified internist, and a fellow in the American College of Physicians. He is the principal author of *The Managed Health Care Handbook, Second Edition; The Essentials of Managed Care* and coauthor of *The Medical Director's Handbook*.

Jennifer Elston Lafata, PhD
Staff Investigator
Center for Clinical Effectiveness
Henry Ford Health System
Detroit, Michigan

Jennifer Elston Lafata is responsible for designing and conducting statistically rigorous program evaluations and cost-effectiveness analysis for clinical practice improvement efforts. She serves as principal investigator and coinvestigator on foundation and federally sponsored health services research projects.

She has a PhD in health services organization and policy from the University of Michigan with a concentration in economics.

John J. Mayerhofer
Principal
Mayerhofer and Associates
Oakland, California

John Mayerhofer provides financial management advisory services to hospitals and health systems, physician organizations, and industry trade associations. He was previously a practice director of KPMG Peat Marwick and the associate administrator and chief financial officer at three hospitals.

He has an MBA from Cornell University and attended the professional accounting program at Northwestern University. He is a fellow in the American College of Healthcare Executives and a fellow in the Healthcare Financial Management Association. He has published in *Healthcare Financial Management* and is a frequent contributor to *California Medicine.*

Thomas F. McNulty
Senior Vice President
Chief Financial Officer
Henry Ford Health System
Detroit, Michigan

Thomas McNulty directs the fiscal affairs of a multidimensional, vertically integrated health system concentrating on capital development, acquisitions, and managed care models. He is a lecturer at the University of Michigan and was an assistant professor of finance at Rush University.

Daniel J. Merlino
Vice President
ECG Management Consultants
Seattle, Washington

Daniel Merlino directs the firm's general healthcare practice provider network development, financial and business planning, and operations management. He specializes in developing provider network strategies as well as market-based solutions.

He has an MBA in organizational development and marketing from the University of California, Los Angeles.

Michael S. Miele
President
Capitated Disease Management Services
Upper Montclair, New Jersey

Michael Miele develops capitation products and models for prescription benefit managers and pharmaceutical manufacturers. He was formerly the actuarial practice leader for the disease state management group at Price Waterhouse LLP.

He is a fellow of the Society of Actuaries and a member of the American Academy of Actuaries.

John L. Miller
Principal
Integrated Healthcare Development Group
Westlake Village, California

John Miller develops and manages capitated physician organizations, from network models to integrated group practices.

He has an MBA from Pepperdine University, is a certified financial planner, certified professional business consultant, and associate editor of the *Integrated HealthCare Report.*

Christine Profita
Joint Venture Program Specialist
Harvard Pilgrim HealthCare, Inc.
Quincy, Massachusetts

Christine Profita focuses on implementing joint venture financial arrangements and supervises a staff of analysts who develop analytic tools to support joint venture performance evaluation. She held previous positions with the health plan in provider relations and hospital contracting.

William Riley, PhD
Chief Executive Officer
Aspen Medical Group
St. Paul, Minnesota

William Riley heads a 180-provider multispecialty medical group that focuses on managed care and capitation.

He has a PhD from the University of Minnesota department of healthcare administration and teaches graduate courses there in healthcare financial analysis and healthcare management.

Alice F. Rosenblatt
Principal
Coopers & Lybrand LLP
Boston, Massachusetts

Alice Rosenblatt specializes in actuarial analysis of healthcare issues for commercial carriers, Blues plans, HMOs, providers, and employers. She was the chief actuary at Blue Cross and Blue Shield of Massachusetts and at Blue Cross of California, chairs the American Academy of Actuaries' risk adjustment work group, and previously chaired the Academy's federal health committee.

She is a fellow of the Society of Actuaries, a member of the American Academy of Actuaries, and has testified before House subcommittees on the subject of risk adjustment.

Mary Schattenberg
Manager
BDC Advisors
San Francisco, California

Mary Schattenberg concentrates on managed care operations, contract review and negotiation, and hospital and physician network development. She was principal contract administrator for PacifiCare of California and established a licensed network of hospitals, medical groups, IPAs, and ancillary providers in the San Francisco Bay Area.

She has a master's degree in hospital and healthcare administration from the University of Minnesota. She has contributed to The Advisory Board's *Capitation Strategy* and *The Medical Staff Strategy Report*.

Heather Shupe
Financial Manager, Health Plan Services
Stanford Health Services and Lucile Salter Packard Children's Hospital
Stanford, California

Heather Shupe provides fiscal management for more than 300 general service and specialty contracts for an academic medical center, pediatric specialty hospital, and large multispecialty group. She has designed and implemented a managed care decision support system and specializes in pricing strategy, shared-risk partnerships, and global capitation.

She has a degree in finance from Santa Clara University and studied international finance at Loyola University in Rome.

Jonathan Solomons
Director, Ancillary Services
Independence Blue Cross and Keystone Health Plan East
Philadelphia, Pennsylvania

Jonathan Solomons manages subcontracting relationships including a full risk arrangement with a hospital system and carve-out laboratory and dental contracts. He was previously director of operations at Aetna Health Plans, responsible for provider relations and contracting, and a consultant for American Health Management and Consulting Corporation, focusing on HMO development for providers.

He has an MBA from Wharton Graduate Division, Univerity of Pennsylvania and has published in *Home Care* magazine.

Edward Thomas
Manager of Clinical Information
Blue Shield of California
San Francisco, California

Edward Thomas manages corporate clinical information and reporting activities for the company including provider profiling and system installations. He serves on the advisory panel for a three-year research effort by the Agency for Health Care Policy and Research on the impact of data reports on physicians' practices. He serves on the clinical subcommittee of the Health Data Information Corporation project and is on the board of the Health Partnership Institute. He was the corporate consultant for utilization management and practice issues at Kaiser-Permanente and has conducted research on practice variation for physicians in Canada and the United States.

He is a registered nurse and received an MBA from St. Mary's College.

David Yauch, MD
Medical Director
Aspen Medical Group
St. Paul, Minnesota

David Yauch is a medical director and a practicing internist with previous experience as a site chief at the medical group. He currently manages physician compensation, performance review, recruiting, quality improvement, and assists with managed care operations.

He has a medical degree from Baylor College of Medicine.

Alan R. Zwerner, MD, JD
Chief Executive Officer
The Medical Quality Commission
Seal Beach, California

Alan Zwerner heads a national nonprofit organization that develops programs for improving the quality of healthcare and administers a medical group accreditation program that includes a component for prepaid healthcare services. He was formerly senior medical director for FHP and has practiced obstetrical and gynecological medicine and healthcare law.

He received a medical degree from Georgetown University and a law degree from Western New England School of Law. He is a frequent lecturer on quality, utilization, and risk management under capitation.

Glossary of capitation and managed care terminology

AAPCC. Average adjusted per capita cost, the basis of the payment formula used for Medicare HMO plans.

access to care. The ability to obtain medical care easily on a timely and local basis without significant financial or other barriers.

actuary. 1. An insurance professional trained in the calculation of risk in insurance coverage. The actuary also develops guidelines for underwriters, who apply the guidelines to individual risks and premium rates. 2. A person trained in statistics and other insurance skills who assesses risk, develops policy premium rates, calculates and reserves dividends, and conducts various other statistical studies, typically for an insurance carrier or HMO.

add-on. The addition of specified benefits to an existing benefit package without requiring re-enrollment of the insured population.

adjusted community rating. Community rating that takes into account group-specific demographics and the enrollee/employer group's prior experience, (i.e., use of health services).

administrative costs. 1. In a health plan, all operational and nonoperational (i.e., investment) expenses other than direct medical costs, including general management and accounting, information systems, quality management, and marketing costs. 2. In a healthcare organization or institution, all costs not directly related to the provision of medical care.

administrative loading. Also known as administrative retention, an amount added by a health plan or HMO to the estimated cost of providing actual health services to a defined population, in order to cover administrative expenses of the plan. The estimated health services cost, the administrative retention, and a percentage added for profit together make up the entire premium rate.

administrative cost ratio. In a health plan or HMO, the proportion of administrative costs to premiums paid; this does not include profit or surplus. *See also* medical loss ratio; surplus.

administrative services only (ASO). The provision of claims processing and related administrative services to a health plan, typically a self-insured employer plan; the ASO contractor takes on no risk for the insured group (i.e., is not liable for the costs of providing care to a plan member).

admissions rate. The rate at which inpatients are admitted for a hospital stay.

adverse selection. 1. A phenomenon in which the members of a health plan generally use more services and are more expensive to care for than expected. 2. A situation in which a health plan attracts sicker-than-average members (i.e., the disproportionate enrollment of high-risk individuals).

age/sex rating. A process of setting premium rates that takes age and gender categories, along with their expected claims or utilization experience, into account.

aligned incentives. Financial incentives that encourage stakeholders to achieve shared organizational goals (e.g., a risk-sharing/gain-sharing arrangement among network providers and a health plan).

ALOS. See average length of stay.

alternate delivery system. A now outdated term referring to HMOs and other managed care plans, so named because of their emphasis on finding alternatives to inpatient care and thereby reducing hospitalizations.

alternative care. Also known as alternate delivery, a term describing noninpatient medical treatment that is a medically justified substitute for hospitalization. This term is becoming outmoded, however, as the medical interventions it represents (e.g., outpatient surgery, home healthcare, or adult day care. become part of standard medical practice). *See also* complementary medicine.

ancillary services. Supplemental medical services that are provided in conjunction with inpatient or ambulatory care (e.g., clinical laboratory, radiology, or physical therapy services).

anniversary date. The day on which a benefit year for an insurance plan or policy begins.

ASO contract. See administrative services only.

assignment. The process by which an insured person requests that the insuring health plan pay a claim directly to a designated provider (e.g., a physician or hospital) rather than reimburse the patient or claimant. This means the provider bills the health plan directly for its portion of the bill rather than billing the patient for the full amount.

at-risk contract. See global capitation.

average length of stay (ALOS). The average number of days that a hospital's patients are hospitalized. Sometimes used as a comparative measure of the severity of illness of a hospital's patient load or of a hospital's efficiency.

balance billing. The process by which a healthcare provider (e.g., a physician, hospital, or independent clinical lab) bills a patient for the excess amount that the patient's health plan does not cover. Balance billing is limited under programs such as Medicare and prohibited by Medicaid.

behavioral health services. Also known as mental and behavioral health or psychiatric care; the assessment and treatment of mental illness, behavioral disorders, and substance abuse.

benefit option. See coverage option.

benefit package. The specific benefits (i.e., covered health services and supplies) included in an insurance policy and the terms under which they are covered.

block grant. A method by which all federal financing for related programs is consolidated under a single grant, so that the state or other recipient of the grant can allocate funding to those programs in the manner it desires, as opposed to receiving specific dollar amounts for each separate program. Typically used for consolidating federal funding to states, counties, or municipalities.

capital and surplus requirements. Minimum reserves of capital and surplus funds to be maintained within a health plan that are required by law and by sound fiscal practice in order to avoid the insolvency of the plan and subsequent loss of coverage for members. *See also* surplus.

capitation. 1. A flat rate per person, paid in advance for providing specified care to a health plan member for a specified length of time (e.g., an amount paid per member per month to a primary care practitioner for the entire range of physician services that person may require for that month) regardless of how many or how few services are actually required or rendered. Most often used by HMOs to pay primary care providers but also used by purchasers to pay HMOs. 2. A flat rate per student paid to medical schools by the federal government to help support medical education.

capitated rate. Same as capitation.

carve out. A set of services, usually for specified types of care (e.g., psychiatric or long-term care), that is excluded from covered care under a health plan and made the responsibility of a separate organization or vendor (e.g., a managed behavioral healthcare firm or mental health PPO).

case management. 1. The systematic organization and coordination of health services and resources in order to optimize clinical outcomes and manage risk associated with chronic, complex, and catastrophic cases. 2. A process by which patients in need of medical care are matched by primary care practitioners or other case managers with providers and services to bring about the best result for the patient with the most efficient use of services, at an acceptable level of cost; usually reserved for higher-cost cases or more severe illness rather than routine, low-cost cases. *See also* case manager.

case manager. An experienced healthcare practitioner responsible for coordinating a patient's care to bring about the best result of treatment while making sure that optimal medically necessary care is provided in a prompt and cost-effective manner.

case mix. A measure that reflects some aspect of the severity of illness, diagnoses, resource use, use of services, or type of patients that typically characterize a provider's patient caseload; often used to compare caseloads among providers or to adjust provider payment or aggregate patient data.

catastrophic case. Any single high-cost medical condition or complication arising from same for which the total cost of treatment exceeds a given level, typically set between $25,000 and $50,000. For stop-loss coverage the trigger level may be higher, for example $100,000 per case.

chemical dependency. Another name for substance abuse or addiction (e.g., drug abuse, alcoholism and alcohol abuse, and nicotine addiction).

claim. 1. A request for payment under an insurance policy. The submission of an itemized bill for services or covered items (e.g., prescription drugs or medical devices) provided to an insured person. 2. The bill itself.

clinical algorithm. A method of describing a clinical practice guideline that uses a structured flowchart of if-then decision steps and preferred clinical management pathways. *See also* practice guidelines.

closed formulary. A specified list of prescription drugs, generally compiled by a health plan's pharmacy and therapeutics committee, that are covered by the plan's benefit package. Exceptions from this list generally are not allowed without prior consultation between the prescribing physician and the health plan's medical director or utilization management consultant. *See also* open formulary.

closed panel. A provider panel or network that is limited to specific selected medical practitioners or hospitals; sometimes used as a synonym for group/staff-model HMOs. *See also* provider panel.

coinsurance. The percentage of an insurance claim that an insured person must pay before reimbursement applies (e.g., in an 80/20 plan, the plan member pays 20 percent of the claim and the plan pays 80 percent).

community rating. 1. A method of setting premium rates that takes into account only the aggregate projected experience of an entire health plan population rather than the projected experience of an individual or employer group. 2. A method of premium setting in which an individual's or group's premium rate is based on the actual or anticipated cost of care for all members of a health plan in a specific service area. 3. A premium rate-setting method that reflects the experience of an entire population or community (e.g., a city, metropolitan statistical area, state, region, or nation).

community rating by class. 1. Community rating that takes into account the expected use of services of an entire class of members rather than expected use of services by specific enrollees or employer groups. 2. Community rating that adjusts premiums based on factors such as individuals' age, gender, marital status, and the industry in which they work. This formula is defined for federally qualified HMOs in the 1981 amendments to the federal HMO Act.

competitive medical plan (CMP). An HMO-like organized provider group that is not a federally qualified HMO but does meet other specific criteria that allow it to participate in Medicare risk contracting. CMPs are often HMOs that are state qualified but can also be capitated multispecialty medical groups that otherwise meet HCFA regulations.

complementary medicine. A generic term used to categorize treatment modalities that are currently outside mainstream Western medicine (e.g., homeopathy, traditional Chinese medicine, and massage therapy). *See also* alternative care.

completion method. A method of determining the dollar value of outstanding claims. This method divides claims paid by a factor representing the estimated percentage of claims paid to date.

compositing. A method of converting a multitiered rate structure into one with fewer tiers.

concurrent review. A determination made by a health plan, at the time care is being sought, that the care is medically necessary and covered under the plan.

conformance request. A written request issued to a participating provider asking that provider to comply with the health plan's rules of participation and practice guidelines. A refusal to conform can result in automatic case review by the plan, denial of payment, or termination of the provider's participation in the plan's provider panel or network.

consensus guidelines. Practice guidelines that reflect the consensus of the panel writing the guidelines rather than the state of the art or best medical practice. A serious shortcoming of consensus guidelines is the significant risk that they may reflect and institutionalize common practice rather than best practice and, as such, may discourage optimal care.

coordination of benefits (COB). The act of reconciling the liabilities of the primary payer's coverage with those expenses to be paid or covered by secondary payers, in order to avoid redundant payment; such coordination is an issue whenever an insured person is covered by more than one health plan (e.g., Medicare and a supplemental policy. In such cases, Medicare has determined that it generally will be the secondary payer).

copayment. The specified out-of-pocket amount that a health plan member must pay for a specific service provided under the plan (e.g., a fixed dollar amount per physician office visit or per drug prescription).

cost accounting. 1. A systematic process of recording and reporting on the cost of production. 2. The accumulation of cost and related data to be used for financial reporting and business decision making.

cost contract. Under federal TEFRA law, a contract between an HMO or CMP and the Medicare program that compensates the plan for services provided to Medicare members under the limits of cost payments specified by Medicare; typically allowed or chosen by participating plans in areas where provider costs are lower than average when compared to other regions. *See also* risk contract.

cost effectiveness. The degree to which a service meets a specified goal at an acceptable cost, where the emphasis is first on meeting the goal and only secondarily on cost; not the same as getting the best results for the price, which puts the emphasis on cost and makes the result secondary.

cost sharing. A situation in which the employer and the health plan member or insured person share the cost of coverage; may be limited to cost sharing of a premium or may also include deductibles, coinsurance, and copayments as well as amounts exceeding a plan's payment limits.

coverage. The provision of insurance under a policy to cover specific reimbursable costs. In health insurance, this means the financing of health services obtained by insured persons. Coverage helps enable but does not guarantee the provision of health services, which also depends on the availability of such services in the insured's service area. *See also* access to care.

coverage option. A rider that specifies coverage beyond that required by an insurance policy. This additional coverage is not automatic but may be added (at additional cost) at the discretion of the insured.

CPT-4. Current Procedural Terminology, fourth edition; a coding and classification system describing medical services and procedures, used by clinicians and by administrators and payers. CPT-4 codes are also used for billing purposes and in payment formulas that use relative value units. *See also* RBRVS.

credentialing. The formal process of examining the professional credentials, abilities, and qualifications of physicians (and, possibly, other healthcare practitioners such as pharmacists, chiropractors, nurse practitioners, and midwives) before approving them for participation in a hospital staff or the provider panel of a health plan or other organized delivery system. The professionals in question must be licensed and must meet certain other specified criteria (e.g., certification in a particular specialty or evidence of continuing professional education).

days per 1,000. Also known as bed days per 1,000; 1. A health plan's total number of inpatient days per 1,000 plan members for a specific 12-month period. 2. A hospital's average number of inpatient days per 1,000 inpatients. A measure typically used to compare hospital use across health plans.

deductible. The out-of-pocket cost that a health plan member must pay for care before the health coverage applies, usually a set dollar amount per benefit year.

diagnostic related groups (DRGs). 1. A classification system, developed for Medicare, that categorizes a hospitalization according to the patient's primary diagnosis and assigns a DRG code. 2. A per case reimbursement mechanism for hospital stays, developed for Medicare but also used by other payers, that pays a flat rate per diagnosis according to the DRG category to which the patient's case is assigned; usually paid per episode or hospital stay, regardless of how many days the patient is actually in the hospital.

direct contracting. An agreement between an employer and providers to render care to employees or retirees without the involvement of an insurer or health plan; not to be confused with a self-insured health plan. *See also* self-insured plan.

direct-pay member. A nongroup member of a health plan who has purchased the coverage independent of an employer (i.e., a member who pays his or her own premiums in full).

disability management. A strategy that tries to prevent the occurrence of a disabling illness or injury, ensure safe and appropriate return to work after the occurrence and treatment, and promote optimal possible functioning for the ill or injured person.

discharge planning. The act or process of evaluating the need for and arranging any necessary posthospital care and services in advance of an inpatient's discharge or release; may also be available for patients in other inpatient facilities such as nursing homes and rehabilitation care facilities.

discounted fee-for-service payment. A discount from the usual fee-for-service payment or fee schedule payment paid to a provider, typically in exchange for a promise of volume (i.e., an increased number of patients); often used for physician payment by PPOs and point-of-service plans and for specialists by HMOs.

disease management. The process of treating a specific illness, injury, or condition, usually chronic or severe, by first studying the disease life cycle and then designing aprropriate interventions for each stage of the condition. Such a program manages a patient's care against the normative model of care developed by the aforementioned process. The program also targets potentially affected patients and takes a comprehensive approach to treating them, including patient education and training in self-care, so that the disease is optimally managed over time (i.e., the patient suffers the fewest ill effects and health status is stabilized or improved).

disenrollment. The act or process of leaving a health plan, so that the person is no longer covered by the plan.

DRG-based payment. A per case payment system for reimbursing hospitalizations that is based on DRG categories. *See also* diagnostic related groups.

drop-in center. In psychiatric care, a consumer-operated and consumer-staffed center that provides peer support for persons with mental or behavioral illnesses.

dual choice. 1. The ability of an insured employee to choose between at least two types of employer-sponsored health plans, one of which is an HMO; not to be confused with an employee benefit program that merely offers two health plan choices. 2. A requirement under the federal HMO Act that employers offering their workers or retirees insured health coverage also offer HMO coverage, so long as there is at least one federally qualified HMO operating within the employer's service area. (Applicable only if the HMO approached the employer. The employer was not otherwise obligated to approach the HMO, nor was the HMO obligated to contact the employer.) The provision expired on October 31, 1995 and did not apply to ERISA-exempt plans (*see* ERISA). Also referred to as the employer mandate provision of the HMO Act.

eligibility verification. The process of confirming a person's eligibility for coverage under a health plan, usually before providing health services or filling a prescription.

employer group. 1. All of the plan members or enrollees covered through a given employer (i.e., the company's eligible employees, retirees, spouses, and dependents). 2. A component of the private or commercial enrollment of a health plan, as opposed to enrollees sponsored by public payers (i.e., Medicare, Medicaid). Commercial enrollment in a health plan that is not self-insured usually includes many different employer groups.

encounter data. Information describing an encounter or visit between a patient and a healthcare provider (e.g., an office appointment). Data include identification and a description of the patient and provider, the diagnosis, services rendered, charges (if any), and the outcome or prognosis of treatment.

enrollee. 1. A member of a managed care plan. 2. An HMO member.

enrollment. 1. The act or process of joining a health plan with a defined population such as an HMO or point-of-service plan. 2. The membership of (i.e., insured persons covered by) an HMO or point-of-service plan; total enrollment includes covered spouses and dependents.

EPO. *See* exclusive provider organization.

ERISA. Employee Retirement Income Security Act of 1974; federal pension reform law that also regulates other employee benefits and exempts self-funded (self-insured) employer plans from state regulation, the sole exception being workers' compensation plans.

exclusive provider organization (EPO). 1. A health plan that restricts members to using providers in its provider network but does not capitate the providers. 2. An HMO-like plan that does not have an HMO license.

experience rating. A method of determining insurance rates that takes into account the previous experience and claims history of the person or entity to be insured.

family coverage. A coverage option that includes all eligible family members as opposed to single coverage, which covers only one person; not to be confused with group coverage.

favorable selection. 1. A phenomenon in which the members of a health plan generally use fewer services and are less expensive to care for than expected. 2. A situation in which a health plan attracts healthier-than-average members (i.e., the disproportionate enrollment of low-risk individuals).

federally qualified HMO. One that meets the requirements of the federal HMO Act and has been certified as such by HCFA's Office of Managed Care (formerly known as the Office of Health Maintenance Organizations).

fee for service (FFS). A reimbursement system in which persons are paid for each encounter or service provided; the more encounters or units of service, the greater the payment.

fee-for-service plan. An indemnity plan that uses fee-for-service payment to pay providers

FEHBP. Federal Employees' Health Benefits Program.

FTE. Full-time equivalent; a statistical proxy for a full-time employee or position, most often used to describe or determine staffing levels and resource use.

full-replacement plan. A health plan offering coverage options that replaces an employer's entire range of previous health plan offerings and enrolls the company's entire eligible population with a single insurer or HMO company. One example of a full-replacement plan would be a traditional HMO plus a point-of-service plan using that HMO's provider network.

full-risk contract. See global capitation.

gatekeeper. A primary care practitioner who coordinates all medical care provided to a patient and through whom all services beyond primary care must be channeled (i.e., to see a specialist or obtain other services, the plan member must obtain a referral from the primary care practitioner).

gatekeeper model. Also known as a gatekeeper plan or system, a health plan that uses primary care practitioners as gatekeepers to authorize and control the use of specialists, ancillary services, and hospitalizations.

global capitation. Also known as a fully capitated arrangement or contract, this represents a single capitation payment made by a health plan to an institutional provider or provider organization that is responsible for the full scope of services to be provided to plan members. The provider (often a hospital or joint venture between a hospital and a physician organization) then must divide the capitated payment on its own among individual practitioners and institutional or organizational providers and must also pay for services rendered by other providers that it cannot itself provide. A fully capitated hospital contract requires the contracting hospital to have far more management and underwriting skills than does a typical HMO or point-of-service capitation contract for hospital care.

global fee. A type of flat-rate payment wherein a single charge or payment is made for a complete set of services covering an entire episode of care (e.g., a global fee for an organ transplant may include all related pre- and posthospitalization services and follow-up visits in addition to the direct procedure-related costs of the transplant).

group coverage. Insurance coverage that is obtained through an employer-sponsored plan, wherein the insured person is part of the employer group; not to be confused with family versus single coverage. *See also* individual coverage.

group-model HMO. An HMO that uses one multispecialty physician group practice for its provider network.

group practice. 1. A contractual arrangement in which two or more physicians practice medicine together in a collegial fashion, share the assets of the practice including a single set of medical records, and care for and share liability for each other's patients; invented by physicians William Mayo and his two sons in Rochester, Minnesota, between 1888 and 1890. 2. The basis of group-model and network-model HMOs.

group/staff model. A generic reference to two kinds of HMOs that, because they use physicians who practice exclusively with a given HMO, function organizationally in a very similar manner; may also refer to a similarly structured physician panel for an HMO-based point-of-service plan.

guaranteed renewal. A provision that ensures a plan member may renew insurance coverage for the next and following years. Employer-sponsored group coverage may feature guaranteed renewal for eligible employees, retirees, spouses, and dependents for as long as the employer maintains coverage with the insurer or HMO, but this provision is usually excluded for individual direct-pay policies.

HCFA. Healthcare Financing Administration, the agency within the federal Department of Health and Human Services that operates the Medicare and Medicaid programs.

healthcare delivery system. 1. An organized system that provides healthcare services in a given service area or region. 2. The entire healthcare infrastructure that provides health services to people of a given nation; may be referred to as *the* healthcare delivery system (national) rather than *a* delivery system (local).

health education. *See* patient education, health promotion.

health maintenance organization (HMO). 1. A state-licensed health plan that offers prepaid, comprehensive coverage for both hospital and physician services but also manages care and restricts members to using only healthcare providers affiliated with the plan. Members are enrolled for a specified period (i.e., a month, year, or calendar quarter). HMOs are characterized by selective contracting with providers, the use of managed care and provider incentives, and prepaid per-member-per-month premiums. 2. A type of prepaid, state-licensed health plan that combines the financing or insurance aspect of coverage with the actual provision of medical care.

health plan. 1. A contractual arrangement that provides health coverage and specified benefits (i.e., financing or reimbursement for same) for insured persons, as individuals or as members of employer groups. 2. An organized delivery mechanism that provides health coverage and health services to insured persons, such as an HMO, PPO, or point-of-service plan.

Health Plan Employer Data and Information Set (HEDIS). A data set of health plan performance indicators and other information, created and updated by the National Committee for Quality Assurance. Different versions for Medicare and Medicaid enrollments are under development. Primarily used for reporting HMO data, HEDIS provides plans a uniform format for reporting data to purchasers and the public, so that they may compare performance across plans and plans can compare themselves to each other. PPOs and indemnity plans do not report similar data, whereas point-of-service plans may report HEDIS data if they are HMO-based POS plans.

health plan member. 1. Also known as an enrollee, a person who is covered under a health plan. 2. The person in whose name the insurance policy is issued as opposed to that person's covered dependents and spouse. In an employer health plan, the employee, retiree, or surviving spouse in whose name coverage is provided. *See also* insured; policyholder.

health promotion. A range of activities, sponsored by a health plan or provider, aimed at encouraging and helping people improve their health and well being; may include patient education programs and materials, wellness activities such as exercise classes and smoking cessation programs, health fairs, and medical literature search services.

health risk assessment. An analysis of the health status and risk factors affecting a particular patient or health plan member.

high-option plan. One that offers an enhanced or more comprehensive benefit package under the same insurance policy. *See also* low-option plan.

HMO. *See* health maintenance organization.

HMO-based point-of-service (POS) plan. 1. An open-ended HMO; a point-of-service plan that uses as its provider network the provider panel of an affiliated HMO. 2. A POS plan offered by a traditional HMO.

horizontal integration. 1. The acquisition and consolidation of like organizations or business ventures under a single corporate management, in order to produce synergy, reduce redundancies and duplication of efforts or products, and achieve economies of scale while increasing market share. 2. In healthcare, the linkage of hospitals or other institutional providers and organizations that are alike or similar in nature, such as acute care facilities, to form a system. *See also* vertical integration; virtual integration.

hospitalization rate. The rate at which plan members are hospitalized (i.e., the admissions rate); typically used to compare hospital use among plans. *See also* days per 1,000.

IBNR. See incurred but not reported expenses.

ICD-9-CM. International Classification of Diseases, ninth edition; a diagnosis-oriented coding and classification system used largely by clinicians and medical and health services researchers.

incentive compensation. Compensation that includes financial rewards or penalties for specified performance, used to encourage desired performance. Rewards represent incentives, whereas penalties are disincentives. Compensation may be modified by incentives and disincentives or based entirely upon them, and the incentives/disincentives may be direct or indirect. Pure capitation, for example, provides an indirect incentive to avoid unnecessary provision of health services (conversely, a disincentive to provide all necessary care) because the amount of payment does not increase with the amount or type of services rendered. In contrast, a withhold repayment based on specified criteria would be a direct incentive for desired performance as described in the criteria.

incurred but not reported expenses (IBNR). For an HMO or fully capitated provider, medical costs that have already been incurred for an insured plan member but for which claims have not yet been submitted by providers. The HMO must continuously estimate the amount of such expenses and reserve funds adequate to cover these anticipated expenses. IBNR expenses are a critical issue for HMOs, which typically cannot retroactively readjust their premiums at year-end to make sure that premiums cover expenses, but not for fee-for-service indemnity plans or PPOs, which pay providers as covered services are incurred and typically do receive year-end retroactive readjustments. *See also* global capitation.

indemnity plan. 1. Traditional insurance plan that reimburses the insured person when a claim is made. 2. In healthcare, a fee-for-service plan (i.e., one that pays for services rendered).

independent practice association. 1. An association of solo practitioners or independent physicians who have joined together to negotiate managed care contracts. 2. A provider network consisting entirely of independent physicians who practice in their own offices rather than at a clinic site.

individual coverage. Insurance coverage that is obtained by the insured person independently of an employer group, for which the insured person pays the entire premium (i.e., not employer-sponsored coverage); not to be confused with single versus family coverage. *See also* direct-pay member.

insured. (v) 1. Covered under an insurance plan; reimbursed. (adj) 2. Reimbursable under an insurance plan. (n) 3. The insured persons(s) in whose name(s) an insurance policy is issued. 4. Any person(s) covered under an insurance policy. *See also* policyholder.

integrated delivery system. An organized delivery system that provides comprehensive health services to a defined population and combines the delivery of services, through owned, salaried, or contracted providers, with the financing of care through an ownership or close contractual relationship with a health plan. In an integrated system, the different parts of the system work in concert to achieve economies of scale and other synergies to a degree not achieved by other delivery mechanisms; however, few organized delivery systems achieve such a high level of integration. The hallmark of an integrated delivery system is that the health plan drives the rest of the system: the other parts of the system operate primarily to support the activities of the plan and the needs and desires of the plan's membership. The term is often misused to describe any system that combines some aspects of delivery with financing. *See also* organized delivery system; vertical integration; virtual integration.

involuntary disenrollment. The act or process by which an individual is dropped from a health plan without having requested it (i.e., not by his or her choice); typically occurs when a member loses eligibility for participation, such as when an employer stops offering a particular health plan or a Medicaid member loses Medicaid or AFDC eligibility, or for nonpayment of the premium.

IPA. *See* independent practice association.

IPA-model HMO. An HMO that uses one or more IPAs or unaffiliated solo practitioners for its physician panel.

lag factor. *See* incurred but not reported expenses.

low-option plan. A plan that offers a basic or less comprehensive benefit package under the same insurance policy. *See also* high-option plan.

managed care. A systematic approach to providing organized healthcare services that manages the cost and use of services while measuring and monitoring the performance of the plan and its providers, with the object of providing cost-effective care to the plan members. The approach uses an organized, selectively contracted provider panel to supply health services.

managed Medicaid. *See* Medicaid managed care.

market penetration. In health insurance, the percentage of all insured individuals in a given geographic market or service area enrolled in a specific health plan or type of health plan (e.g., HMO, PPO, or point-of-service plan); HMO penetration refers to the percentage of the insured persons in a market who are enrolled in any HMO operating in that market.

matrix pricing. A form of prospective hospital payment that uses multiple per diems; the highest per diem rates occur early in an admission, and rates decrease as the hospitalization progresses (i.e., as length of stay increases). *See also* per diem.

medical loss ratio. Also known as medical cost ratio; in a health plan or HMO, the proportion of direct medical expenses or costs incurred for the provision of care (i.e., payment to individual and institutional or organizational providers and related costs for services provided by medical labs, pharmacies, and durable medical equipment vendors) to total premiums paid to the plan. The medical cost ratio does not include the resources a health plan spends on clinical quality improvement or quality surveillance activities. *See also* administrative cost ratio.

medically necessary. Care clinically judged to be required (i.e., not optional) in order to preserve the life or health of a patient, with the expectation that the benefits of such care generally outweigh the risks to the patient.

Medicaid managed care. A range of programs that applies managed care to Medicaid programs; may include use of HMO risk contracts, primary care case managers, or cost contracts.

Medicare risk contract. *See* risk contract.

medical underwriting. Using a person's medical history and potential for future illness or injury to determine eligibility for coverage or set a premium rate for that person (e.g., a preexisting conditions clause); an integral part of experience rating.

mixed-model HMO. An HMO that uses any combination of staff physicians, group practices, IPAs, and solo practitioners for its provider network.

network-model HMO. An HMO that uses two or more group practices or a group practice plus staff physicians, possibly with a few solo practitioners, for its provider network.

occupancy rate. The percentage of hospital beds filled with patients on a given day or the average percentage of filled beds for a given period.

open-ended HMO. An HMO that permits its members to receive some health services from physicians or hospitals that are outside the HMO's provider network in exchange for higher out-of-pocket costs for the plan member. In an open-ended HMO, the member is automatically enrolled in the HMO and has little or no out-of-pocket cost for seeing in-network providers. *See also* point-of-service plan.

open enrollment. A period during which people may join or switch health plans without penalty. In an employer group, this occurs a few weeks or months before the start of a new benefit year.

open formulary. A list of preferred prescription drugs that a health plan's participating providers are encouraged to use in treatment. Exceptions are allowed and covered under the plan but may require a higher copayment, depending upon the plan member's specific benefit package. *See also* closed formulary.

open panel. A provider panel or network that uses selected medical practitioners or hospitals but will accept for participation any other provider that agrees to follow the plan's rules of participation, which may require signing a contract with the plan; sometimes used as a synonym for IPA-model and mixed-model plans.

organized delivery system. A generic name for networks of healthcare delivery organizations and institutions that (1) provide or arrange for a broad range of coordinated care for a defined population, (2) are clinically and financially accountable for the outcomes and health status of the population(s) served, and (3) own, are owned by, or are closely allied with a health plan (i.e., are tied to an insurance mechanism in some manner). The organized system and its affiliated practitioners should be put at-risk by the health plan, and the system should achieve a significant degree of integration; however, in practice, many systems and their practitioners are not capitated yet, the systems vary in the degree to which they have achieved either vertical or virtual integration, and they also vary in the degree to which such integration has achieved the desired synergies. Thus, the presence of a continuum of care, accountability, and connection to a health plan, rather than full integration, are the defining characteristics of organized delivery systems. *See also* capitation; integrated delivery system; vertical integration; virtual integration.

outcomes research. The study of the health effects that patients experience as a result of medical care. These results may include short-term and long-term effects upon the patient.

outcomes study. A systematic study undertaken across a group of patients to observe the effects of treatment for a specific illness, injury, or condition. The study may or may not take into account the comparative cost/benefit of competing treatments.

out-of-area care. Care that is provided when a plan member is outside the health plan's geographic service area (e.g., while traveling in another state or country).

out-of-network care. Medical care received by a plan member from providers that are not included in a health plan's provider network. Such care is not reimbursed in a traditional HMO but is covered with greater out-of-pocket cost to the plan member in a PPO, point-of-service plan, or open-ended HMO.

out-of-pocket cost. The portion of medical costs that a plan member or insured person must pay for receiving care as opposed to the portion paid by the plan; may include copayments, deductibles, and coinsurance amounts as well as balance billing, premium contributions, and uncovered services.

P and T (P&T) committee. *See* pharmacy and therapeutics committee.

participating provider. A practitioner, medical group, or institutional provider that has contracted with a health plan and is included in that plan's provider panel or network.

per diem. A set per day rate paid by a health plan for hospitalizations or other inpatient or residential care.

per member per month (PMPM). A unit of premium payment for a managed care plan, literally a flat rate per member (i.e., capitation).

pharmacy and therapeutics (P&T) committee. A multidisciplinary team of healthcare professionals, typically consisting of pharmacists, physicians, and nurses, that meets periodically to review and update a health plan's or provider's drug formulary. New pharmaceutical agents are reviewed by the committee before being added to the formulary, and any additions or revisions are typically based on prior experience and current medical literature and research. *See also* closed formulary; open formulary.

physician-hospital organization (PHO). A legal entity that includes at least one hospital and at least one physician organization, such as a group practice or an IPA, and is empowered to negotiate or contract with health plans on behalf of both the hospital(s) and the physicians. The PHO may or may not be legally structured as a joint venture between physicians and a hospital or multi-hospital system.

plan member. *See* health plan member.

PMPM. *See* per member per month.

point-of-service (POS) plan. Also known as non-HMO point-of-service plan, a type of fee-for-service health plan that permits members to choose at the time they need care whether to receive it from a provider in the plan's network or from one outside the network; if a member sees a provider outside the plan's network, there is greater out-of-pocket cost to the member. Also, the provider network used is not an HMO network but one either borrowed from an affiliated PPO or specially assembled for the POS plan. A POS plan may have lower out-of-pocket costs than a PPO, but this is neither the rule nor required.

policyholder. Under a group health plan, the policyholder is the employer, labor union, trustee, professional association, or other organization to which the group coverage contract is issued. Under a direct-pay contract, the policy-holder is the individual or family to whom the contract is issued. *See also* enrollee; health plan member; insured.

population-based care. Provision of health services that focuses on the current and long-term needs of populations within a health plan or geographic area rather than only on individual patients' requirements; care that uses popula-tion-based measures of health status to ascertain progress and providers' or health plans' performance. Population-based care may focus on the entire enrolled population or classify subsets of the population according to target group characteristics such as demographics, geographic area, clinical condi-tions (e.g., the incidence and prevalence of a given condition), and risk fac-tors or charateristics.

POS. *See* point-of-service plan.

PPO. *See* preferred provider organization.

practice guidelines. 1. Rules or guidelines developed to help healthcare practi-tioners decide on the best treatment for specific illnesses or injuries; often formulated as standardized treatment protocols or if-then decision trees. 2. Systematically developed statements to assist practitioners' and patients' decisions about healthcare to be provided for specific clinical circumstances; this definition is the one used by the federal Agency for Health Care Policy and Research. *See also* clinical algorithm; protocol.

practice patterns. Overall characteristics of a provider's practice over time, usu-ally analyzed by specific procedure or diagnosis in order to indicate the fre-quency with which given treatments or procedures are used and the degree of effectiveness of treatment. Comparative analysis of practice patterns can be undertaken for individual practitioners, individual institutional providers, or both.

preauthorization. *See* precertification.

precertification. The process of a health plan approving coverage for the use of services before the fact (e.g., approval for a hospitalization in advance of the admission).

preexisting condition. A medical illness or condition already present or previ-ously treated before a new member joins a health plan. Payment for treating such conditions is often excluded, typically for a limited length of time, under a plan's preexisting conditions clause. *See also* preexisting conditions clause.

preexisting conditions clause. The exclusion of preexisting conditions from coverage under a health plan, for a specified length of time or altogether; sometimes classified as a form of medical underwriting.

preferred provider organization (PPO). A type of fee-for-service health plan in which members may obtain care either from an affiliated network of physicians, hospitals, and other providers or from any other providers they choose; however, if a member sees an affiliated provider (i.e., stays in the network to receive care), the member's copayments and deductible (out-of-pocket costs) are lower than if the member goes outside the provider network for care. PPOs are characterized by the use of discounted provider fees, incentives for both providers and plan members, and some degree of utilization management. *See also* managed care.

premium. 1. The cost of obtaining health insurance coverage. 2. The payment for an insurance policy, which may be paid on a monthly, quarterly, or annual basis. 3. The premium rate.

premium rate. The dollar amount per unit, usually per the insured (e.g., a person, family, or group), of an insurance premium.

prepaid group practice. 1. A physician group practice that provides services to members who pay a flat rate in advance, per person, for a given period of time. 2. Antecedent of group-model HMOs. 3. Another name for a group-model HMO.

primary care. Basic or general healthcare, typically provided by physicians and nurse practitioners who specialize in family or general practice, pediatrics, or internal medicine; sometimes includes obstetrics and gynecology as well. *See also* specialty care; tertiary care.

primary care practitioner (PCP). A physician or nurse specialist who provides most of patients' routine medical care and who is trained in general or family practice, internal medicine, pediatrics, or obstetrics and gynecology.

protocol. The plan or outline of a scientific experiment, study, or medical treatment. *See also* practice guidelines; clinical algorithm.

provider. An individual healthcare practitioner, medical group, or institution/organization (e.g., a hospital or home health agency) that renders healthcare services.

provider panel. The practitioners, hospitals, and other institutional and organizational providers contracted by a managed care plan as the providers of choice for that plan.

provider profiling. Comparative analysis of individual provider performance that includes practice patterns or other performance measures, such as resource use, referral rates, adherence to practice guidelines, or degree of improvement in patients' health status.

psychosocial rehabilitation. Vocational and socialization services aimed at helping seriously and persistently mentally ill adults and seriously emotionally disturbed children achieve a maximum level of self-sufficiency.

quality assurance program. In healthcare, a set of activities intended to determine and monitor the quality of care provided to patients; because it focuses on identifying and preventing inappropriate care or fraud and abuse, quality assurance is generally considered a more passive and rudimentary activity than quality management or quality improvement programs, which involve active intervention in routine care as well as outliers (i.e., exceptions to the norm).

quality management program. Also known as a quality improvement program; 1. In healthcare, a planned, systematic, organizationwide approach to the measurement, assessment, and improvement of organizational performance in order to improve the quality of patient care and service delivery. 2. A set of activities intended to improve the average level of care provided to patients by making such care more effective, efficient, timely, and user friendly to patients while increasing accountability to both patients and plan members and purchasers.

RBRVS. See resource-based relative value scale.

RBRVS-based payment. A payment mechanism for physician reimbursement that is based on the Harvard resource-based relative value scale.

referral fund. Money set aside by a health plan to cover medical expenses incurred by providers other than primary care practitioners as a result of referrals made by PCPs. Referral funds typically do not cover mental health services or routine preventive care such as mammograms, obstetrical care, or care provided to infants during the first 30 days of life.

relative value units (RVUs). Units that represent a standardized measure of work output or resource use; typically part of a relative value scale that measures comparative amounts of work among professionals.

reinsurance. Excess insurance coverage, obtained by an insurance plan from a reinsurance carrier, through which the plan passes on some or all of its risk to the reinsurer; the object is to protect the insured from insolvency due to unexpected catastrophic cases. Also may be purchased by self-funded plans or capitated providers. *See also* stop-loss coverage.

resource-based relative value scale (RBRVS). A scale that measures the relative work effort and resource use by physicians for different procedures and different levels of office visits (i.e., intensity of service); created during the 1980s for the Medicare program by William Hsiao and colleagues at the Harvard School of Public Health.

retrospective review. A determination made by a health plan, after the fact, of the need for medical treatment for a specific episode of care.

risk. 1. In insurance, the amount of uncertainty involved in predicting loss expense or claims under a specific policy. 2. The degree to which an insured person or entity is likely to make a claim; the likelier the claim and the higher the associated expense, the higher the risk to the insurer issuing the policy. Low-risk insureds are those for whom the anticipated risk can be reliably predicted and whose anticipated claims are infrequent and of low cost. High-risk insureds are those for whom claims are expected to be high in total cost (e.g., prematurely born infants with complications) or for whom risk cannot be reliably calculated. By the latter definition, nongroup individual insureds are automatically considered high risk because statistics are unreliable predictors for specific individuals.

risk avoidance. 1. For an insurer or health plan, the act of denying coverage to or otherwise avoiding enrollment of insureds thought to be of higher than average risk (*see* favorable selection; risk skimming). 2. For an employer, the act of denying employment to individuals who may potentially increase the employer's liability exposure.

risk contract. 1. Also known as a TEFRA risk contract, an agreement between an HMO or CMP and the Medicare program (as authorized by the federal Tax Equity and Fiscal Responsibility Act) to provide all specified care and coverage to Medicare members at a prepaid flat rate per member per month (i.e., under capitation); so named because the plan takes the risk that the rate may not cover all the services required by a patient for a given month. 2. Any contract between a health plan and a provider wherein the provider accepts a flat rate for all care to be provided during a given period or for a given episode of care, thereby taking on risk. *See also* cost contract.

risk management. 1. In workers' compensation and property-casualty insurance, the process of actively controlling or changing attitudes, behavior, practices, or environments in order to lower the incidence of work-related illnesses, injuries, or associated losses that would result in insurance claims. 2. In healthcare, the process of educating and working with patients, employers, and others in order to lower insureds' health risks. Managed care, for example, is a risk management process rather than a risk avoidance strategy.

risk pool. 1. An aggregation of insureds, often high risk, or health plans into a single group (*see* risk pooling; risk spreading). 2. The aggregation and segregation of capitation withholds and other incentive or bonus payments intended for providers and to be redistributed at a later date according to a specified formula or predetermined criteria.

risk pooling. The combining of specific insured populations into a single large group to accomplish two goals: (1) to distribute the risk over a larger number of insureds and thereby avoid adverse selection due to fragmentation, and (2) to lower the premium cost to higher-risk insureds; often used for segregating high-risk insureds. *See also* risk spreading.

risk skimming. Also known as cream skimming or cherry picking (slang); in insurance, the practice of selectively avoiding the enrollment of insureds perceived to be of high risk to the insurer or intentionally attracting only low-risk insureds. *See also* risk avoidance; favorable selection.

risk spreading. The act of distributing risk across a large group of insureds or health plans; the essence of pooling and of insurance itself.

selective contracting. The practice of doing business with a limited number of contractors, usually according to predetermined criteria, in order to concentrate or increase market share for those contractors and thereby increase the influence of the organization offering the contracts upon the contractors; a key principle of managed care.

self-administered plan. One in which the employer or welfare fund itself handles claims administration and reimbursement without the assistance of an insurer or other intermediary; under such a plan, some benefits may be insured or sub-contracted (e.g., to a provider group, as in direct contracting, or to a specialized vendor such as a mail-order prescription drug firm, an employee assistance program, or a managed care organ transplant program), whereas others may be self-funded.

self-funding. See self-insured plan.

self-insured plan. An employee benefit, welfare, pension, or other insurance plan for which the employer has set aside funds and taken on the risk (i.e., self-funded) rather than passing on that risk to an insurer. All such plans that benefit employees and retirees are commonly known as ERISA plans because they are exempt from state regulation, with the exception of workers' compensation laws. *See also* ERISA.

shadow pricing. 1. The practice of intentionally setting a price for a product or service just below that of a competitor, regardless of whether the shadow price covers costs; as the competitor's price rises or falls, so does the shadow price. 2. In healthcare, the setting of a managed care plan's premium rate (usually but not necessarily an HMO rate) below the indemnity plan rate in order to undercut the indemnity competitor and attract enrollees to the managed care plan.

single coverage. A coverage option that covers only the person in whose name the policy is issued (i.e., not the spouse or dependents); not to be confused with individual coverage.

solo practitioner. An independent physician who practices alone rather than in a group practice.

specialty care. 1. Healthcare services beyond primary care that are provided by physicians, nurse specialists, and other selected health practitioners (e.g., chiropractors, inhalation therapists, and acupuncturists). 2. Services beyond primary care for which plan members must obtain a referral from their primary care practitioners or from the plan (e.g., hospice care, home infusion therapy). *See also* primary care; tertiary care.

specialty care practitioner. A physician or nurse trained in a specialty other than family or general practice, internal medicine, pediatrics, or, possibly, obstetrics and gynecology; may also include allied health professionals (e.g., physical therapists, occupational therapists, and inhalation therapists) as well as selected other nonphysician healthcare practitioners such as chiropractors, acupuncturists, psychologists, or psychiatric social workers.

staff-model HMO. An HMO that hires and salaries physicians for its provider network (i.e., it owns the provider network).

stop-loss coverage. A form of reinsurance purchased by a health plan that is automatically triggered when a claim exceeds a specified dollar amount. Stop-loss is one form of solvency protection often required for health plans by insurance regulators. *See also* reinsurance.

subrogation. The act of seeking reimbursement from other insurers whose policies may cover a portion of incurred claims submitted to a primary payer. For example, injuries arising from an automobile accident may be covered both by the injured person's health insurance and by the driver's automobile insurance, but if the driver is determined to be at fault for the injury, the automobile insurer becomes the primary payer, not the health plan. The primary payer then must reimburse the health plan for services rendered to the injured person after the health plan makes a subrogation claim.

subscriber. An enrolled employee or nongroup individual or family covered by a health plan.

surgicenter. Freestanding facility that provides outpatient surgery.

surplus. 1. The funds remaining after all costs have been covered; the excess of revenues over expenditures in a budget (budget surplus). 2. In not-for-profit organizations, the equivalent of profit (i.e., another word for profit). The difference between profit and surplus is that in a not-for-profit organization, the surplus remains within the organization instead of being distributed to shareholders because not-for-profits do not have shareholders.

TEFRA. Tax Equity and Fiscal Responsibility Act of 1982; enabling legislation for Medicare HMO and CMP risk and cost contracting that also defined primary and secondary coverage rules for Medicare.

tertiary care. Healthcare services obtained from highly specialized providers such as neurosurgeons, therapeutic radiologists, thoracic surgeons, transplant units, or intensive care units. These services frequently require highly sophisticated technologies and facilities.

third-party administrator (TPA). A company that processes claims and performs other administrative services for a health plan, usually a self-insured employer plan.

third-party payer. 1. An intermediary between an insured employer and a health plan member that actually insures the member and pays for care; the employer pays for heath coverage, the patient uses health services, but a third party—an insurer, HMO, or public payer such as Medicare or Medicaid—pays the medical care provider for services rendered. 2. Any commercial carrier, HMO, or public payer, such as Medicare or Medicaid, that provides health coverage and therefore pays providers.

TPA. *See* third-party administrator.

triple-option plan. A range of health plan coverage options including indemnity coverage, a PPO or point-of-service plan, and an HMO, all offered to an employer group by the same insurer as a unified product; not to be confused with an employee benefit program that merely offers three health plan choices. *See also* full replacement plan.

underwriting. In insurance, the process of determining insurance risk and setting premium rates based on the relative risk characteristics of insured groups or individuals.

urgent care. Medical care for an injury or illness that requires prompt attention but is not life threatening (e.g., an uncomplicated broken leg).

urgent care center. A freestanding facility that provides care for serious injury or illness that requires prompt attention but is not life threatening.

utilization. The use of medical care services.

utilization management. 1. The active management of all aspects of the use of medical care, including but not limited to utilization review, in order to produce optimal results for patients with optimal use of resources. 2. A comprehensive set of strategies and techniques aimed at ensuring appropriate allocation of healthcare resources (i.e., use of health services that take into account medical necessity, timeliness, efficiency, and cost).

utilization rate. The rate at which medical care services are used; may be expressed as a single number (e.g., total annual admissions), a ratio (e.g., hospital days per 1,000), or as a percentage (e.g., a 25 percent cesarean section rate).

utilization review. The process of determining whether or not the provision of care is medically necessary and effective and represents the best use of resources for a specific illness, injury, or condition. The determination may be concurrent (at the time treatment is recommended or sought) or retrospective (after the fact); intended to reduce or eliminate unnecessary, ineffective, and equivocal care (care for which the amount of benefit to the patient is not clear).

vertical integration. 1. The aggregation of dissimilar but related business units, companies, or organizations under single ownership or management in order to provide a full range of related products and services. 2. In healthcare, the combination through ownership or contracts of dissimilar institutional and organizational providers (e.g., hospitals, urgent care clinics, ambulatory surgery centers, home health agencies, nursing homes) and vendors (e.g., a durable medical equipment company) in order to provide a continuum of care. The purpose is to meet as many of a patient's needs as possible within the same organization and thereby keep the patient from going outside the system or network for care. *See also* horizontal integration; virtual integration.

virtual integration. In healthcare, a method of simulating integrated delivery or vertical integration through the use of contracts or formal affiliations rather than ownership. Some management and strategic planning issues may not be resolved by a virtually integrated system because it relies on voluntary participation, which can be withdrawn, and because its independent participants may not be able to delegate legal liability to the umbrella organization, thus preventing some reduction of duplication in areas such as credentialing or utilization management. *See also* horizontal integration; integrated delivery system; vertical integration.

withhold. The amount of a primary care physician's capitation or fee-for-service payment that is withheld by the plan until year-end and either used to pay for incentive payments and bonuses to PCPs or retained by the plan or medical group due to greater-than-expected use of services; usually a percentage of the capitation or a flat dollar amount.

workers' compensation. A no-fault insurance system, regulated by the states, in which all employers must participate and under which workers are compensated by their employers for the costs of work-related injuries and illnesses; consists of two components, (1) medical and related costs and (2) lost wages and disability payments.

Index